The Global Planning Revolution

The Global Family Planning Revolution: Three Decades of Population Policies and Programs

Warren C. Robinson and John A. Ross, Editors

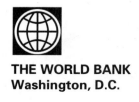

THE WORLD BANK
Washington, D.C.

© 2007 The International Bank for Reconstruction and Development / The World Bank
1818 H Street NW
Washington, DC 20433
Telephone: 202-473-1000
Internet: www.worldbank.org
E-mail: feedback@worldbank.org

1 2 3 4 10 09 08 07

ISBN-10: 0-8213-6951-2
ISBN-13: 978-0-8213-6951-7
eISBN-10: 0-8213-6952-0
eISBN-13: 978-0-8213-6952-4

DOI: 10.1596/978-0-8213-6951-7
Cover design: Quantum Think, Philadelphia, Pennsylvania
Cover photo: Peter Adams/Getty Images

Library of Congress Cataloging-in-Publication Data
The global family planning revolution : three decades of population policies and programs / Warren C. Robinson and John A. Ross (editors).
    p. cm.
Includes twenty-three case studies.
Includes bibliographical references and index.
ISBN-13: 978-0-8213-6951-7
ISBN-10: 0-8213-6951-2
ISBN-10: 0-8213-6952-0 (electronic)
1. Population policy—Developing countries—Case studies. 2. Birth control—Developing countries—Case studies. 3. Contraception—Developing countries—Case studies. 4. Fertility, Human—Developing countries—Case studies. 5. Population—Developing countries—Case studies. I. Robinson, Warren C., 1928- II. Ross, John A., 1934-
HB884.F35 2007
363.909172'4—dc22
                                                    2007003152

Contents

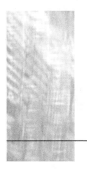

Foreword: The Family Planning Program Revolution in Perspective

The family planning programs carried out in many developing countries from the 1950s through the 1980s represent one of the important social experiments of the post–World War II period, but the details of their operations, their commonalities, and their differences have been insufficiently archived given the programs' day-to-day pressures and the large numbers of people involved. This volume helps fill this gap with much useful information and informed analysis.

The programs were complex undertakings in difficult settings that had little prior experience to draw upon. Not surprisingly, as the case studies described here demonstrate, no single strategy was available that could be employed across these diverse situations, and procedures that were successful in one country did not necessarily function well in another. However, a common thread wove through the multiplicity of approaches: more often than not, an effective starting point was built from insights into a particular country's social, economic, and cultural settings along with a realistic appraisal of resources available and the political will to move forward. Many of these efforts also demonstrate that persistence is important. For a program to encounter unforeseen problems was not unusual, but those countries that adopted a trial-and-error mentality could often overcome these setbacks and get the program back on track.

The case studies also indicate that developing a successful program was as much an art as a science. The key ingredient was being able to distinguish when a somewhat radical new approach was needed and when only some fine-tuning was necessary. That wisdom cannot be taught. However, many countries were fortunate in that their leaders and those who helped develop and run the programs had this skill at crucial times in a program's development.

While not a focus of this book, the family planning programs had several important, indirect effects on the field of population studies that merit attention as part of the record. First, uncertainty about the programs' worth and how to measure the extent of their success spurred a great deal of research on the measuring and modeling of fertility and contraceptive practice, on fecundity issues, on the effect of marriage patterns on fertility, and on a host of related topics. Investigators developed new methods of collecting data and measuring these dimensions, and the challenge of making good estimates in the face of incomplete and fragmentary information spurred a number of advances in formal demography.

Second, the programs greatly advanced the science of evaluation. How did one demonstrate that the programs were working in the face of the social and economic changes also ongoing in most countries? Researchers developed a number of new evidence-based techniques, many built on the new models of fertility and fecundity, while others advanced statistical practice in contextual or multilevel analysis.

Third, the programs led demographers to work with specialists from many other disciplines, including public health, economics, sociology, political science, and psychology. These disciplinary perspectives became key ingredients of population studies and, in turn, the demographic perspective influenced the other fields. The collaborations also widened the subject matter scope of demography, making it much more open to pursuing broader questions of health, economic status, family dynamics, and other facets of societal functioning. For example, a look at the current programs of the annual meetings of the Population Association of America as compared with those of the 1950s reveals how the field has expanded to tackle a wide array of health and societal issues.

Finally, the family planning efforts attracted many new and talented people to the field of population studies. Motivated in part by concern about rapid population growth, which was highly publicized at the time, many students from different disciplines chose to undertake graduate work in demography and population studies.

In addition, the family planning programs helped pave the way for many subsequent health, social, and economic programs. They helped establish the feasibility and legitimacy of mounting large-scale interventions aimed at such objectives as improving maternal and child health, eradicating disease, improving nutrition, enhancing educational opportunities, and undertaking village economic development. Of course, many health efforts were launched before the 1950s and many kinds of programs were motivated by other sources, but the family planning efforts around the world contributed to the development of a mindset that massive, worthwhile efforts were feasible and desirable. The programs also helped train many practitioners who went on to other programs and brought some of the lessons learned to their new endeavors.

We are pleased to see these generally effective early efforts recognized and the lessons adduced passed on to those facing similar challenges in carrying out broadened reproductive health programs in new settings, and more generally to practitioners of the many important social, economic, and health programs ongoing around the world today.

Ronald Freedman
Roderick D. McKenzie Professor Emeritus of Sociology
Research Scientist Emeritus, Population Studies Center,
Institute for Social Research, University of Michigan

Albert I. Hermalin
Professor Emeritus of Sociology
Research Scientist Emeritus, Population Studies Center,
Institute for Social Research, University of Michigan

Preface

This book was conceived with the conviction that the historic emergence of national family planning programs should be brought back to the world's attention. As a new social instrument to address a new social problem, the family planning program swept much of the developing world in the 1960s. We felt that the memory of this vital experience was in danger of being lost; it deserved to be captured in a definitive fashion, partly for young people unaware of the programs' origins, partly for the historical record, and partly for lessons that apply to other spheres of concern. The story of the appearance, for the first time in human history, of organized national programs devoted to the challenge of excessive and unwanted fertility should not be lost but should be mined for the lessons those programs might teach. This collection of essays was undertaken to answer that need.

The years just after 1960 saw the appearance of a new fertility determinant—organized actions by whole societies to bring birthrates down to match falling death rates, and to ease the accompanying dislocations faced by educational, medical, economic, housing, and family system institutions, and others. Those actions were also meant to give women greater control over their own childbearing, and to relieve families from the unexpected burdens of raising more surviving children than in the past. The two results together, societal benefits and personal benefits, flowed from programs based on new contraceptive technologies that could be deployed to whole populations. This book sets forth the stories of those social and technological breakthroughs as they emerged in very diverse country circumstances.

The financial generosity of the William and Flora Hewlett Foundation, supplemented by a gift from John Snow Inc. and a gift from an anonymous donor have made this book possible, while the Population Research Institute of the Pennsylvania State University kindly provided the necessary institutional linkage. We are especially indebted to the World Bank, which made an exception to its usual practice and entertained the inclusion of an outside publishing project, and we thank Tony Measham for recognizing and encouraging the possibility. Many persons have helped with this project in many different ways and we can only list a few of them: Edward Bos, Carol Carpenter-Yaman, Gordon DeJong, Jane Delung, Peter Donaldson, Alice Faintich, Mary Fisk, Robert Gillespie, Gavin Jones, Jack Kantner, Joel Lamstein, Richard Leete,

Tom Merrick, Jim Phillips, Malcolm Potts, Ron Ridker, Carlos Rossel, Patrick Shields, Ruth Simmons, Steve Sinding, and Amy Tsui.

The final tribute must go to the chapter authors, whose immediate enthusiasm for the project encouraged and sustained the editors. The authors worked hard on tight deadlines and freely gave additional time to read and critique one another's efforts, knowing that their only compensation would be the professional satisfaction of setting down their unique experiences in the furthering of something good and new on the face of the Earth, a societal invention intended for the common good, that has endured and continues to evolve. We trust that this book will help confirm that legacy.

Warren C. Robinson
John A. Ross
Editors

About the Editors and Authors

Editors

Warren C. Robinson, Ph.D., has over forty years of experience in economic and population program planning and research. He was a long-term resident adviser to the governments of Bangladesh, Pakistan, and Thailand and has done short-term missions in thirty other countries. He served as the senior policy adviser to the United States Mission to India (1986–89) and Egypt (1993–95), where he had primary responsibility for the preparations for the International Conference on Population and Development, which took place in Cairo in September 1994. He was founding director of the Population Research Center at the Pennsylvania State University and is the author or coauthor of 5 books and more than 100 scholarly papers.

John A. Ross, Ph.D., has several decades of experience in the fields of family planning and fertility, focusing on applied research, evaluation, and program design. His published works include a score of books and over 100 articles on experimental design, evaluation, cost and expenditure issues, guidelines for program statistical systems, program effort, unmet need, and demographic topics such as the modeling of birth intervals. He has also devoted attention to making accumulated knowledge more broadly available, through critical reviews and through a series of statistical compendia of international demographic and program data. He has merged research and writing interests with residencies in Indonesia, the Republic of Korea, and Turkey, where he worked closely with local action programs and demographic agencies.

Authors

Ayşe Akin, M.D., obstetrician and gynecologist, is a professor in the Department of Public Health, Hacettepe University Medical Faculty, and Director of the Hacettepe University Research and Implementation Centre in Women's Issues. She is also Coordinator of the Hacettepe University–WHO Collaborating Centre in Reproductive

Health. The results of Dr. Akin's research with the WHO on fertility regulation were used extensively in the preparation of the second population planning law in Turkey (1983). She also served for five years as the General Director of Maternal and Child Health and Family Planning in the Ministry of Health. In addition to her faculty appointments, she provides national and international consulting in the field of reproductive health.

Jane Bertrand, Ph.D., M.B.A., is Director, Center for Communication Programs, and Professor, Department of Health, Behavior, and Society at the Johns Hopkins Bloomberg School of Public Health, Baltimore, Maryland. She worked in Guatemala from 1976–95 as a technical adviser to APROFAM, and from 1995–2001 on the evaluation of HIV/AIDS programs in the Central African region.

George F. Brown, M.D., M.P.H., is an international health consultant with the William and Flora Hewlett Foundation. Previously, he held senior positions at the Rockefeller Foundation, the Population Council, and the International Development Research Centre. From 1964–66 he served with the Population Council as the first resident advisor in family planning to the government of Tunisia. He then moved to Morocco, where he was that country's first resident adviser in family planning from 1967–69.

John C. Caldwell, Ph.D., Emeritus Professor of Demography at Australian National University, lived in Ghana 1962–64 while he was Senior Fellow in Demography and Associate Professor of Sociology, University of Ghana, Legon, Accra. He continued to visit Ghana from 1965–99. He has traveled, researched, and lived widely in Africa.

Fatma H. El-Zanaty, Ph.D., is Professor, Department of Statistics, and Director of the Center for Surveys and Statistical Applications, Faculty of Economics and Political Sciences, Cairo University. She is also President of El-Zanaty & Associates and has directed the Egyptian Demographic Health Surveys since 1992. She has done extensive research on the Egyptian family planning program as a consultant for the United Nations Population Fund, the U.S. Agency for International Development, the World Bank, and other groups.

Susan Fan, M.B.B.S., M.P.A. is Executive Director of The Family Planning Association of Hong Kong. A graduate of the Medical Faculty of the University of Hong Kong, she is a member of the U.K. Royal College of Obstetricians and Gynecologists. She has served as Senior Executive Manager of Professional Services in the Hospital Authority of Hong Kong and serves on numerous public advisory bodies and non-government organizations related to health, HIV/AIDS, and gender. She teaches as Honorary Clinical Associate Professor in the University of Hong Kong. Dr. Fan received Hong Kong's Ten Outstanding Young Persons Award in 2000.

Oscar Harkavy, Ph.D., directed for many years the Ford Foundation's work in population and family planning and has made numerous visits to India beginning in 1959.

He is also former Chairman and presently a member of the board of directors of the Population Resources Center.

Donald F. Heisel, Ph.D., was a Population Council Field Associate, seconded to the then University College, Nairobi, from 1965–68. He continued his association with the Population Council until 1977, when he moved to the United Nations Population Division and served as the Division's Associate Director. He is currently a Senior Adviser to the Center for Migration Studies of New York City.

Alejandro N. Herrin, PhD., is Visiting Research Fellow at the Philippine Institute for Development Studies. He worked at the Xavier University Research Institute for Mindanao Culture in Cagayan de Oro City from 1972–78 and at the University of the Philippines School of Economics from 1978–2004. In both institutions he was engaged in teaching and research on demographic measurement and on population and development issues and worked closely with the National Economic and Development Authority and the Commission on Population.

Terence H. Hull, Ph.D., has worked on the social and political aspects of the Indonesian Family Planning Program since 1971, conducting field studies on the motivations of Indonesians for adopting contraception, and on the achievements of the program in serving the needs of the community. With Dr. Valerie Hull, he has written political interpretations of the role of the family planning program in the Indonesian governmental system and has advised the government on ways to improve the delivery of quality services. Most recently, Dr. Hull has worked with Indonesian colleagues on the analysis of laws relating to population, abortion, and reproductive rights.

Taek Il Kim, M.D., played a formative role in the design and implementation of the national family planning program of the Republic of Korea, as Director of the Maternal and Child Health Section of the Ministry of Health and Social Affairs, and later as Director of the Bureau of Public Health. He initiated the establishment of the National Family Planning Center and headed it; this Center played a key role in research, evaluation, and training for the national program. He also served with the Population Project Department of the World Bank for seven years, participating in its projects mainly in the Asian region. Later, he served as the first president of Hallym University in Korea.

Timothy King, Ph.D., joined the Population Studies Division of the World Bank in August 1969 and was Chief of that group from 1973 to 1982. He was a member of the team that appraised the first Jamaica Population Project.

Guillermo Lopez-Escobar, M.D., M.S., F.A.C.S., F.A.C.O.G., is President of the Regional Population Center (Centro Regional de Población), Bogota. From 1969–73 he was Head of the Division of Population Studies at the Colombian Association of Medical Schools (ASCOFAME). He served as Professor of Obstetrics and

Gynecology at the National University, Bogota, Colombia, and at the University of South Florida, Tampa. Dr. Lopez-Escobar is an honorary member of the National Academy of Sciences, Colombia.

Anthony R. Measham, M.D., Dr. P.H., is a consultant to the World Bank, the Fogarty International Center of the National Institutes of Health, and the Population Reference Bureau. From 1970–72, Dr. Measham served as Population Council Medical Adviser to the Colombian Association of Medical Schools in Bogota. From 1972–75, he was Population Council Resident Representative in charge of the Latin America Regional Office, responsible for activities in Bolivia, Colombia, Ecuador, and Peru.

Caroline J. Min, M.P.H., is Research Associate at the Mailman School of Public Health, Columbia University.

Richard Moore, Ph.D., retired Vice President, John Snow, Inc., worked for the United Nations Population Fund, the Ford Foundation, and the Population Council and lived and worked in developing nations in every region for over 40 years. From 1971–73, he was a research fellow in the Ministry of Health of Iran and special assistant to the director of the national family planning and maternal and child health program.

Allan R. Rosenfield, M.D., is DeLamar Professor of Public Health, Professor of Obstetrics and Gynecology, and Dean, Mailman School of Public Health, Columbia University. He was in Thailand as the Population Council Representative and as adviser to the Ministry of Public Health from 1967–73 and stayed closely involved for the next decade.

Krishna Roy, Ph.D., taught at Allahabad University and at the Indian Institute of Technology and served on the India Planning Commission, where she was principal assistant to V.K.R.V. Rao, the member for population and health. From 1968–76 she held an assignment in Latin America for the United Nations and later taught at Columbia University's School of Public Health. She returned to the United Nations in 1979 as Special Technical Adviser in Population and then as Interregional Adviser. After 1995 she managed technical assistance to 10 Latin American countries for women's reproductive rights and reproductive health and has since worked in community-based organizations in Washington, D.C., concerned with assistance to immigrant populations.

Fred Sai, M.B., B.S., F.R.C.P., M.P.H, is Adviser to the President of Ghana on Reproductive Health, HIV/AIDS. He was Professor of Preventive and Social Medicine in the University of Ghana Medical School and Director of the Ghana Health Services, as well as one of the founders of the Planned Parenthood Association of Ghana, Assistant Secretary General and later President of the International Planned

Parenthood Federation, and Senior Population Advisor at the World Bank. He chaired the Main Committees that produced the Programs of Action of both the International Population Conference held in Mexico in 1984, and the International Conference on Population and Development (ICPD) held in Cairo in 1994.

Hernán Sanhueza, M.D., M.Sc., made contributions to the Chilean program in three stages. He was a practicing obstetrician-gynecologist providing family planning services in the early 1960s. He was later an evaluator working in collaboration with the Latin American Demographic Center (CELADE) to assess the effects of the program; finally, he was the Regional Director of IPPF for the Western Hemisphere, providing international input and contributions to the program.

Roberto Santiso-Gálvez, M.D., is an obstetrician-gynecologist who trained in Brazil, Guatemala, and Uruguay. He served as a founding member of APROFAM (the private family planning association of Guatemala), was its first President in 1965, Coordinator of Programs from 1966–75, and Executive Director from 1976–96. He also established family planning services in the Guatemala Social Security Institute (IGSS).

Steven W. Sinding, Ph.D., is former Director General, International Planned Parenthood Federation (IPPF). He worked for 35 years at the U.S. Agency for International Development, the World Bank, the Rockefeller Foundation, Columbia University, and the IPPF. He lived and worked for 10 years in developing nations, including Pakistan, the Philippines, and Kenya.

Nai Peng Tey is Associate Professor at the Department of Applied Statistics, Faculty of Economics and Administration, University of Malaya. Prior to joining the university in 1992, he was the director of the Population Studies Centre of the National Population and Family Development Board (NPFDB) where he worked for 18 years. He is now a member of that board.

Jayanti M. Tuladhar, Ph.D., was associated with the national family planning program of the Nepalese Ministry of Health from 1969 to 1990, also as Program Associate with the Population Council working in Indonesia and India from 1992 to 1999, and is currently Adviser on Reproductive Health/Family Planning Management Information System and Logistics of the United Nations Population Fund (UNFPA), as part of the Country Technical Services Team (CST), in Bangkok.

Nicholas H. Wright, M.D., M.P.H., a medical epidemiologist, is retired and serves as an adjunct professor at Williams College. He helped develop and evaluate family planning services at Grady Memorial Hospital and the Georgia Department of Health, Atlanta, while associated with the Centers for Disease Control and Prevention (CDC), 1963–66, and then was Representative, the Population Council, in Sri Lanka, 1967–1970, and in Thailand, 1973–1976. Currently he is developing a leadership course in international health and the health professions for undergraduates.

Mui Teng Yap, Ph.D., is Senior Research Fellow at the Institute of Policy Studies, a public policy think tank in Singapore. She worked as a statistician in the Research and Evaluation Unit of the Singapore Family Planning and Population Board from 1975–79, before pursuing graduate studies at the University of Hawaii. She also worked at the Population Planning Unit, Ministry of Health, Singapore (1987–89) before joining the Institute of Policy Studies.

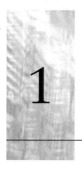

1 Overview and Perspective

STEVEN W. SINDING

A large body of literature about the international family planning movement has appeared over the past 20 to 25 years. The purpose of this overview chapter is not to recapitulate or summarize that literature (instead see, for example, Donaldson 1990; Donaldson and Tsui 1990; Harkavy 1995; Kantner and Kantner 2006). Rather, the chapter's purpose is to highlight what I believe to be the movement's major characteristics and accomplishments and the most important debates that surrounded it, some of which persist to this day and have important implications for the future of reproductive health services. The country chapters that comprise the bulk of this volume illustrate and provide solid evidence to support the generalizations put forward here.

Origins of the Movement

Two separate streams of thought and action came together to form the family planning movement that flourished from the mid-1960s to the mid-1990s. The first was the birth control movement of Margaret Sanger, Marie Stopes, and other pioneers that began in the first years of the 20th century. These innovators were concerned primarily with women's rights and empowerment, particularly the right to avoid unwanted pregnancies, as well as the many social pathologies that, in the reformers' views, accompanied unwanted childbearing. The primary focus was on the individual woman and her well-being.

The second stream originated later, although it had its origins in late 18th century British social philosophy as exemplified most prominently in the writings of the Reverend Thomas Malthus, who during the Industrial Revolution worried about the imbalance between the rapidly growing numbers of people in increasingly prosperous Western Europe and the problem of stagnating agricultural production. The modern manifestation of Malthusianism was the recognition in the decade following the end of World War II of the extraordinarily rapid growth in human populations in the developing regions of the world. Concern about rapid population growth was particularly notable in the United States, especially among a small elite that shared concerns about the shape of the postwar world and the institutions that would determine its development. John D. Rockefeller III was an exemplar and a leader of this second population control movement,[1] whose primary concern was less the well-being of individuals than of entire societies, a well-being that, in the view of these neo-Malthusians, was threatened by a growing imbalance between human numbers and a wide variety of natural and other resources, including food supplies. High on the list of concerns of the neo-Malthusians was the potential for political instability resulting from impoverishment and deprivation induced by rapid population growth in poor countries.

One can date the beginning of the modern family planning movement from various starting points: Sanger's opening of the first birth control clinic in 1916; the nearly simultaneous establishment in 1952 of the first national population policy in India, the International Planned Parenthood Federation, and Rockefeller's Population Council; or the beginning of significant transfers of financial and technical assistance for population programs from industrial to developing countries in the mid- to late 1960s. My own preferred starting date is 1952, as it was then that the two streams that formed the torrent that was to become the family planning movement first began to merge.

Building of a Consensus, 1952–66

As nearly all the national case studies in this book demonstrate, the convergence of the birth control and the population control movements has not always been smooth or easy. Many in the older movement, which promoted expanded access to contraception and individual control over fertility, resisted joining forces with those who were promoting national policies to reduce high rates of population growth. The former feared that the population movement would lead governments to condone, or even promote, restrictions on individual decision making with respect to reproduction. The latter, many of the most fervent proponents of population control, were convinced that such limitations on individual reproductive freedom were indeed essential to achieve the goal of reducing population growth rates.

To be sure, many believed that common ground existed in the proposition that voluntary birth control programs would be sufficient to bring about significant declines in fertility, and hence in population growth rates. Sanger was among those who took this view, and even though she never liked or accepted the term family planning, which she regarded as a distracting euphemism, she nevertheless became an early proponent of the convergence principle. She was able to champion both individual reproductive freedom and reduction of population growth rates. Indeed, it was this convergence view that drove the formation of the International Planned Parenthood Federation in 1952 and that lay behind Rockefeller's vision of the Population Council as a producer of research that could inform intelligent policy formation and program action. Deeply imbedded in the thinking of both institutions was the principle of voluntarism alongside an understanding of the political risks associated with any policies that smacked of coercion. This commitment to noncoercive approaches to policies and programs naturally led to what came to be called the family planning approach, and later the family planning movement.[2]

The period following the historic events of 1952 was one of slow expansion of both family planning services—as the International Planned Parenthood Federation gradually added member associations to the founding eight members—and policy-relevant knowledge, as the Population Council's research program expanded understanding of the underlying dynamics of demographic change. The work of the member associations of the International Planned Parenthood Federation, which gradually expanded in number from eight at its founding in 1952 to dozens by the mid-1960s, was seminal in many developing countries, as these nongovernmental family planning associations demonstrated both the high level of demand for services, especially on the part of women, and the political acceptability of family planning among large segments of the public.

During this period, a number of private foundations in the United States, led by the Ford Foundation, underwrote many of the costs of the expanding field. Funds were provided not only for undertaking research and for expanding family planning programs in developing countries, but also for building the training programs that prepared the first generation of family planning leaders in developing countries and public agencies. However, it was not until the mid-1960s, when large-scale funding became available from international development agencies, that what we now think of as the family planning movement really took off. The first of these was under the Swedish government, which supported early family planning efforts in Ceylon (now Sri Lanka), India, and Pakistan as early as 1962.

While the decision by funding agencies to enter the population field had many progenitors, the consensus that began to solidify in the mid-1960s probably had its principal origins in neither formal demography nor public health. Rather, development economists, impressed by the writings of economist demographers Ansley Coale and Edgar Hoover, economist Stephen Enke, and Swedish Nobel Prize–winner Gunnar Myrdal (Coale and Hoover 1958; Enke 1960; Myrdal 1968), played the critical role when they persuaded policy makers in the United States and some European governments, and soon thereafter in the World Bank, that rapid population growth was a major hindrance to economic development. (Indeed, the Bank financed the book by Coale and Hoover even though it did not begin to make loans for population programs until many years later.) By 1966, strong consensus had developed in international development policy circles on the imperative to reduce the high population growth rates of developing countries, a consensus that included a growing number of ministers of finance and development planning in those countries.

Early Program Disappointments and the Resulting Debates, 1966–74

The earliest national family planning programs were launched in South and East Asia, with India, Pakistan, and Sri Lanka leading the way in South Asia and Hong Kong, the Republic of Korea, Singapore, and Taiwan (China) doing so in East Asia, even before the new international consensus had fully taken hold. The near simultaneous invention of the modern intrauterine device and the oral contraceptive pill around 1960 permitted realization of the dream that easy-to-use and effective contraception could be made available to nearly all married couples. However, as the country studies in this book demonstrate, some of the early programs, particularly those in India and Pakistan, were bitterly disappointing to their champions, producing little or no change in fertility, or even in continuing rates of contraceptive use. Plagued by service delivery naïveté and incompetence, cultural resistance, and even outright fraud, the early program failures in South Asia resulted in deep skepticism in many quarters about the efficacy and prospects for success of national family planning efforts.

At the same time, the striking progress in the smaller East Asia economies, sometimes referred to as demonstration programs, gave hope, as contraceptive use rose rapidly and signs of fertility declines were evident. Nevertheless, the disappointments elsewhere remained and drove a wedge between the two academic disciplines—demography and public health—that were most directly engaged in the design of early policies and programs because of their quite different explanations of why programs were failing. Demographers increasingly came to believe that deeply embedded cultural inhibitions, as well as the economic and emotional value of children to poor households, were the primary causes of program failure. This explanation led to the belief that only far-reaching socioeconomic transformations—such as major reductions in infant and child mortality and in illiteracy, as well as educational and employment opportunities for women, increased incomes, and modern old-age economic security systems—would create conditions that were conducive to fertility decline. Social scientists were skeptical that family planning alone would lead to significant fertility reduction. Kingsley Davis of the University of California–Berkeley was one of the earliest and best-known adherents to this position (Davis 1967).

Public health professionals, by contrast, ascribed the early program disappointments to factors intrinsic to the programs themselves: poor planning, inadequate training of fieldworkers, inappropriate selection of field staff members, inadequate safeguards against fraudulent reporting, and so on. They believed that programs could be made more effective by revising and redesigning them.[3] Thus was born one of the two "great debates" in the population field: disagreement about the proper approach to reducing high fertility, or what I call the "debate about how" (Sinding 2000). This debate did not begin to be resolved for many years, but it was at its most fevered during the late 1960s and most of the 1970s. It was not until family planning programs outside of South Asia, most notably in East and Southeast Asia and in some countries in Latin America, showed a marked demographic impact that the debate about how began to recede.

A second, and older, debate was also causing major problems for champions of national population programs. This was the debate that had existed in one form or another since Malthus's time about whether rapid population growth had an important negative impact on human welfare. Over the ages, Malthus's pessimism about the relationship between human reproduction and food production (and, by extension, any number of natural and humanmade systems) had engendered passionate opposition, ranging from optimism that all systems can and do adapt to changing circumstances—the prevailing view of mainstream economics—to the more ideological view that population growth is not so much a cause as it is a symptom of poverty, the so-called Marxist position. Thus, the contemporary debate was about whether or not efforts to reduce rapid population growth were a necessary aspect of efforts to promote social and economic development. I call this the "debate about whether."

By the early 1970s, international efforts to reduce rapid population growth in the developing world were well advanced. The U.S. Congress had earmarked substantial foreign assistance funds for population programs; many other industrial countries were providing assistance for family planning programs in developing countries; the World Bank was actively seeking to make loans for population projects; and the United Nations (UN) had agreed to create a fund, the UN Fund for Population Activities (today known simply as the UN Population Fund, although it retains its original acronym, UNFPA). Developing countries were coming under fairly intense pressure, particularly from the U.S. government, to adopt population policies and to mount family planning programs. Many private foundations in the United States had joined the Ford Foundation in promoting and supporting population projects around the world.

One individual who stands out for special mention is William Draper, the author of an influential report (Draper 1959) that first advocated U.S. development assistance for population programs, the founder of the Population Crisis Committee in the United States (known today as Population Action International), and an indefatigable champion of global efforts to reduce population growth rates. Throughout the 1960s, Draper worked almost single-handedly first to persuade the U.S. Congress to earmark funds in the foreign aid budget for population activities, then to substantially increase those funds, then to lobby European governments and Japan to support the International Planned Parenthood Federation, and finally to create the UN Population Fund (Piotrow 1973). In other words, as the Ford Foundation and the Population Council played the leading roles in establishing the intellectual foundation of the movement, Draper did much to create the essential financial architecture to enable its full implementation. The U.S. contribution to overall external funding for population and family planning programs amounted to well over 50 percent of global resource transfers between the late 1960s and the late 1990s, and U.S. leadership, including funding, played a hugely influential role, particularly from the early 1950s until the mid-1980s. R. T. Ravenholt was the sometimes controversial, but undeniably effective, director of the U.S. Agency for International Development's enormously important program and the person who provided its basic direction.

Perhaps equally influential, but less widely recognized, was the venerable Spurgeon (Sam) Keeny, who, after a long and illustrious career with the UN, joined the Population Council and served as leader of its many pioneering family planning program efforts in Asia. Indeed, Keeny and his corps of enthusiastic young field professionals played a critical role in testing and perfecting the program approaches that would form the basis of many of the program successes that followed.

A Decisive Point: Bucharest 1974

All this energy and activity, including much of the underlying tension, came to a head in August 1974 with the World Population Conference in Bucharest, where both the debate about whether and the debate about how burst out in full. Many developing countries, encouraged by the socialist bloc and full of fervor for a new international economic order that was then the subject of hot debate within the UN, expressed deep reservations both about whether population programs were a necessary or desirable thing and about how population policies should be framed. The developing country view was best encapsulated in an aphorism voiced by the head of the Indian delegation. "Development," said Dr. Karan Singh, "is the best contraceptive," thereby seeming to renounce more than 20 years of vigorous attempts by the Indian government to reduce population growth through sterilization and the provision of contraceptive services. In other words, forget about family planning programs; invest instead in programs that address the underlying causes of high fertility: poverty and want. Take care of the people, this argument went, and population will take care of itself.

Much of this rhetoric was in response to a perception that the Western powers, especially the United States, was pressing too hard for population control through its advocacy of global demographic goals and targets. Many countries viewed the U.S. pressure as a naïve shortcut to economic development that ignored the critical importance of a broader (and hugely more costly) approach that would address the underlying causes of high fertility. President Lyndon B. Johnson had reinforced this suspicion with his unfortunate statement some years earlier that a dollar spent on family planning was equal to five dollars spent on economic development. Moreover, the policy and approach of the Office of Population of the U.S. Agency for International Development, under Ravenholt, had acquired a well-earned reputation for promoting family planning programs to the exclusion of other investments to reduce fertility. In this, the United States was largely isolated from other nations that were arguing for a more balanced approach to population policy.

So much for the debate about how. The debate about whether, while somewhat less contentious, was also the subject of considerable skepticism, with countries such as China and the former Soviet Union, joined by Algeria, Argentina, and many Sub-Saharan African states, arguing against the Malthusian view and insisting that rapid population growth was a red herring invented by the Western powers to keep developing countries' populations under control and that population growth was more a symptom than the cause of underdevelopment.

Meanwhile, most of the East Asian economies were quiet nonparticipants in these ideological showdowns. These future "tigers"—Hong Kong, Korea, Singapore, Taiwan (China), and Thailand—as well as Indonesia and the Philippines, had decided that fertility reduction through family planning needed to be an integral component of their economic development strategies, which also gave high priority to the very investments the development-is-the-best-contraceptive proponents were touting, that is, reducing infant mortality, raising the level of education of women, providing guarantees for old-age economic security, and the like. The pragmatists of

East Asia did not see family planning and investments in other aspects of development in either/or terms. Sensibly, as it turns out, they saw them as complementary.

Bucharest was something of a catharsis: a chance for countries to blow off some steam and to get a set of grievances toward the United States and its allies off their chest. I say this because, after all the rhetoric, the World Population Plan of Action that emerged as the consensus document called for a mix of family planning and other development investments that would help reduce the demand for children. Indeed, during the following few years, a large majority of the countries that had participated in the Bucharest conference proceeded to enunciate and implement population policies, most of which were principally comprised of voluntary family planning programs.

Perhaps the most influential advocate of a balanced approach was the president of the Population Council, Bernard Berelson. A strong advocate of family planning programs who stressed that they represented the most direct and least costly route to lower fertility, Berelson nonetheless recognized that the upper boundary on what family planning programs could achieve in terms of fertility control was set by the socioeconomic setting in which they operated. Thus, Berelson called for an approach that blended family planning programs with measures beyond family planning that would reinforce a small family norm. In time, the Berelson approach, which was widely accepted by the UN Population Fund, the World Bank, and other development agencies, as well as most governments, did indeed become the blueprint according to which most national programs operated.

Launching of a Reproductive Revolution, 1974–94

The vast majority of countries adopted voluntary family planning programs, which in most cases were part and parcel of their maternal and child health or primary health care systems. Thus was ushered in, following the *sturm und drang* of Bucharest, a golden era of family planning—a period of 20 years during which a reproductive revolution occurred in every region of the world except Sub-Saharan Africa.[4]

Of what did this revolution consist? Two statistics help answer the question. Between the mid-1960s and the mid-1990s, average fertility in the developing world, including China, fell from around six children per woman over her reproductive lifetime to around three, a 50 percent decline. During the same period, the prevalence of contraceptive use among women increased from less than 10 percent to nearly 60 percent. Establishing how much of the decline in fertility was due to organized family planning programs and how much would have occurred as the natural byproduct of other influences on childbearing behavior is, of course, difficult, but two facts suggest that programs, and the broader population policies of which they were a part, played an important role. The decline in fertility that occurred over a single generation in the developing countries took roughly a century to achieve in today's industrial countries, and this rapid decline in developing countries is unlikely to have happened in the absence of public policies designed to bring birthrates down and organized programs to help implement them. By the same token, countries that developed strong and robust programs saw their fertility rates decline far faster in most cases than countries that lacked such programs or whose programs were weaker (Ross and Mauldin 1997). One highly respected analysis ascribes half of the fertility decline of the modern era to organized family planning programs (Bongaarts, Mauldin, and Phillips 1990).

The remarkable success of programs began in East Asia in the 1960s and spread relatively quickly through most of the rest of the developing world during the 1970s and 1980s. Even two countries that were thought to be highly unlikely sites for family planning success stories saw remarkable progress: Bangladesh, which was desperately poor and the scene of half of Pakistan's failed program of the 1960s, and Kenya, which in the 1970s had the dubious distinction of possessing the highest birthrate in the world, more than eight children per woman. Both countries cut their fertility rates in half between 1975 and 1995. In Latin America, many countries began to approach the replacement level of a fraction over two children per woman by the 1990s, and in the Middle East and North Africa, Algeria, the Arab Republic of Egypt, Morocco, and Tunisia joined the Asian countries of Bangladesh, Indonesia, and Malaysia in showing that Islam is not necessarily a barrier to successful family planning programs. Even Sub-Saharan Africa had more bright spots than Kenya. Indeed, both Botswana and Zimbabwe brought their birthrates down earlier and further than Kenya, joining South Africa in moving southern Africa toward low fertility. More recently, Ghana appears to be headed in the same direction. Nonetheless, most of Sub-Saharan Africa, particularly Central and West Africa, has had little success in lowering fertility. Indeed, most countries have barely tried.

The existence of an inverse relationship between the overall level of development and the rapidity of fertility decline does not appear to be in question. Thus, the relatively more prosperous, literate, and healthy countries of Latin America experienced rapid fertility declines at relatively low levels of public program effort, while the governments of poorer, unhealthier, and less educationally advanced countries, such as Bangladesh and Kenya, needed to push somewhat harder to achieve comparable results. In a few places, including Bangladesh and Indonesia, governments put considerable pressure on couples, women in particular, to have fewer children. Some observers have argued that these programs were actually coercive, compelling women to limit childbearing beyond their real wishes. While differing views on whether the reimbursement payments to sterilization acceptors in Bangladesh represented an incentive and, if so, were a form of coercion, and on whether the pressure on village leaders and program staff members in Indonesia to achieve predetermined contraceptive targets led to coercion in some communities, particularly on Java, are reasonable, no one would dispute that Indira and Sanjay Gandhi's forced sterilization campaign in India in 1976, or China's rigidly enforced one-child policy that began in 1979–80 and continues to the present, represented coercion. In other words, in places where socioeconomic conditions were not especially conducive to rapid and sustained fertility decline, public action to achieve lower birthrates skirted, and sometimes crossed, the line between pure voluntarism and coercion. This approach enraged human rights activists and women's health advocates and led to a quite different political orientation toward population policies and programs by the early 1990s.

Thus, despite the intense ideological and empirical debates of the Bucharest era, the vast majority of countries adopted population or family planning policies during the 1970s and implemented these policies with varying degrees of enthusiasm and vigor through the 1980s and beyond. The result was a global decline in fertility that could hardly have been imagined and that few had predicted in the pre-Bucharest era.

Emerging Harbingers of Change, 1984–94

A global conference held in Mexico City in 1984 on the 10th anniversary of the Bucharest conference served mainly to reaffirm the basic principles of the World Population Plan of Action that had been adopted at Bucharest. It also provided an opportunity for the community of nations to recommit itself to voluntary family planning programs and other policy initiatives designed to bring about eventual population stabilization. However, a dark cloud hung over the Mexico City conference that came to have a serious, long-term impact on the family planning movement. This was the announcement by the United States that it had abruptly shifted from its longstanding commitment to population and family planning policies and programs to one of neutrality as far as population growth was concerned, along with a categorical opposition to abortion. The U.S. announcement came as a shock to delegations accustomed to the United States urging them to take more vigorous action to curb high fertility. Crafted by the Reagan administration to deliver on a campaign promise to the religious right in the United States, this "Mexico City policy," as it came to be called, ushered in 12 years of U.S. exceptionalism in international population affairs and foreshadowed an even deeper antipathy toward international cooperation in relation to population with the advent of the George W. Bush administration in 2001.

By 1994, the world was a very different place than it had been in 1974. As the UN began to prepare for a third global population meeting, the International Conference on Population and Development to be held in Cairo, several factors were moving the international consensus in new directions. First, the global demography had changed since 1974. Rapid and massive fertility declines had occurred across Asia and Latin America and in much of the rest of the developing world, encouraging the impression that the population problem was largely solved. At the same time, fertility in the industrial world, which demographers had confidently predicted would stabilize at replacement level, had fallen well below replacement and appeared to be stabilizing at such low levels as to call into question the sustainability of the indigenous populations of most European and some East Asian countries. In other words, fear of a global population explosion had almost completely disappeared.[5] Second, a strong and determined international women's movement had concluded that the population movement as implemented in many countries with the assistance of international development agencies represented a significant threat to women's health and rights. These women's groups were determined to transform the population and family planning movement into a reproductive health and rights movement, that is, one that explicitly rejected demographic targets and focused instead on improving the rights and health of individuals while respecting their reproductive freedom.

The 1994 International Conference on Population and Development and the Paradigm Shift

At the Cairo conference, the combination of a lack of macro-level urgency on the question of population growth and an intense micro-level concern with reproductive health and rights led to what became an almost complete reformulation of global population policies and strategies. The International Conference on Population and Development Program of Action explicitly called for dropping demographic and family planning program targets in favor of a broader policy agenda that included a range of reproductive health measures, including family planning, that would cater to women's overall reproductive health needs, as well as a series of social and economic policy measures designed to empower women and to strengthen their rights. While population issues were mentioned, they were not a prominent part of the Cairo agenda and were almost entirely forgotten once the conference was over. Family planning became an almost forgotten term after Cairo. Indeed, the main chapter of the Program of Action on service delivery programs, which had been entitled "Family Planning and Reproductive Rights and Health" in preconference documents, was simply called "Reproductive Rights and Reproductive Health" in the final version adopted by the more than 180 delegations present.

Cairo was truly a watershed. Some have already seen it as the end of the family planning movement, an event celebrated by many feminists and women's rights and human rights activists as a paradigm shift and equally regretted by traditional population advocates, including many demographers and others concerned about high fertility rates, as abandonment of a decades-long commitment to population stabilization. In the years since the conference, global attention has increasingly shifted away from population growth as a central political or development concern, while the rising toll of HIV infection and AIDS deaths has captured the attention of policy makers. The UN's Millennium Development Goals, agreed to by nearly all nations in 2000, did not include any mention of population growth or of reproductive health or family planning. Indeed, the Cairo goal of universal access to reproductive health services was the only goal among those emerging from a series of global conferences in the 1990s that did not make the final list of eight Millennium Development Goals. In addition, beginning in 2001, the United States joined the Vatican in a determined effort to oppose abortion, an opposition that so conflated abortion with sexual and reproductive health issues that it turned the earlier political consensus into an arena of contention and controversy to the extent that it began to frighten many governments away from reproductive health at all. Not surprisingly, resources to provide family planning and related sexual and reproductive health services have declined markedly over the past decade (Population Action International 2005; Speidel[6]).

Conclusion

So what are we to make of the remarkable movement that has spanned the better part of four decades? Can it be called a success or a failure? Has it achieved the goals that its founders had hoped for? What sort of a legacy has it left? The country cases that follow provide a rich tapestry of experience, much of it positive, some of it less so. In my view, the family planning movement has been one of the most successful examples of development cooperation in history. For all the underlying cultural and political conflict that attended it, the movement stands alongside the Green Revolution in agriculture as a demonstration of what collective political will and strong international cooperation can achieve. As such, it should serve as a beacon of hope to those who despair about the prospects for effective global action to reverse such pressing contemporary problems as global warming or the AIDS pandemic.

Notes

1. The term *population control,* still in widespread use by the media and others outside the movement itself, has been effectively banned from use within the movement since around the time of the first World Population Conference in Bucharest in 1974. Many developing countries saw in the term the shadow of neocolonialism. I use it here because it was still in vogue during the period under discussion.
2. Many of the early advocates of birth control, particularly in the United Kingdom and the United States, came from the eugenics movement, which was quite strong in both countries in the early decades of the 20th century. That movement had a certain intellectual respectability until the horrors Nazi Germany perpetrated in the name of racial policies destroyed it.
3. Indeed, R. T. Ravenholt, an epidemiologist and the head of the U.S. Agency for International Development's population program between 1966 and 1978, also published a trenchant rebuttal to Davis's argument in *Science,* a rebuttal that also foreshadowed the agency's well-known family planning program approach (Ravenholt 1969).
4. Meanwhile, in yet another dramatic and ironic about-face, India, within two years, had initiated one of the most draconian programs of coercive birth control the world has ever seen: the forced sterilizations of hundreds of thousands of people, mostly men.
5. This fear had abated despite the addition of 600 million people in India from 1965 to 2005, equal to the entire population of Sub-Saharan Africa in 1995.
6. Speidel, J. Joseph. "Population Donor Landscape Analysis." In *Review of Packard Foundation International Grantmaking in Population, Sexual and Reproductive Health and Rights.* David and Lucile Packard Foundation. http://www.packard.org.

References

Bongaarts, John, W. Parker Mauldin, and James Phillips. 1990. "The Demographic Impact of Family Planning Programs." *Studies in Family Planning* 21 (6): 299–310.

Coale, Ansley, and Edgar Hoover. 1958. *Population Growth and Economic Development in Low-Income Countries: A Case Study of India's Prospects.* Princeton, NJ: Princeton University Press.

Davis, Kingsley. 1967. "Population Policy: Will Current Programs Succeed?" *Science* 158 (10): 730–39.

Donaldson, Peter J. 1990. *Nature against Us: The United States and the World Population Crisis, 1965–1980.* Chapel Hill, NC: University of North Carolina Press.

Donaldson, Peter J., and Amy Ong Tsui. 1990. "The International Family Planning Movement." *Population Bulletin* 45 (3).

Draper, William H., Jr. 1959. *Report of the President's Committee to Study the U.S. Military Assistance Program.* Washington, D.C.: Government Printing Office.

Enke, Stephen. 1960. "The Economics of Government Payments to Limit Population." *Economic Development and Cultural Change* 8 (4): 339–48.

Harkavy, Oscar. 1995. *Curbing Population Growth: An Insider's Perspective on the Population Movement.* New York: Plenum Press.

Kantner, John F., and Andrew Kantner. 2006. *The Struggle for International Consensus on Population and Development.* New York: Palgrave Macmillan.

Myrdal, Gunnar. 1968. *Asian Drama: An Inquiry into the Poverty of Nations.* New York: Pantheon.

Piotrow, Phyllis T. 1973. *World Population Crisis: U.S. Response.* New York: Praeger.

Population Action International. 2005. *Progress and Promises: Trends in International Assistance for Reproductive Health and Population.* Washington, DC: Population Action International.

Ravenholt, R. T. 1969. "A.I.D.'s Family Planning Strategy." *Science* 10 (163): 124–27.

Ross, John, and W. Parker Mauldin. 1997. *Measuring the Strength of Family Planning Programs.* Washington, DC: Futures Group International.

Sinding, Steven W. 2000. "The Great Population Debates: How Relevant Are They for the 21st Century?" *American Journal of Public Health* 90 (12): 1841–47.

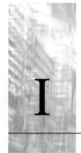

I Middle East and North Africa

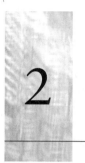

2

The Evolution of Population Policies and Programs in the Arab Republic of Egypt

WARREN C. ROBINSON AND FATMA H. EL-ZANATY

At the beginning of the 20th century, neither the ruling Egyptian elite nor the elite's numerous foreign experts and advisers seem to have been worried about the Arab Republic of Egypt having too many people. Lord Cromer, the British consul general in Egypt from 1883 to 1907 and the effective ruler of country wrote, "One great advantage of Egypt's situation is that no hidden economic problem lurked between the pages of the budget. The Finance Minister had not to deal, as in India, with a congested population, of whom a large percentage were in normal times living on the edge of starvation. He never had to refer to the pages of Malthus" (Shanawamy 1973, p. 189).

This began to change, however, not long after the beginning of the 20th century. A series of modern population censuses began in 1897 and, over time, these decennial counts revealed a steady increase in population. Articles were written in the press and awareness of the longer-run implications of such growth began to dawn on some academics and the medical profession.

Wendell Cleland, a sociology professor at the American University in Cairo, was drawn to the topic by his concern for the obvious and growing poverty of rural villagers and presented his findings in a number of publications (Cleland 1936, 1937, 1939). Using the series of decennial censuses taken since 1897, Cleland presented statistical evidence that the population was growing at an increasing rate. Egypt, he observed, was already a desperately poor country and any sustained increase in the population would pose a serious threat to the country's economic viability. Indeed, Cleland concluded that Egypt was already overpopulated, as he estimated that the country could provide an adequate standard of living for 12 million people, but already had more than 16 million people. In response, he developed a plan (Cleland 1939) that called for (a) increasing and conserving natural wealth, including all available arable land, which would involve the destruction of some new, high-rise housing developments for the middle class so as to return some land to cultivation; (b) encouraging emigration to newly irrigated areas and also to Sudan; and (c) reducing births by implementing public provision of contraceptives, raising educational and

---

This essay draws heavily on an earlier, somewhat more detailed work on the same topic (Robinson and El-Zanaty 2006). See also the recent historical survey by Makhlouf (2003) and Moreland's excellent 2005 review.

social standards, introducing legislation to raise the age of marriage, and promoting other measures to reward low fertility and penalize high fertility. Cleland had no official government standing, but he presented his findings at numerous meetings in the late 1930s, both in Egypt and abroad, and his work generated controversy. His suggestion that a birth control program was needed stirred up even more controversy, reflecting the prevailing conservative moral and religious attitudes of the day.

Somewhat later, Ammar studied economic and social development in the province of Sharqiya and concluded that "the real problem is a population one. The trend has been rising rapidly since the beginning of the century without an equivalent increase in incomes" (Ammar 1942, p. 55).

According to Dr. Zahia Marzouk, one of Egypt's family planning pioneers (Houston 1991, p. 121):

> In 1937 we began to think about the population explosion. University professors, gynecologists, statisticians, all sorts of people were interested in the future population of Egypt. We formed a small, unofficial association to discuss demographic issues. We wanted to hold a conference but thought it best to consult a religious person. Fortunately, the religious authority we contacted did not disapprove of family planning. He believed it was necessary if the woman's health or life was in danger or if they were afraid of being in a very poor, needy situation. Based on his opinion, we went ahead and held a conference on population in 1937. It was sponsored by the medical association.

Egypt's organized efforts to deal with family planning date to these beginnings. Box 2.1 provides a timeline of key events.

First Steps toward a Government Policy

The Egyptian government had also begun to think about the population question. It created the Ministry of Social Affairs in 1939 partly to study the population question and its social implications. Several government reports of that time highlighted the relationship among land, resources, and population growth. The creation of an expanded public health program built around so-called health bureaus in rural areas was due, at least in part, to the belief that high death rates were linked to high birth rates, a notion Cleland stressed in his book (Cleland 1936). This notion reflected the theory implicit in Cleland's plan, namely, that high death rates and high birth rates were both premodern. He saw modernization as consisting of a series of interconnected changes that would, by first reducing death rates, later reduce birth rates as well.

This, of course, is the essence of the theory of the demographic transition, a notion that was already finding its way into the thinking of population specialists. First propounded by Thompson, Wilcox, and others in the late 1920s, Notestein, Davis, and others in the late 1930s refined and focused the concept (Kirk 1996), which took final shape in the years after World War II. Cleland and other scholars in Egypt were no doubt aware of this literature, and were guided by it, at to least some extent, in thinking about Egypt. In 1942, Cleland actually participated in a Milbank Fund workshop on these issues, along with many of the luminaries responsible for developing the theory. Kiser wrote a detailed analysis of Egypt's demographic situation

---

BOX 2.1 Timeline of Key Events in the Evolution of Egypt's Family Planning Program

1937:	Wendell Cleland and other scholars document Egypt's rapid population growth.
	A private family planning association is organized in Cairo.
	Al-Azhar University issues an Islamic fatwa approving spacing methods.
1953:	President Nasser endorses population limits.
1957:	The Ministry of Social Affairs begins to study the population issue.
1960:	The semi-official Egyptian Family Planning Studies Association begins work in cities.
1962:	The new government charter lists population as a major problem.
1965:	The Supreme Council for Family Planning is created.
	Some foreign technical assistance is provided by the Ford Foundation, the Population Council, and others.
	The Ministry of Health adopts family planning as an incremental program.
	The contraceptive prevalence rate begins to rise mainly in relation to use of the oral contraceptive pill; medical practice constrains use of the intrauterine device (IUD).
1974:	Following the Bucharest conference doctrine, revised policy sees population as part of broader development issues.
	The Population and Development Program is launched.
1979–80:	The Egyptian fertility survey reveals the failure of the Population and Development Program and policy wavers.
1981:	A social marketing program, Family of the Future, is launched.
1985:	The National Population Council is created; Dr. Maher Mehran becomes Secretary-General
	Management, logistics, and research components are strengthened.
1985:	Constraints to IUD use are removed, the copper-T IUD is introduced, and the contraceptive prevalence rate rises sharply.
	The U.S. Agency for International Development becomes a major donor.
1988–90:	The State Information Service begins expanded, sharply focused, mass media campaigns nationwide.
	The Clinical Services Improvement Project is expanded and becomes nationwide.
	The Ministry of Health launches the Gold Star Program to enhance service quality.
1992–95:	The program reaches a turning point.
	A series of surveys show continued rises in the contraceptive prevalence rate and declines in fertility.

for this workshop and concluded that "Egypt is in a demographic jam" (Kiser 1942, p. 122). Egypt was a major battlefield for much of World War II, and all other concerns were put on hold.

Ambivalence during the Postrevolutionary Period

Egypt's modern political history dates from 1952 and the overthrow of the monarchy. The new government, soon to be headed by Gamal Abdel Nasser, a leader of the so-called young officers group, launched strong, far-reaching policy and program interventions in many areas of Egyptian economic and social life. Their approach was progressive, but also centralist and authoritarian, which was in keeping with long Egyptian traditions of governance (Goldschmidt 1990).

The new approach was also explicitly socialist, which was not in the Egyptian tradition, but the socialism that emerged was more pragmatic and paternalistic than the Eastern European and Asian versions and had a distinctly Egyptian flavor. This circumstance helped spare Egypt some, but not all, of the costly and painful mistakes that the European socialist model of development inflicted on many developing countries, especially in the agriculture sector.

The new government also took the first tentative steps toward a population policy. In November 1953, the minister of social services submitted a memorandum to the Permanent Council for Public Services entitled "The Population Situation in Egypt and the Necessity for Planning a Population Policy for the Country." Following this, in January 1954, the National Commission on Population Matters was created with subcommittees dealing with the demographic, medical, and economics aspects of population growth. Beginning in 1955, the medical subcommittee set up clinics, initially 8 and later expanded to 15, to provide services for couples in relation to both fertility and sterility (Farag 1970; Gadalla 1968; Ibrahim 1995; Ibrahim and Ibrahim 1996; Rizk 1955). In 1957, in the National Assembly, the same minister of social services raised the question of whether a national population policy was desirable, stating that the government had not yet made any firm decision.

Even these cautious first steps were controversial and provoked strong comments from conservative groups, including the then-powerful Moslem Brotherhood. Religious opinion was mixed, however, with the prevailing interpretation of Sharia law being that a woman's efforts to terminate childbearing were not consistent with Islam, but that a woman could space her births in the interest of her own health or the well-being of her family. This interpretation remains, in essence, the prevailing religious doctrine still in place today.

The top leaders of the new government were not opposed to family planning, but seemed skeptical about its effectiveness. The first president, General Mohammed Naguib, wrote, "The realization of our hopes will depend on a number of factors, the most important of which is Egypt's rapidly increasing population . . . but, birth control by means of contraception is hardly feasible in villages whose homes are lacking in running water, toilets and electric lights. A more effective means of controlling births, we feel is to provide the villages with the rudiments of modern civilization"(Naguib 1955, p. 160).

Naguib's successor, Nasser, displayed similar ambivalence. In 1953, he said, "The total number of Egyptians is 22 million. 350,000 are added annually. In 50 years the population of Egypt will reach 44 million. The heavens do not rain gold or silver. If we are earnest about raising our standard of living we should not be forgetful of this fact. The standard of living is deteriorating, the population is increasing and you are familiar with the limits to our wealth"(Shanawamy 1973, p. 193). Yet in a frequently quoted 1959 interview, Nasser said, "Instead of concentrating on birth control, we would do better to concentrate on how to make use of our own resources. We live in and make use of only four percent of our country. The rest is neglected and all desert. If we direct our efforts to expanding the area in which we live, instead of reducing the population, we will soon find a solution" (Shanawamy 1973, p. 194).

Many other influential Egyptians felt the same way. Family planning seemed like a negative policy, and this was a time of positive thinking. The first five-year plan had been announced, the new dam on the Nile at Aswan was being planned, and the country was optimistic about the rapid industrial and economic growth that would follow the dam's completion. The growing labor force would become educated, industrial workers who would power the planned industrial growth of the new Egypt. Other, more subtle elements provided unarticulated support for this position. Birth control was thought of as "Western" and the West was seen as declining. Egypt's already powerful position in Arab and Middle Eastern politics could only be strengthened if Egypt became more populous.

Given this atmosphere, the population policy initiative languished and no program was launched. In 1960, the National Commission on Population Matters was transformed into a nongovernmental organization (NGO), the Egyptian Family Planning Studies Association, which was in reality quasi-governmental, because it received financial support from the government and government officials served on its various committees and assisted with its clinical work. However, its NGO status meant that its activities were outside the sphere of official policy. The association was a compromise between an active program and no program at all. In response to hostile questions raised in parliament during this period, the government continued to state that it had not yet defined its position on population growth.

Nevertheless, the pendulum had begun to swing in the other direction. In 1962, the government promulgated a new national charter that laid out the basic assumptions and guiding principles for the new Arab Republic of Egypt. This charter clearly identified rapid population growth as a threat to the economic betterment of the Egyptian people: "Population increase is the most dangerous obstacle that faces the Egyptian people in their drive toward raising the standard of production in their country in an effective and efficient way." (translation from Makhlouf 2003, pp. 236–37) The government set up a ministerial committee to study what should be done, and parliament discussed and debated the issue. Islamic scholars at Al Azhar University formally considered the matter and again ruled that family planning to space births was not inconsistent with Islamic law and custom.

This change of heart on the part of government leaders came about because the new regime had raised popular expectations to an unrealistically high level. After a decade of high hopes and lofty speeches, people were realizing that no significant increase in the standard of living was likely for some time to come. Rising aspirations had become rising frustrations, and the regime turned to population control in something approaching desperation. The top leaders probably still did not really believe it would work, but it might, and trying would do no harm. By the mid-1960s they were more serious about creating a service delivery program.

Family planning organizations were created in both Cairo and Alexandria, and the Egyptian Family Planning Studies Association changed its name to the Egyptian Family Planning Association and then became affiliated with the International

Planned Parenthood Association, which was based in London. Funds for the organization's operations were initially obtained by shifting them from other social welfare projects unrelated to family planning under the Ministry of Social Affairs, under whose auspices the association operated and continues to operate. In 1964, the Population Research and Family Planning Division was created in the Research Section of the Ministry of Health, the ministry's first foray into the field of family planning. Modern contraceptives became available during this period, largely though the private sector. Local manufacture of oral contraceptives began in 1965, and the new foreign-manufactured intrauterine device (IUD) was introduced in 1964.

The First Family Planning Program

In 1965, the government set up the Supreme Council for Family Planning to serve as the top policy-making body for population and family planning. This also marked the first time that family planning had a line item in the national budget and was thus an administrative reality. The council's mandate was to be responsible for overall planning for family planning; to study the relationship among population and economic, social, and medical issues; and to coordinate the activities of all pertinent ministries and private groups.

The council consisted of the ministers of health, education, cultural and national guidance, local government, cabinet affairs, religious affairs, and social affairs and the head of the Central Agency for Public Mobilization and Statistics. The prime minister acted as the ex officio chair. Similar groups, known as governorate family planning advisory committees, were formed in each of the country's 21 governorates. Each of these was chaired by the governor and composed of local directors of the various ministries represented on the Supreme Council for Family Planning, along with representatives of the Arab Socialist Union, which was the ruling political party, and representatives of other interested local groups. A regional executive bureau worked under each governorate committee to supervise program implementation. The Executive Family Planning Secretariat was created at the national level to implement family planning policy.

The Ministries of Health and Social Affairs were responsible for actual service delivery, as they already had staff members and facilities in place across the country. The Ministry of Health established the National Family Planning Project within its existing organizational structure, and the Ministry of Social Affairs continued to supervise the NGOs, including, in particular, the Egyptian Family Planning Association. The new Family Planning Board was to coordinate the ministries' activities and to undertake research, training, and educational activities. It was given a budget of LE 1 million per year and came into effect in 1966.

Egypt's official policy and program preceded any significant financial involvement by foreign donors by a decade, although limited technical assistance was provided along with some commodity aid supplied by the International Planned Parenthood Federation (formerly the International Planned Parenthood Association) and several

U.S.-based groups, including the Ford Foundation, the Rockefeller Foundation, and the Population Council. At that time, the major government bilateral and international multilateral aid agencies were not yet involved in the fields of population and family planning. This began to change dramatically in the late 1960s. The Swedish International Development Cooperation Agency began providing technical assistance for family planning in the mid-1960s. The United Nations Fund for Population Activities was created in 1968, and shortly thereafter the U.S. Agency for International Development (USAID) was authorized to provide aid for family planning activities. The World Bank's interest in population dates from about this same time. All these donors came to play a role in Egypt later during the evolution of the program, but only the NGOs (the Ford Foundation, the Population Council, and the Rockefeller Foundation) actually helped shape the original policy (Croley 1969; Husein 1977).

By 1966, Egypt had both a policy and a program aimed at reducing fertility and population growth. The program seemed to have straightforward and sensible goals and a coherent organizational structure. The government decided to make use of existing Ministry of Health and Ministry of Social Affairs facilities and staff members to actually deliver services and contraceptive supplies and viewed the entire scheme as incremental in relation to other health-related activities already under way. As a result, all the members of the numerous committees created were already fully occupied with other duties, and thus the existing Supreme Council for Family Planning was constituted as such a committee. This council rarely, if ever, actually met, and the real leadership was vested in the Family Planning Executive Board. Personnel assigned to the staff of this body, its subcomponents, and the local implementing agencies were selected from among regular Ministry of Health staff members and paid an addition 30 percent of their base salaries to cover their new duties. Family planning services were clinic based, with clinics being open for family planning activities three afternoons a week, after their regular clinic hours, and the physicians and other personnel providing services being paid on an overtime basis. They were also allowed to impose modest charges for supplies (LE 0.10 per packet of oral contraceptive and LE 1 per IUD), with half the money going to the doctor and half to the other staff members.

The approach adopted was an attempt to build a program quickly while economizing on the use of scarce personnel and clinical resources. On the positive side, a nationwide system of more than 2,000 clinics, hospitals, and other service delivery points was created virtually overnight. Moreover, the use of Ministry of Health facilities seemed to ensure that family planning would be fully integrated into regular health activities, a tactic that most family planning experts favored. However, the reality that emerged over time was somewhat different. What had actually been created was the appearance of a program, much of which existed on paper only, not a fully functioning service delivery operation. The shortcomings of this structure quickly became apparent. In his sympathetic review of the program, Omran (1973, p. 127) warned that "the strengths of the program may become its weaknesses" and noted that while the program's design was admirable, its implementation left much to be desired.

Criticisms of the First Program

A particularly analytical criticism by Gadalla (1968, pp. 215–20) found many major problems with the program, including the following:

- *The program was inadequately funded.* From 1965 to 1970, the average annual budget allocated to the Family Planning Board was approximately LE 5.50 per married woman aged 15 to 45, with much of this amount consumed by overhead and administrative expenses.

- *The top leadership changed frequently.* The chair of the Family Planning Executive Board changed five times in the first four years of the program, and similar turnovers occurred in many governorate committees. Continuity was lacking, and the program's direction was uncertain.

- *The program's leaders lacked knowledge of and experience in organizing and running family planning activities.* No model existed that could easily be copied, and efforts by some foreign donors to furnish advice and technical assistance were not always welcomed. By starting immediately with a nationwide program, the Family Planning Board denied itself the opportunity to begin small, on a trial-and-error basis and to develop a locally appropriate structure that could be shown to work. Once launched nationwide, the program was difficult to modify or to reduce in scale.

- *The division of labor and responsibilities between the Ministry of Health and the Family Planning Board caused confusion.* Most staff members were full-time employees of the ministry and part-time employees of the Family Planning Board, but which entity was really responsible for them and their activities was unclear.

- *The staff were inadequately trained.* The Ministry of Health physicians and others recruited to work on family planning received little or no special training, and the members of local implementing agencies, who were supposed to play an important outreach function, received no training at all.

- *The supply of contraceptives was inadequate.* Only one method of contraception was generally available, the pill, and supplies came from several sources in an unreliable fashion. IUDs were in demand, but only a fraction of even government hospitals had sufficient trained staff members and supplies to meet this demand.

- *The quality of services was often poor.* When IUDs were available in clinics, they were inserted with no client counseling or follow-up, and workers were not equipped to deal with problems and erroneous client perceptions. Clients receiving the contraceptive pill were also inadequately briefed, and service providers did not worry about switching clients from one brand to another, which can lead to complications and side-effects that staff members were not prepared to deal with.

- *The leadership's commitment to the program fluctuated.* Even though the president had endorsed the program in 1965, he seemed to have second thoughts and seldom mentioned it after it was under way. Midlevel and lower-level political and administrative leaders gave no indication of being in favor of the policy or the program, and clients and field workers were aware of this. Opposition to the whole philosophy of family planning continued to be loud and recurrent in the media and from some conservative religious and political groups.

- *The program lacked a concerted information, education, and communications component and, for all practical purposes, remained "hidden."* Given that the government was advertising and promoting its other development goals and programs, this lack suggested to many that the family planning policy was not being taken seriously.

The inadequacy of funding for field activities was largely a management failure, as international donors had been ready to help the program if asked. Following a visit by a United Nations evaluation team in 1969, the newly created United Nations Fund for Population Activities began to provide contraceptive supplies and technical assistance. In 1971, the United Nations Fund for Population Activities and the government signed a five-year agreement for US$6.4 million, which doubled the budget of the Family Planning Executive Board, and the United Nations Children's Fund, the World Health Organization, the Ford Foundation, and other international groups also provided funds. However, the aid was poorly used, and funds frequently went unspent because of administrative delays.

Some accounts of the first program are even more negative. Potts (Malcolm Potts, private communication to Warren C. Robinson, December 10, 2002), for example, wrote:

> I was on a World Bank team . . . I was appalled by the desire to put more money into government health centers. The ones I saw were poorly staffed or actually physically locked up. A poor person might go with a broken bone but there was no trust of the government system and very few people would ever go to such a place for preventive medicine. I had seen the results of the first phase. It was a top-down bureaucratic effort that was meaningless to the general population. It cannot by any stretch of the imagination be called a supply-side effort.

Conflicting Strategies for Population Control

Persistent ambivalence at the top levels of government also accounted for the failure of the first program. The Egyptian development strategists never saw family planning as a top priority. President Nasser and the country's political and administrative leaders never really believed that family planning would work, and the documents pertaining to the government's economic five-year development plan reflected this skepticism (and continue to do so). While the formal five-year economic plans accepted that population growth was becoming a problem, the goal of reducing fertility was typically submerged in official development plans and strategy papers as one of four lines of action to deal with the problem of excess numbers, with the other three being resettling people in new communities, reorganizing existing villages, and increasing the skills and productivity of the labor force. None of the government's plan documents conveyed any sense of urgency about the country's high fertility, and this lack of urgency was quickly clear to the midlevel and lower-level government officials charged with implementing the new population control policy.

Economic planners stressed increasing the resource base rather than reducing population. The authorities have undertaken land reclamation projects, and the amount of cultivated and/or inhabited land has risen by 25 percent since 1952. The government's economic policies have made strenuous efforts to reclaim desert land to build new settlements in previously barren areas, and many new towns have been created in the Nile Delta region. However, elsewhere cultivable and habitable land has been lost to the relentless encroachment by the desert. One recent policy paper comments, "A second objective of the population policy, a more balanced spatial distribution, was introduced in the mid-1970s. On this objective, there is yet to be any marked success" (Ibrahim and Ibrahim 1996, p. 31).

The deliberate policy effort to reduce the rate of growth of large urban areas by redirecting the increase to new towns or rural areas has probably been somewhat more successful in Egypt than in other developing countries and continues today. The most recent economic plan includes a massive new reclamation effort in Upper Egypt, the Toshika or New Valley Project, but the policy has not had a major impact on crowding in already existing areas. In Cairo as a whole, the population density is more than 25,000 people per square kilometer, and in some wards of Cairo and Alexandria, the density is more than 100,000 people per square kilometer, compared with the national population density of 50 people per square kilometer.

The Second Phase of the Family Planning Program

Some critics saw the first family planning program as hopelessly simplistic. Human fertility is, after all, they argued, embedded in a sociocultural setting. This view held that deeply rooted cultural and psychological resistance to family planning was prevalent in traditional rural and agricultural societies such as Egypt. They claimed that people could not be induced to adopt family planning unless the underlying culture was modified, and until this had changed, nothing could be accomplished by distributing family planning supplies. Thus, to succeed, the family planning effort would have to be merely one part of a major effort to totally restructure village life in Egypt. This was a widely held point of view and seemed to be both intuitive and sensible. Thus, what was required was a new program strategy based on this premise, and the outcome was known as the Population and Development Program approach.

Thus, by 1970, the program had moved into a totally new phase motivated by the new policy philosophy: the Population and Development Program. The new approach made no effort to address the specific shortcomings of the existing supply system pointed out by Gadalla and other critics. It represented a completely different approach, not a reform of the existing one. It also took a soft-sell, low-profile approach to information, education, and communication to avoid offending groups and individuals who were opposed to family planning. The key was a newly recruited cadre of young, female, multipurpose, village field workers, one per village, who worked under the supervision of a local village council. These workers were charged with undertaking family planning motivation and a range of other development activities and community improvements.

The Population and Development Program approach proved to be another false start. Following some 10 years of effort and ample funding, objective evaluations showed clearly that contraceptive prevalence was not rising and fertility was not falling. The new approach had been no more successful than the earlier one. Indeed, a modest decline in actual usage and impact seems to have occurred.

The situation in the mid-1980s appeared to be that, after nearly 20 years of having an official policy and program aimed at reducing fertility in place, little had been accomplished. By most standards, the government's efforts had been both persistent and pragmatic. When one approach did not work, it had tried another, but neither had worked. Experience seemed to prove what many people had been saying all the time: that family planning simply was not Muslim or Egyptian and that it would not catch on in this part of the world (Warwick 1982).

Changes in the Socioeconomic Infrastructure

Along with its attempts at fertility control, the government was making strenuous efforts to achieve overall economic and social development, and the latter programs proved more successful. Health programs reduced mortality sharply; education levels rose, including among women; and housing, transport, and communications infrastructure all improved dramatically.

The changes in economic infrastructure and social services almost certainly benefited population control. The structural transformations achieved and the increased investment in the human capital base through education and health undoubtedly influenced the public sector's ability to deliver family planning services and the public's awareness and acceptability of the use of such services, and perhaps also changed people's values and aspirations (Cleland and Wilson 1987; Moreland 2005). While the social developments facilitated and enhanced the spread of contraceptive knowledge and practice, they did so with a considerable time lag.

Key Program Changes in the 1980s

In the mid- to late 1980s, when many had written off the Egyptian program, it turned the corner. Contraceptive prevalence rose and fertility fell sharply between 1985 and 1988, beginning a trend that continued to 2000 and beyond (Makhlouf 2003; Moreland 2005). The history of this period suggests that a series of improvements and developments, as discussed in the following paragraphs, occurred that together had a major cumulative effect on program coverage and effectiveness and on the supply of contraceptive services.

Improving Program Organization and Leadership

In 1985, an important organizational change occurred with a presidential decree that created the National Population Council (NPC) to replace the Supreme Council for

Family Planning. The membership remained much the same, except that a new secretary-general was named, Dr. Maher Mahran, who was also the director of the Family Planning Executive Board. Mahran was an obstetrician and gynecologist by training and a university professor by background, and he quickly became a familiar, and controversial, figure in the media. He spoke out often and loudly, and the press criticized him extensively, and even mocked him. Under his leadership, the visibility of the program was sharply elevated and family planning became impossible to ignore (Rakia 1994).

The NPC benefited from the support of President Hosni Mubbarak, who personally interested himself in the program's fortunes and, from 1982 onward, spoke out often and strongly in favor of family planning. The NPC became the lead agency for all family planning activities by donors, and the USAID, in particular, invested heavily in the NPC. The USAID's Institutional Development Subproject was developed within the NPC to train and upgrade the NPC staff, to help create an NPC planning and coordination office in each of the 21 governorates, and to help develop effective management and research capacity in the NPC.

The NPC received support for the first Egyptian demographic and health survey carried out in 1988 and for the second such survey in 1992. The NPC undertook research projects with the Central Agency for General Mobilization and Statistics to ensure timely and complete publication of the 1986 population census and worked with the Cairo Demographic Center in relation to the conduct and analysis of other surveys. These surveys involved contracts with international technical assistance groups paid for by the USAID but using local Egyptian agencies and staff members.

Involving the Private Sector in the Supply Effort

In 1979, the quasi-private Egyptian Family Planning Association launched the Urban Community Distribution Program, and this program was officially chartered in 1980 by the Ministry of Social Affairs. Beginning in Cairo and then spreading to Alexandria and other cities of the Nile Delta, this program was aimed at bringing private sector medical care providers into the business of supplying family planning services and commodities. In 1981, the program was expanded with USAID funding and renamed the Family of the Future, a social marketing scheme for contraceptive distribution. Family of the Future was an NGO but was indirectly controlled by the government through appointments to its board. Family of the Future obtained contraceptive commodity supplies free of charge from the USAID and made them available to private sector and NGO service providers at less than what would have been the usual private sector market prices. Family of the Future quickly became the major source of contraceptive pills for commercial pharmacies and of IUDs for private physicians. Its initial focus was in urban areas, where it worked closely with the existing network of private NGO clinic facilities, but it soon established a distribution mechanism in rural areas as well, and Family of the Future supply networks covered most of the country. Contraceptive supplies, particularly pills, became available in the most remote rural areas where none had previously been available.

Launching Sharply Focused Mass Media Programs

Mass media activities date from 1978, with the creation of a family planning communications center within the government's State Information Service with United Nations Fund for Population Activities support. (Egypt has two nationwide and several regional television channels, as well as several radio stations serving various market areas, but all are controlled by the State Information Service.) The radio and television messages in the late 1970s and early 1980s were broadly educational, stressing the theme of excessive population growth as a national problem, but made little effort to relate this national problem to listeners' and viewers' day-to-day social and economic concerns. The messages also lacked any specificity concerning contraceptive methods, benefits of use, sources of supply, or possible problems (Bogue 1983).

Acting on a survey-based evaluation of the impact of the communication program that indicated that a more specific focus on methods and sources of supply was needed, the government launched a new higher-visibility campaign in the mid-1980s. This was a multimedia campaign in that it employed posters, leaflets, and active outreach by field workers, but it emphasized the use of electronic mass media, especially television. The second demographic and health survey had revealed that television ownership was widespread, with more than 90 percent of urban households and 70 percent of rural households owning a television in 1992. Television ownership was even higher than radio ownership nationwide, and studies showed that most women relied on television as their main source of new information.

The new State Information Service program began with a campaign to make people generally aware of family planning; moved on to a discussion of how having many children complicated efforts to feed, cloth, and educate one's family; and then later turned to frank discussions of specific contraceptive techniques. Radio spots, dramas, and message inserts in other programs were also employed, and open discussions of contraceptive techniques and their possible side effects followed during 1995 to 1997. The emphasis became behavior change rather than just the provision of information (Robinson and Lewis 2003).

Expanding Choices

The single most popular method of contraception quickly became the IUD, but making it widely available entailed a considerable struggle within the Egyptian medical profession. Until the mid-1980s, the Egyptian Medical Association had ruled that only fully trained obstetricians and gynecologists working in hospitals or large clinics could insert IUDs, which ruled out the majority of physicians. Changing this archaic rule and making the IUDs generally available required strong pressure from the government. The Population and Development Program had been an oral contraceptive program, to the extent that it was a service-oriented program at all, but Egyptian women seemed to prefer a method of longer duration, and demand for the IUD rose sharply after it became more readily available. The improved IUD, the copper-T 380A, which had fewer side effects than older types and could remain in place almost indefinitely, was introduced in the mid-1980s and quickly proved popular with clients. Considerable staff retraining was required, but this was accomplished. The new IUD was made available to private sector physicians through the social marketing program, and they accounted for a significant portion of total insertions.

Enhancing the Quality of Services

In 1987, the USAID funded the Clinical Services Improvement Project, which involved upgrading a group of Egyptian Family Planning Association clinics, setting up new ones, and expanding in-service training for service providers at these and other facilities. The Clinical Services Improvement Project was ultimately planned to extend to some 112 clinics in all the urban areas of 20 governorates, including some, for the first time, in relatively remote Upper Egypt. These training services were provided to local clinics on a fee basis, with the proceeds then being used by the Clinical Services Improvement Project for further improving and expanding the project. The Clinical Services Improvement Project clinics became models for quality improvement efforts throughout the system and convinced the Ministry of Health to take more of an interest in its own clinical quality, with the outcome being the creation of the Gold Star Clinic Program. Under this program, the ministry developed a checklist of points for measuring and rating service quality. Clinics were then evaluated using this list, and those that passed the evaluation were given cash incentives and a gold star award to display.

USAID subprojects funded many new initiatives that also provided training and supplies to numerous private sector groups and institutions to bring them into family planning service provision and to improve quality. These included the Private Practitioners Family Planning Project with the Egyptian Junior Medical Doctors Association to train young physicians and their assistants in family planning, the Comprehensive Family Care Project with the Coptic Association for Social Care to establish and maintain clinics and outreach activities, the Rural Community-Based Family Planning Project with the Coptic Evangelical Organization for Social Services for community-based work in 50 villages, the Governors' Council for Women for the Development and Family Planning Training Project with the Institute for Training and Research in Family Planning to develop leadership skills and family planning knowledge among women leaders from across Egypt, the Training Professionals in Family Life Education and Counseling Project to train family planning counselors for work with the Egyptian Family Planning Association in 12 governorates, and three small demonstration projects on family planning implemented by Family Planning International. The flow of donor funding during this period is also important, as most of the new and/or improved tactics were connected with specific donor-funded projects. The outcomes were clearly visible in the increasing contraceptive prevalence rates (Mahran 1995; Mahran, El-Zanaty, and Way 1995; Robinson and El-Zanaty 2006).

Lessons Learned

The following conclusions can be drawn from Egypt's experience:

- Rapid economic growth in household income and consumption are not prerequisites for fertility decline, but improvements in basic social and economic infrastructure are important elements leading to a less traditional outlook and the rise of the small family norm.

- Programs that focus on villages or that are gender oriented do not seem to be important to changing attitudes and contraceptive acceptance.

- Programs must be visible and must welcome debate and discussion, as this is the best way to attain general legitimacy with the public.

- Public support from top political leaders is useful for motivating program workers, if not clients.

- Programs must be sufficiently funded to allow a trial-and-error approach to implementation.

- Program-oriented research plays a vital role in identifying problems and solving them.

- The private sector must be made responsible for a major share of service delivery.

- Quality of services, including a wide range of choices in relation to methods of contraception, is more important than the number of personnel or clinics.

- Programs work best when they are voluntary and noncoercive.

In one sense, the lukewarm support by midlevel government bureaucrats may have been a good thing. Egypt avoided the mistake of overly ambitious goals, never pushed clients and staff members too hard, and thus never ran the risk of a sharply negative backlash. Crash programs that treated high fertility as an epidemic that required emergency measures have proved to be disasters in other countries, and Egypt avoided this trap even when faced with apparent failure.

Final Observations on the Program's History

The Egyptian program was never a total failure. Contraceptive prevalence has risen, and fertility has been falling slowly but steadily since about 1960. In 1960, the estimated contraceptive prevalence rate for Egypt as a whole was some 5 percent of all married women. Initiation of the family planning program in 1965 had a modest impact, and contraceptive use rose to some 10 percent of married women by 1970. From 1975 onward, a series of national contraceptive and fertility surveys is available, and these surveys provide somewhat different estimates for some years from those reported by the program's statistics, while supporting the general trend. The first national prevalence survey in 1975 reported usage as 26 percent. Prevalence did level off—and even declined slightly—during the Population and Development Program period, to 24 percent by 1980. By the mid-1980s, the rate was rising again and reached 37.8 percent in the first demographic and health survey (1988) and 47.1 percent in the second survey (1992). Thus, prevalence only failed to rise for a brief period during the program's 30-year history (Moreland 2005). As time passed, policy-focused research identified weaknesses and program managers made gradual improvements. People seem to have expected too much too soon of the program and to have given up on it just as its cumulative efforts were beginning to bear fruit.

References

Ammar, Abbas M. 1942. *A Demographic Study of an Egyptian Province: Sahrqiya.* London: Percy Lund and Humphrey.

Bogue, Donald J. 1983. *How to Evaluate a Communications Campaign for Family Planning: A Demonstration Based on Data from the SIS Program in Egypt, 1980–82.* Research Report 6, Carolina Population Center. Chapel Hill, NC: University of North Carolina Press.

Cleland, John, and Chris Wilson. 1987. "Demand Theories of Fertility: An Iconoclastic View." *Population Studies* 41 (2): 237–59.

Cleland, Wendell. 1936. *The Population Problem in Egypt.* Lancaster, PA: Science Press.

————. 1937. "Egypt's Population Problem." *L'Egypte Contemporaine* 28: 67–87.

————. 1939. "A Population Plan for Egypt." *L'Egypte Contemporaine* 30: 461–84.

Croley, H. T. 1969. *The United Arab Republic.* Country Profiles Series. New York: Population Council.

Farag, M. 1970. "The Origin and Development of Family Planning in the U.A.R." In *Report of Cairo Demographic Center Annual Meeting, 1969,* 55–87. Cairo: Cairo Demographic Center.

Gadalla, S. 1968. "Population Problems and Family Planning in Egypt." Paper presented at the Eighth International Conference of Anthropological and Ethnographic Sciences, September, Tokyo. Also published as Reprint 14 by the American University in Cairo.

Goldschmidt, Arthur E. 1990. *Modern Egypt.* Cairo: American University in Cairo Press.

Houston, Perdita, ed. 1991. *The Right to Choose: Pioneers in Women's Health and Family Planning.* London: Earthscan Publications.

Husein, Hassan M. 1977. "United Arab Republic." In *Family Planning in the Developing Worlds: A Review of Programs,* ed. W. B. Watson, 143–50. New York: Population Council.

Ibrahim, Barbara, and Saad Eddin Ibrahim. 1996. "Egypt's Population Policy: The Long March of State and Civil Society." In *Do Population Policies Matter?,* ed. Anrudh K. Jain, 19–52. New York: Population Council.

Ibrahim, Saad Eddin. 1995. "State, Women and Civil Society: An Evaluation of Egypt's Population Policy." In *Family, Gender, and Population in the Middle East: Policies in Context,* ed. Carla Makhlouf Obermeyer, 57–89. Cairo: American University in Cairo Press.

Kirk, Dudley. 1996. "Demographic Transition Theory." *Population Studies* 50 (3): 361–88.

Kiser, Clyde V. 1942. "The Demographic Position of Egypt." In *Demographic Studies of Selected Areas of Rapid Growth,* ed. Clyde V. Kiser, 99–122. New York: Milbank Memorial Fund.

Mahran, Maher. 1995. "The National Population Council's Huge Achievement for the Last Ten Years" (in Arabic). *Al Wafd,* January 23.

Mahran, Maher, Fatma H. El-Zanaty, and Ann Way, eds. 1995. *Perspectives on Fertility and Family Planning in Egypt.* Calverton, MD, and Cairo: National Population Council and Macro International.

Makhlouf, Hesham H., ed. 2003. *Population of Egypt in the Twentieth Century*. Cairo: Cairo Demographic Center.

Moreland, Scott. 2005. *Egypt's Demographic Transition: Assessing 25 Years of Family Planning*. Washington, DC: Futures Group International.

Naguib, Mohammed. 1955. *Egypt's Destiny*. London: Victor Gollancz.

Omran, A. R. ed. 1973. *Egypt: Population Prospects and Problems*. Chapel Hill, NC: University of North Carolina Press.

Rakia, Nina. 1994. "We Will Solve the Problem: An Interview with Prof. Maher Mahran of Egypt." *Integration* (41): 4–7.

Rizk, Hanna. 1955. "Population Policies in Egypt." In *Fifth International Conference of Planned Parenthood, Tokyo, Japan, October 1955*, ed. G. Pincus. London: International Planned Parenthood Federation.

Robinson, Warren C., and Fatma H. El-Zanaty. 2006. *The Demographic Revolution in Modern Egypt*. Lanham, MD: Lexington Books.

Robinson, Warren C., and Gary Lewis. 2003. "Cost-Effectiveness Analysis of Behaviour Change Interventions: A Proposed New Approach and an Application to Egypt." *Journal of Biosocial Science* 35 (3): 95–110.

Shanawamy, H. 1973. "Stages in the Development of a Population Control Policy." In *Egypt: Population Problems and Prospects,* ed. A. R. Omran, 189–219. Chapel Hill, NC: University of North Carolina Press.

Warwick, Donald P. 1982. *Bitter Pills*. New York: Cambridge University Press.

3

Family Planning in Iran, 1960–79

RICHARD MOORE

In the early to mid-1960s, Iran was among the first wave of developing countries to initiate a national population and family planning program. In doing so, it became a pioneer in a historic and enormously complex undertaking for which relatively little experience, few lessons learned, or tools and methods on which to rely were available. Most developing countries viewed family planning as a culturally and politically sensitive initiative, especially traditional Muslim countries. From 1967 to 1979, through major efforts and the provision of adequate resources, international assistance, and strong political support, Iran's program developed quickly, learned rapidly, and had many promising attributes and achievements. That period is the focus of this chapter and is referred throughout as the first stage of the program. However, when the Islamic Revolution swept Iran in early 1979, it quickly became evident that the shah's family planning program and his social modernization initiatives had few supporters among religious groups and also among many lay groups. Furthermore, at that time the leaders of the Islamic Revolution were essentially pro-natalist. This period, 1979–88, is referred to as the second stage of the program. However, in an about-face in 1989, these same leaders reversed themselves and produced remarkable and ongoing achievements in family planning. This period, 1988 to the present, is referred to as the third stage of the program. For a timeline of major events covered in this chapter, see box 3.1.

Setting

Iran is a large and geographically heterogeneous country, with high mountains; vast deserts; tropical lowlands; and hot, dry plains. Historically, it has been an agricultural and rural country, with low population density, that has only intermittently

The author wishes to acknowledge his debt to John Friesen, Bob Gillespie, Joel Montague, and Steve Solter—all "old Iran hands"—for their numerous and helpful comments and wise counsel during the preparation of this chapter. Thanks are also due to Sandy Lieberman for his creative ideas on content. Editorial support from Warren Robinson was especially helpful and much appreciated.

BOX 3.1 Time Line for Family Planning in Iran

1961:	Restrictions on the importation of contraceptives are lifted, initiating the role of the commercial sector.
1962:	The shah initiates social reform by means of the White Revolution, including creation of the Health Corps and other "revolutionary corps."
1966:	Results of the 1966 census are released. A mission from the Population Council reviews program options and makes recommendations.
1967:	The shah signs the Tehran Declaration as the basis for a national population and family planning program.
	The Family Planning Division is created as part of the Ministry of Health.
	The High Council for the Coordination of Family Planning is created.
	Family planning services are initiated and expand rapidly.
1968:	The Population Council assigns resident advisers to the Family Planning Division until 1975.
1969	A resident population program adviser (later known as the senior population adviser) is posted to Tehran by the United Nations Development Programme. In 1973, the adviser is replaced by a United Nations Population Fund coordinator.
1970:	The government sets a fertility reduction target to reduce the annual population increase to 1 percent within 20 years.
	The model communications project is initiated in Isfahan province and is gradually expanded in scope and replicated in other provinces.
1972:	A Westinghouse study shows that the private sector was responsible for half of all contraception.
1973:	The Fifth Economic Development Plan (1973–78) increased funding for the family planning program to US$100 million for the plan period.
	A World Bank project is initiated, then canceled in 1977.
1974:	A dramatic increase in oil revenues begins to transform society.
Mid-1970s:	The government initiates a national mass communications campaign.
Late 1970s:	More than 2,000 program clinics provide family planning services.
Early 1979:	The revolutionary government overthrows the shah and suspends official population and family planning policies and programs.
1981–88:	The Iran-Iraq War takes place.
1989:	The Islamic Republic of Iran resumes and dramatically expands family planning policies and programs.

---

been tied together into a discrete national entity. Modernization efforts in the late 1960s and early 1970s included dramatic upgrading of mass communications, access to education, and transportation.

The country's first national census in 1956 reported a total population of 19.0 million, up from an estimated 15.9 million 10 years earlier. By 1966, the population had grown to 25.8 million and by 1976 to 33.7 million. Urban-rural fertility differentials were dramatic: in 1966, the total fertility rate in urban areas was 7.0 births per woman, while the total fertility rate in rural areas was 8.2 births per woman, and this difference would persist (Bulatao and Richardson 1994).

Changes in the distribution of the population were equally dramatic. For example, in 1956, 32 percent of the population was urban, but by 1966, the urban population had grown to 38 percent of the total population, and by 1976, it was

47 percent, nearly half of the total population (Bulatao and Richardson 1994). The population of Tehran increased by a staggering 80 percent during 1956 to 1966 (Moore, Asayesh, and Montague 1974). In rural areas, 60 percent of the women of reproductive age lived in the country's 66,500 villages and another 12 percent lived in towns with fewer than 50,000 people. Moreover, 40 percent of Iranian villages had a population of 250 or fewer (World Bank 1973). Creating services fast enough to keep up with the rapidly growing urban population while also creating access to services of all kinds for the majority of widely dispersed rural citizens clearly posed a daunting problem.

The urban-rural divide is also important, as it was highly correlated with many other factors. These factors included important differences in beliefs, literacy, and wealth as well as the links between these factors and the modern economic system; access to and use of information; access to health and other social services; health status and fertility; status of women; and openness to contemporary influences and thinking. Even though the benefits of modernization and public services began to spread into rural areas in the mid- to late 1960s, the gap in attitudes and lifestyles between the urban middle-class and the rural majority widened. For example, in 1966, literacy levels were 51 percent in urban areas, but only 15 percent in rural areas.

Overall, the status of Iranian women has traditionally been low. One indicator of this is that in 1966, female literacy was only 18 percent, while male literacy was 41 percent (Friesen and Moore 1972). Another indicator of women's status was that only 7.5 percent of the listings in the 1974 *Who's Who* in Iran were women, despite efforts by the royal family going back to 1935 to even the score through a variety of measures.

Per capita income rose from US$192 in 1962 to US$420 by 1972 (Friesen and Moore 1972). Between 1972 and 1990, it rose from US$420 to more than US$2,000. The cause of this major jump in income was the rise in oil prices in 1974–75: Iran's oil revenues increased from about US$2.6 billion in 1972 to about US$20 billion in 1974–75. Among other effects, the oil price boom resulted in rapid expansion of the economy along with a number of important socioeconomic changes. Rapid economic growth fostered accelerated development of infrastructure and industry and gave rise to an even more rapid rate of urban in-migration.

While religious leaders were willing to go along with the government's antinatalist policies and programs, they did oppose sterilization and any form of contraception that would result in an abortion, even at the start of conception. Oral contraceptives were not perceived to be an abortifacient. Religion, traditional views, and the influence of religious leaders carried considerable weight in rural areas and among traditional elements in urban areas, such as bazaar merchants and the poor. These traditional views contrasted with the values and behavior of the far more secular and modern middle-class in the cities and big towns. People were also aware that the shah was using various coercive methods in a major effort to control the Muslim religious establishment to avoid the rise of competing power centers. As part of this effort, the shah, in effect, appointed all the important Muslim leaders. In actuality, all Iranians knew that the religious establishment at all levels was totally against any change that might affect the legal and personal status of women. Those aligned with the shah (including the upper classes and the well-educated in Tehran) viewed the clerics as an embarrassment and a conservative hindrance to progress. However, they ignored or were unaware of the strongly held views that permeated the bazaar and the poorer classes, in both rural and urban areas.

To his credit, since the early 1960s, the shah had striven to impose a broad program of socioeconomic and legal reforms—part of his so-called White Revolution—that would improve social services, would enhance living conditions and the status of women, and would create the foundations of a modern national infrastructure and a modern state. Unfortunately, how these reforms were carried out was at least as important as what was done, and the operative word is "impose." While the shah and his influential, but unpopular, sister Princess Ashraf had many supporters for these changes, primarily among those who would benefit directly or who had the vision to see how the country would benefit, the shah's modus operandi was to order things done and to discourage any opposition. Given that these constraints to his family planning program existed and that the crude birth rate was 49 live births per 1,000 population in 1966 and was still in the 40s by 1976, the fact that as late as 1978 the Population Council placed Iran in the group of countries that were unlikely to achieve a crude birth rate of 20 by 2000 was perhaps not surprising. This put Iran in the same league as Afghanistan, Nepal, Nigeria, and Sudan despite its commitment, its efforts, and its large expenditures on family planning throughout the previous 10 years (Berelson 1978).

Motivating Factors, Enabling Policies, and Implementing Mechanisms

As the number and seriousness of demographic and socioeconomic concerns grew, the government responded. These responses took the form of policies that would create the goals and resources to respond. A formal family planning services and information organization was created to implement the policies.

Concerns

The International Planned Parenthood Federation initiated family planning services in Iran in the early 1950s. These consisted exclusively of counseling until 1957, at which time the International Planned Parenthood Federation introduced contraceptives through the commercial sector. Note, however, that until the early 1960s, the government of Iran was moderately pro-natalist.

The first indication that Iran might face a demographic problem resulted from studies based on the 1956 census, which showed a rapid population increase. Alarmed, the government formed a population committee. However, the 1966 census, which showed that population growth was in excess of 3 percent per year, shocked the government into action. The possibility of a population of more than 100 million, that is, a doubling in population in only 23 years; the need to achieve contraceptive use at twice the rates that the United Nations had forecast; and the economic and social implications of a very young population and of a dramatic increase in the urban population prompted a rapid shift to a fertility reduction policy and the initiation of a national program (Friesen and Moore 1972).

In 1966, the government invited the Population Council to make recommendations on how Iran might deal with its population problem (Keeny and others 1967). In addition, the government sent several Ministry of Health officials to study population programs in the Arab Republic of Egypt and Pakistan. Iranian officials, and even members of the royal family, became active participants in international and regional United Nations and other forums devoted to population and family planning issues.

Iran's demographic and economic concerns were no doubt reinforced by the growing international alarm about population growth in the developing world. For example, the concerns and actions included in the World Population Plan of Action adopted at the Bucharest conference in 1974 were well known in Iran, and Iran's exposure to such internationally disseminated concerns, policies, and plans continued to grow throughout the 1960s and 1970s. The government carefully studied international developments and influences, and these had an important impact on Iran's own policies and programs.

The environment in the country at the time the government launched the national family planning program was not favorable to efforts to limit fertility. The majority of the population was illiterate; conservative; traditional, especially in rural areas; and pro-natalist, or would at least have had difficulty grasping the concept of over-population. Moreover, infant mortality was still high and the country did not yet have a social security system, so most couples favored high fertility, as they saw children as a source of social and economic support. Also many couples no doubt had a religious, or simply conservative and traditional, rationale for high fertility.

Policies

Official policy was first enunciated in the Tehran Declaration in 1967, which asserted that family planning was a human right and sought to promote it to enhance the social and economic welfare of families and the nation. In 1970, the government issued a more aggressive and focused policy that set forth the ultimate goal of the population and family planning program, which was to reduce the annual increase in population to 1 percent within 20 years.

To implement the program, the government passed a number of pieces of legislation and adopted various policies. The most visible and important of these policies was to assign responsibility, in 1967, for the national population and family planning program to the Ministry of Health under the control of an influential undersecretary for family planning. Within months, a specific plan for the family planning program with budgetary estimates was submitted via the Ministry of Health to the government for approval. Under this plan, the ministry's Population and Family Planning Division (henceforth referred to as the Family Planning Division) would provide services and information in all of the ministry's clinical and primary health care facilities, train medical and paramedical staff members, support health education activities, and encourage research. Laws were passed to repeal restrictions on sterilization and abortion, to incorporate population issues into high school and university curricula, and to further improve the status of women.

The overall objective of the family planning program was to help couples control the size of their families, that is, to strike a balance between the number of children in a family and its economic circumstances. More specifically, the program sought to change fertile couples' knowledge, attitudes, and practices in relation to contraception. The intent was to achieve this primarily by means of information and motivational messages and by increased access to and use of modern means of contraception.

Like many other family planning programs at the time, the Iranian program focused primarily on urban, clinic-based services, although it did use some mobile clinics in rural areas. In effect, the family planning program inherited this services infrastructure, as these clinics and their associated staff already fell under the auspices of the Ministry of Health and a range of other organizations, and because this largely urban infrastructure was already in place, it served to influence, or even dictate, the population that would be served. The clinics provided contraceptive services and information within the context of their preexisting primary care services. Outreach was limited, and because of the vagaries of transportation, physical access to services was highly variable (Moore 1974). Over time, auxiliary health workers, midwives, and village health workers were made responsible for delivering supplies of oral contraceptives to rural women and, on a trial basis, some were taught to insert intrauterine devices (IUDs). Preventive health care, including family planning, was provided at no cost except for a small registration fee for those able to afford it.

The program relied almost entirely on a single type of contraceptive—the pill—and 90 percent of acceptors were given this method. The program placed little emphasis on condoms, IUDs, sterilization, or abortion. Strategists and demographers did not favor such heavy reliance on a single method, especially the pill, because the greatest demand and need for contraception came from women who had had the number of children they wanted and were older than 31. At this time in those women's lives, with many fertile years ahead of them, only longer-acting methods made sense. The rationale behind the emphasis on the pill reflects the state of contraceptive technology at that time. IUDs were still being field tested, and the one large-scale effort to introduce the loop—a Ford Foundation initiative in India in the mid-1960s—had mixed results. The Iranian program was also pill centered because of the almost total absence of female physicians; of midwives trained in IUD insertion; and in rural areas, of the clinical infrastructure needed to manage the more complex clinical methods. In addition, the opposition by religious leaders precluded a serious effort to introduce sterilization.

One attempt to increase access to services was the assistance provided by the Population Council to implement a postpartum family planning program, which initially seemed promising. However, like most postpartum programs initiated in a number of countries, this one never really took off and was never replicated to any extent. While the reasons for this are not clear, they may have had to do with the fact that most of these programs were judged largely in terms of their potential demographic impact, rather than as a strategy for meeting the reproductive health needs of women. Despite the program's promotion of modern methods, the prevalence of traditional methods of contraception remained high.

In contrast to current views about abortion, the mind-set during this period was such that some international observers and Iranian officials urged the program to use all possible means of fertility limitation, including expanded use of abortion (Moore Asayesh, and Montague 1974), and until the late 1970s, the United Nations Population Fund (UNFPA) was providing governments with large numbers of so-called menstrual regulation (abortion) kits. In practice, however, abortion was never a widely available official option in Iran, though nonprogram abortions were common, with an average of about three abortions per woman (Bulatao and Richardson 1994).

The overreliance on a single method of contraception constrained the growth of the program, especially given its high-fertility target group. At the same time, given the program's formative nature, the providers' inexperience with contraception, and the relative ease of procuring pills and managing this method, this was not an irrational decision. More difficult to explain is why the program's leaders did not make an earlier and greater effort to promote and provide condoms and to begin to lay the groundwork for the eventual introduction of long-acting and terminal methods, while at the same time promoting spacing of children.

The target population of the family planning program was primarily younger, urban women who had not completed their preferred family size. The almost exclusive reliance on temporary spacing methods for women meant that, in practice, older women (who had completed their family size and were more motivated to initiate contraception), rural women, and men were less assertively targeted to receive information and services. No explicit policy appears to have been in place regarding the eligibility of unmarried couples or youth for official contraceptive services. Presumably, such clients would have had to purchase contraceptive supplies from the private sector.

The Government's Program

Any national health or family planning program is, inevitably, a highly complex undertaking. A number of organizational elements have to be created, provided with human and other resources, coordinated, and managed for such programs to function at all, much less function effectively.

Organization, Management, and Capacity

The Family Planning Division of the Ministry of Health was organized into five major units: the Office for Population Affairs; the Office for Women's Health Corps Affairs; the Directorate for Technical Affairs, which included motivation and communications, clinical services, and technical training; the Directorate for Research and Planning, which included evaluation; and the Directorate for Maternal and Child Health and Nutrition. Three directors general headed the three directorates.

The inclusion of the division of maternal and child health and nutrition (MCHN) services and the national Women's Health Corps was intended to help integrate family planning services with more mainstream MCHN services and to provide the program with a national health and family planning information and motivation capacity over which it had control. The author is not aware of any studies undertaken to assess whether the program may have benefited from the, at the time, rather innovative pairing of family planning and MCHN services.

The Family Planning Division was represented at the provincial level by a director of family planning who was appointed by and reported to the director general of the provincial health department. Senior officials at Family Planning Division headquarters made the decisions on most important matters.

An important role of the Family Planning Division was to set standards and to set basic patterns for all government-operated clinics where family planning services were provided. These standards and patterns included staffing, equipment, drugs, the way that contraceptive services were delivered, and records management. The ministry delegated the procurement and supply of contraceptives to a nonprofit company, which supplied government health centers with the necessary commodities and also provided oral contraceptives to other government organizations and to some nongovernmental organizations. The Population Council provided IUDs, and the Swedish International Development Cooperation Agency provided some condoms. Oral contraceptives were also available through numerous commercial outlets.

The Ministry of Health family planning program was implemented primarily through a network of ministry and other clinics. Stating the number of fixed and mobile clinics for any given year with any accuracy is impossible, as estimates vary so widely. The major problem is that some sources include only the ministry's own clinics, while other sources include clinics operated by both the ministry and other organizations. The Family Planning Division itself kept poor records on the number of clinics available to it. Friesen and Moore (1972) estimate that as of 1967, only about 160 clinics were providing family planning services, but by 1974, Zatuchni (1975) estimates that 2,200 clinics were providing services. To put these numbers in perspective, in 1972, the Family Planning Division estimated that providing good access across the country would require a total of 2,450 clinics by the end of the Fifth Economic Development Plan in 1978.[1] These would need to be supplemented by part-time clinics and the private sector. The mobile teams operated as extensions of the fixed clinics. To the degree that this analysis is reasonably accurate, the program already had most of its clinic infrastructure in place by 1974. Numbers alone, however, do not speak to the important issue of clinic siting to ensure good access, but as the program had inherited clinics from the Ministry of Health and other agencies, siting was not an option.

Choosing to implement the program primarily through fixed facilities gave the program a clinic versus a field delivery orientation, a policy that had important implications for physical access to services, counseling, and information. Most clients had to go to clinics for all pre-contraceptive screening and for initial and resupply of contraceptives, usually one cycle of pills at a time, which meant that acceptors had to return to the clinic every month. This created a barrier to access and resulted in dropouts, particularly among women in rural areas. In addition, supplies of the most popular pill brands ran out fairly regularly, further reducing access (Moore 1974).

Aware of the program's inadequate presence in rural areas, the Family Planning Division sought to increase the number of paramedical village and clinical personnel, mainly midwives, and to devolve less technically demanding tasks to lower-level staff members. Plans also included expanding the number of home visitors, non-medical personnel who would visit clients' homes to provide counseling and contraceptive re-supplies. The division was also considering using local nonprogram personnel, such as village heads and traditional midwives, as sources of referrals and contraceptive distributors.

Financial Resources

In 1967, the program began with an initial allocation of only US$500,000. Government financial support continued to increase, reaching US$9.2 million by 1972. The Fifth Economic Development Plan (1973–78) allocated US$100 million for the national family planning program, plus an additional US$700 million for a major expansion of the overall health services system (World Bank 1982). Note that much of the program's physical infrastructure and human resources were not charged to the family planning program, but were budgeted via their parent agencies or other parts of the Ministry of Health. As a result, the program was well, even lavishly, funded by the standards of most family planning programs of that time.

Foreign donors provided most of their contributions in kind in the form of studies, short- and long-term advisers and overseas fellows, fellowships and study tours, training, communications equipment, contraceptives, and vehicles.

Interorganizational Relationships

One of the most interesting things about Iran's family planning program was the number and range of organizations that claimed to be active in providing services, information, or both. In practice, no doubt some did so far more than others. The High Council for Coordination of Family Planning, established in 1967, included at least 12 organizations, not counting the Women's Health Corps, which was an integral part of the Family Planning Division, but a number of other organizations were also active in relation to some aspect of the program. These included a host of other ministries, including the Ministries of Education, Labor, Housing and Development, Agriculture, and Land Reform. Each of these claimed to provide briefings and training for their staff members on family planning and encouraged their staff members to disseminate information on family planning. The Ministry of Labor, through the Workers Insurance Scheme, provided family planning services to industrial workers and their dependents as part of an overall package of health services. The gendarmerie (responsible for security in rural areas and along the borders), the armed forces, the police force, and the National Oil Company did the same for their employees. Added to these were the efforts of the various so-called revolutionary corps. The shah initiated these corps in 1962 to implement social reform and development activities, including family planning. Corps members were assigned to various functional units, such as the Literacy Corps, the Men's Health Corps, the Women's Health Corps, and the Extension and Development Corps (Friesen and Moore 1972).

Human Resources

The Family Planning Division did not recruit, directly supervise, or pay for the majority of family planning workers. Instead, the Ministry of Health or other agencies involved in the program employed most family planning workers. For the ministry staff who manned the clinics, the division acted as trainer, adviser, standard setter, motivator, contraceptive supplier, planner, and coordinator. In addition, more than 700 young Health Corps women with special training in family planning information and motivation worked in the clinics and as field workers.

While this arrangement had its positive aspects, it also meant that the Family Planning Division had little operational or technical control over the facilities or the personnel who provided the services, so even though the division was responsible for the performance of the national family planning program, it was in the impossible position of having little effective control over its key assets.

A shortage of doctors and nurses posed an early and continuing constraint to the expansion of services. This was true for a number of reasons, including that few doctors or nurses were willing to move away from the big cities, that the program was over-medicalized, that too many doctors went abroad for study and either stayed away when they were needed or did not come back at all, and that clinics' staffing patterns in terms of the numbers and types of staff members bore little relationship to demand and the work load. The program was over-medicalized in the sense that it demanded too much unnecessary medical screening and imposed too many barriers on access to relatively simple methods like the pill. These policies also meant a heavy, and largely impractical, reliance on medically trained personnel.

To fill the need for the appropriate staff to motivate and counsel married women where the latter lived, the leadership of the family planning program developed a special category of "mature" field worker. These mature field workers were over 25 years old, were married, had at least six years of schooling, and lived in the areas where they would work. By 1971, 455 workers of this kind had been trained and posted. The goal was to train and field 5,000 such workers.

Given the number and types of family planning workers, the provision of a great deal of training by the Family Planning Division, including short term and long term, technical and nontechnical, was not surprising. To achieve this, the training section of the division operated a number of training centers throughout the country.

Communications and Education

To deliver information about family planning, and to link family planning with the education system, the Family Planning Division created a special section overseen by the director general for technical affairs. The principal means of providing information and motivational messages was via a combination of mass media; clinic counseling; and a number of other formal and informal channels (for example, social workers, teachers, shop floor peer educators, and a plethora of rural health and development cadres). Perhaps the major cadre providing information about family planning in rural areas was the Women's Health Corps. Members of the corps worked in family planning clinics and maternal and child health centers throughout the country and are believed to have helped increase acceptance rates (Ziai 1974).

Although family planning information and education campaigns were used periodically throughout much of the country, they focused mainly on urban areas. A huge mass media campaign began in the mid-1970s, but it did so without creating the necessary information base or laying the strategic groundwork by means of extensive market research and evaluative tools for rapid feedback (Aghajanian 1994). To put this into perspective, most family planning programs have found that modifying people's attitudes and behaviors in such an important and complex area of their lives is extremely difficult. This may have been especially true in Iran in the program's early days, given the country's conservative Muslim traditions. To seek guidance on the best approaches, the government and the Population Council carried out a large-scale model communications project in Isfahan beginning in 1970. This operations research project generated a great deal of useful knowledge about the program's target groups and tested ways to have the desired impact on knowledge, attitudes, and practices in relation to family planning (Moore, Asayesh, and Montague 1974).

Surprisingly, as late as 1972, the program rarely attempted to directly recruit clients. While the hope was that the heavy use of MCHN clinics would expose women to family planning information and services in a positive context, there is no record of any assessment of how best to take advantage of this opportunity (Friesen and Moore 1972).

As concerns the population side of the equation, the government implemented an extensive program of legally mandated education activities in schools. These activities were carried out by the Ministry of Education with major inputs from the Family Planning Division. Efforts included revising school curricula and textbooks. The division also initiated a program to introduce and explain population concepts and concerns to public school teachers. By the end of 1971, some 20,000 teachers had attended these one-day sessions.

In collaboration with the United Nations Educational, Scientific, and Cultural Organization, the government and the Population Council initiated a work-oriented adult literacy project in Isfahan that included a family planning–oriented literacy text for women. To promote implementation, the program was backed up with specific directives to the Literacy Corps and to schoolteachers and included family planning training programs and a mass media effort relying primarily on the use of radio (Bob Gillespie, personal communication, 2006).

Monitoring, Evaluation, and Research

Despite some efforts to improve them, the monitoring and program evaluation capabilities of the Family Planning Division remained weak from its creation until the end of the first stage of the program in 1979. The limitations to the program's ability to evaluate its progress towards its objectives meant that program managers and policy makers lacked much of the information they needed to learn from experience and to make needed midcourse corrections (World Bank 1982). The chronic nature of this problem is documented by studies done in 1972, 10 years earlier, that noted the same problems (Moore 1974; Moore, Asayesh, and Montague 1974). The studies hypothesized that a possible reason for failing to gather and disseminate results and to set planned targets was due to the extreme politicization of government operations, whereby engaging in evaluation and planning in such an environment could be risky. However, the same lack of evaluation and planning was common to nearly all family planning programs in developing countries. Remarkably, this still remains the case for many otherwise effective programs.

In contrast to the weak monitoring and program evaluation capabilities of the national family planning effort, few national family planning programs in the 1960s and 1970s can have enjoyed the ferment of evaluative research and trials that took place in Iran. The focus of these was diverse and included a number of large-scale operations research projects. These included projects that focused on expanding the cadres capable of providing information and services to remote rural populations in southern Iran (Economic and Social Commission for Asia and the Pacific 1977; Ronaghy 1976; Ronaghy and others 1976; Zeighami and Zeighami 1976; Zeighami and others 1976, 1977). Other projects demonstrated how to conceptualize, design, and implement a large-scale services program to determine how to solve health problems through better approaches to health delivery systems (Assar and Jaksic 1975).

By far the biggest, most innovative, and most influential operations research undertaken in Iran during this early period was the government and Population Council communications project, mentioned earlier, that began in Isfahan, which also introduced and tested many components of family planning services delivery. For example, the so-called model project introduced and tested the use of integrated approaches to communications and services, which were virtually unknown outside Iran at that time; the expansion of primary health services in rural areas to prevent pregnancy among adolescents and raise the age of marriage; the incentives for birth spacing and ways to reinforce a desire for families with only two or three children; the mobilization of physicians and paramedical personnel to deliver IUDs and oral contraceptives; the use of depot distribution; the use of functionaries such as mullahs, health and literacy corps members, village leaders, traditional village midwives, and schoolteachers to support family planning activities; the elimination of prescriptions for the pill and, instead, provision by government facilities of the full range of modern family planning methods; and the implementation of a social marketing program. The project also conducted extensive surveys in relation to knowledge, attitudes, and practices. Later, most features of this integrated model project were replicated throughout Isfahan, as well as Shiraz, Khuzistan, and Iranian Azerbaijan.

The project demonstrated significant improvements in knowledge, attitudes, and practices in the pilot districts. The project's findings also made important contributions to the program's knowledge about the characteristics of its target group (Gillespie and Loghmani 1972; Lieberman, Gillespie, and Loghmani 1973; Treadway, Gillespie, and Loghmani 1976). For example, the model project and other studies showed that Iranian women did little in the way of contraceptive use until they approached or exceeded their desired family size. In Isfahan, the average woman accepting family planning was 31, had five living children, and did not want any more children (Gillespie and Loghmani 1972). Experience elsewhere in Iran indicates that this was fairly typical (Ajami 1976).

Dozens of other studies were also carried out, many of which had the potential to contribute to the program's ability to create better demand for and access to services and to enhance the coverage of target populations. The extent to which the program's leadership used the studies' findings and recommendations to enhance learning, develop policy, and make midcourse corrections is unknown.

The number and range of these studies were the most remarkable and creative feature of Iran's family planning program. Other national programs at that time were
unlikely to have matched this performance, even though evaluative research into
family planning probably reached its apogee internationally during the 1960s and
1970s.

The Private Sector

By the 1960s, Iran had a number of influential and well-established nongovernmental agencies. Most of those with a social welfare orientation ended up playing an active
role in the family planning program. These included the Red Lion and Sun Society
(Iran's version of the Red Crescent or Red Cross), the Imperial Organization for Social
Services, the Women's Organization of Iran, the Institute for Protection of Mothers
and Children, the Community Welfare Center of Iran, the Family Planning Association of Iran (an International Planned Parenthood Federation affiliate), and numerous
universities. Note that nearly every one of these organizations was closely associated
with or overseen by a member of the royal family or had other close ties with the government. In addition, most, if not all, of these organizations received funds from the
government, in addition to whatever other funds they may have received (Friesen and
Moore 1972).

Prior to 1961, importing contraceptive pills into Iran was illegal. Legalization
finally allowed the commercial sector, mainly pharmacies and private practitioners,
to become active participants in providing contraceptive services. Other than that,
little was known about the role of the commercial sector in providing family planning services until a 1972 study by the Westinghouse Population Center (1973). This
study concluded that the commercial sector supplied half the couples using contraceptives in Iran; concluded that the growth potential was enormous; and made a
number of recommendations on how this growth could be realized via a series of
actions at the government, importer, manufacturer, retailer, and consumer levels.
The author is not aware whether the recommendations of the Westinghouse study
were acted upon.

In mid-1971, the United Nations sent a fact-finding mission to Iran headed by
Lord Caradon. The Caradon mission estimated that between 90,000 and 100,000
pill cycles were sold each month through commercial channels, representing 39 to
43 percent of all estimated pill cycles distributed. If correct, this corresponds roughly
to the Westinghouse findings.

Program Effects

Except for the results unequivocally generated by the program, such as the number
of pill cycles distributed, the attributable impact of the program on most of the
effects summarized here, especially the demographic ones, is unknown. This basic
problem is made worse by the lack of agreement among those who have gathered,
analyzed, and reported the data on a given effect. Moreover, some surveys and

TABLE 3.1 Number of Oral Pill Cycles Distributed Per Month by the Program and Those Purchased Commercially, Selected Years

Method	1968	1971	1974	1978
Distributed by the program	1,433	21,000	—	389,000
Purchased commercially	50,000	100,000	225,000	—

Source: Friesen and Moore 1972; Mehryar and others 2000.

Note: — = not available.

censuses produced unlikely results on one or more indicators, for example, figures cited for the total fertility rate in 1976 range from 5.5 to 6.8 live births per woman, depending on the source (Bulatao and Richardson 1994). Oddly, these figures come from a common database, the census. In such cases, the author simply took the number that seemed to make the most sense. For present purposes, program effects are broken out into three sets of categories: oral contraceptives distributed and bought, new acceptors, and number of users and prevalence of use. In addition, a summary of demographic effects is provided. As the Iranian program was overwhelmingly a pill program, only this method will be reported here. Even though urban-rural differentials are substantial for every effect discussed, for the sake of brevity, they are not reported here except in relation to traditional methods.

Distribution and Purchase of Oral Contraceptives

Table 3.1 shows the numbers of oral cycles distributed by the program per month versus those purchased commercially. As the table shows, between 1968 and 1978, the number of pill cycles distributed by the program increased dramatically. In addition, according to Zatuchni (1975), at least 800 specialists and other private practitioners were inserting IUDS. Given the poor state of data and information about the commercial sector, its role in providing services is no doubt underreported.

New Acceptors

Zatuchni (1975) estimates that between April 1970 and September 1974, the program served about 2.31 million new acceptors. The average number of new acceptors per month served just by the program (note that some may have been new acceptors more than once) increased from 7,700 in 1968 to 46,100 in 1972, to approximately 50,000 in 1974 (World Bank 1982). The year 1974 saw approximately 600,000 new acceptors, up 4 percent from 1973.

Contraceptive Prevalence

Table 3.2 shows the percentage of married women aged 15–49 using family planning services from all sources during 1972 to 1978. As of 1969, prevalence was estimated to be only 3 percent (Bulatao and Richardson 1994).[2] Such estimates are difficult to rely on or to compare. For example, a study by the Economic and Social Commission for Asia and the Pacific (1974) estimated prevalence for that year to be 44.9 percent,

TABLE 3.2 Contraceptive Prevalence, Selected Years

Year	Percentage of married women aged 15–49 using contraception
1972	8
1974	14
1976–77	36
1978	36–38

Source: Bulatao and Richardson 1994.

which seems too high. The latter study also estimated, by way of comparison, that 1974 levels were 30 percent in the Philippines and 42 percent in urban India.

Table 3.3 presents information about the use of traditional methods, such as withdrawal, within the overall contraceptive prevalence rate. Clearly, traditional methods have played a major role in contraception, and their prevalence changed relatively little in urban areas from the early 1970s through the early 1990s. Surveys in Tehran from the mid-1960s to the early 1970s show that use of traditional methods as a percentage of overall contraceptive prevalence ranged between 45 and 55 percent. Data from a knowledge, attitudes, and practice study done with mainly rural women in 1971 reported that withdrawal was the preferred method for 24 percent of the respondents (Friesen 1969; Friesen and Moore 1972).

Two things are remarkable about these results. First, traditional methods have continued to be popular despite the growing availability of affordable modern methods and the urging by authorities to use them. Second, and most remarkable, is that the use of traditional methods has consistently been higher among urban residents than rural residents. Indeed, urban residents relied more on traditional methods than on any single modern method, whereas traditional methods ranked second in popularity among rural residents (Bulatao and Richardson 1994). This finding defies all obvious explanations. Also curious is the lack of attention to this anomaly in the literature. The answer could have something to do with urban residents being more forthcoming and more willing to mention withdrawal than rural respondents, who may be more embarrassed about the whole subject. Alternatively, being better educated, perhaps urban residents were more likely to comprehend the question and have a better understanding of what a contraceptive method is. However, these are all guesses, with no empirical basis whatsoever (Steve Solter, personal communication, September 2006).

TABLE 3.3 The Use of Traditional Methods of Contraception, Selected Years
percentage of overall contraceptive prevalence

Location	1972	1976	1989	1992
Urban	35.3	37.4	48.8	36.4
Rural	37.1	25.5	32.8	20.2

Source: Bulatao and Richardson 1994.
Note: The numbers here are based on survey data and are mostly likely overstated.

TABLE 3.4 Total Fertility Rates, Crude Birth Rates, and Population Growth Rates, Selected Years

Category	1956	1965	1966	1975	1976	1985	1986
Total fertility rate (average number of children born during a woman's lifetime)	—	7.6	—	6.5	—	7.0	—
Crude birth rate (live births per 1,000 population)	50	—	50	—	42	—	48
Population growth rate (%)	1.74	—	>3	—	2.68	—	3.83

Source: Bulatao and Richardson 1994.

Note: — = not available.

Demographic Effects

Table 3.4 provides information on total fertility rates, crude birth rates, and the population growth rate during 1956 to 1986. Bulatao and Richardson (1994) note that the crude birth rate followed a pattern similar to that of the total fertility rate. While the drop in the crude birth rate from 50 live births per 1,000 population to 42 represents good progress, this rate was still higher than the government's crude birth rate target of 38 live births per 1,000 population. With regard to the population growth rate, while the reduced rate of 2.68 percent for 1976 shows progress, it was higher than the government's target rate of 2.60 percent. The failure to meet the target was due to the slower-than-expected decline in the birth rate. In line with the total fertility rate and the crude birth rate, the population growth rate jumped to 3.83 percent in 1986. As the foregoing numbers indicate, Iran experienced high fertility throughout the 1950s and 1960s, which declined substantially during the 1970s, and then rebounded, or experienced slower decline, in the 1980s.

Summary of Program Effects

The program started up rapidly and began to show progress early on. Steady increases were apparent in the number of contraceptives distributed or purchased, in new acceptors, and in prevalence, along with decreases in fertility and the crude birth rate. The results were respectable for a program that was just starting up and were achieved during a relatively brief period. Nevertheless, as noted throughout this chapter, any assessment of the program's performance must take into consideration the many constraints and challenges this new initiative faced.

External Assistance and Influence

Iran's nascent family planning program enjoyed a great deal of external assistance and support. Indeed, such assistance helped to bring attention to the demographic problem in the first place, then played an important role in helping to inform policy as well as many of the features of the national program. The vast majority of foreign assistance was oriented toward technical issues and human resource development rather than being financial or material. Different organizations played different roles in terms of the amounts and kinds of support they offered. While judging which organizations were more important than others is difficult, during the program's formative period, the most active and influential foreign organizations included the Population Council; a number of United Nations agencies (the United Nations itself; the United Nations Educational, Scientific, and Cultural Organization; the United Nations Fund for Population Activities; and the Economic Commission for Asia and the Far East [later changed to the Economic and Social Commission for Asia and the Pacific]); and the U.S. Agency for International Development. Others included the Swedish International Development Cooperation Agency, the International Planned Parenthood Federation, the World Bank, and the United Nations Children's Fund.

The Population Council

Many observers believe that the Population Council was easily the most influential of all the external agencies working in Iran during 1960 to 1979. Several key factors allowed the council to play its unique and important role. To begin with, the council already had a worldwide reputation as the premier repository of technical expertise in population and family planning. Thus, it was no surprise when, in 1966, the government asked the council to review Iran's demographic and services situation and make recommendations in relation to the new population and family planning program. The report by Keeny and others (1967) provided the country with extraordinary guidance on population that dramatized the need for population programs. It also provided a template for exactly how to design and implement such a program based on the somewhat modest experience gained at that time and remains as a wonderful snapshot of the state-of-the-art approach 40 years ago. The congruence between the council's recommendations and the major aspects of Iran's eventual family planning policies, services, and information program is striking.

In addition, the two Population Council advisers resident in Iran from 1968 through 1975 enjoyed a unique level of access to and influence over the program's leadership and across the government.

Finally, the council initiated, largely paid for, and provided technical support to many of the major research initiatives carried out at that time, including the model project. More than any other agency, the council helped create the large number of evaluative research studies and trials that took place in the 1970s. In addition, the council provided important support in the form of training programs, a four-year postpartum family planning services program at Farah Maternity Hospital, a resident consultant for the model project, numerous short-term consultants, assistance with the national communications effort, data processing equipment, and all the IUDs for the national family planning program (Friesen and Moore 1972; Joel Montague, personal communication, September 2006).

United Nations Agencies

In 1969, the United Nations Development Programme appointed a population program officer, later designated as a senior population adviser. In 1971, the United

Nations carried out a comprehensive review of the Iranian program via a team that also included the World Health Organization and the United Nations Educational, Scientific, and Cultural Organization. The findings and recommendations of the team's report became the basis for a series of project requests that were sent to the newly created UNFPA. By 1973, UNFPA had expanded its role and its presence in key countries like Iran, and by the end of that year had posted one of its 17 UNFPA coordinators to Tehran to oversee its growing program (UNFPA 1973). The Economic Commission for Asia and the Far East provided training programs and, like a number of other agencies, sponsored conferences and workshops in which Iranian officials participated (Friesen and Moore 1972).

U.S. Agency for International Development

The U.S. government contributed to the family planning program via the provision of three population interns recruited by the University of Michigan, the University of North Carolina, and Johns Hopkins University. The U.S. Agency for International Development also contributed to the funding of numerous research projects, fellowships, and other forms of support via the same three American universities as well as others. In addition, it provided support to the Population Council to help fund the postpartum family planning program, research grants, and additional fellowships (Friesen and Moore 1972).

The World Bank

The Work Bank attempted only one population project in Iran. The project was approved in May 1973 and was canceled in March 1977, during which time only US$640,000 of the approved US$16.5 million loan had been disbursed. Like many Bank projects, this was primarily a bricks-and-mortar project intended to extend health and family planning services to smaller towns. The project's objectives also included improving the management of the national program, increasing the capacity and the quality of training, and laying the groundwork for a subsequent nutrition project. Project monies financed only two studies, a management assessment and a nutrition study needed to prepare for the nutrition project. A frank internal Bank report offers a number of reasons for the failure of this population project, some of them quite damning. These included delays in construction and procurement, cost overruns, and alleged low commitment to the project on the part of Ministry of Health officials (World Bank 1982).[3]

Assessment of the 1960–79 Program

Like many national family planning efforts, Iran's program achieved a great deal, but also had its share of problems and weaknesses. This section seeks to present a balanced picture of the program's performance in the context of its time and setting.

Achievements

As of early 1967, Iran had virtually no family planning activity aside from some private sector purchases of contraceptives in urban areas and services offered by a few nongovernmental organizations services. Within just a few years, family planning activities had become an important component of the national five-year plans, adequate (even lavish) financing had been made available, a national program had been created and staffed and was providing services and information involving many multisectoral agencies, and a broad range of social measures beyond family planning had been added to those already in place (Zatuchni 1975). From the outset, the program enjoyed unequivocal support from the highest levels of government. Moreover, given the formative nature of the program and the constraints of the setting, it achieved measurable progress in contraceptive distribution, in acceptance and use rates, and in reduction of fertility. Examples of its achievements include the following:

- To deal with the shortage of physicians in rural areas, the Family Planning Division sought to compensate for an inherited clinic infrastructure with poor coverage in rural areas by introducing services and information via a number of paramedical and volunteer cadres. The recruitment of thousands of medically trained and other educated and service-oriented young people to the Health Corps was a social reform of great significance, especially for a developing country in the early 1960s.

- To deal with the need for long-acting methods, the program experimented with postpartum family planning services (which tended to emphasize IUDs) and with the use of paramedics to insert IUDs.

- To improve communications with older women, the program fielded a cadre of older, married women as field motivators.

- Rather than waiting to create its own services infrastructure, the program took advantage of existing infrastructure and staff, which permitted its rapid start-up.

- While the program itself was demographically focused, it was part of an overall national effort to upgrade the status of women and to enhance social welfare.

- The program's leadership was open to outside advice and, as a result, received invaluable technical support and encouragement from the international community and from other family planning programs.

- Family planning services were being provided through more than 2,000 clinics nationwide by the late 1970s.

- Contraceptive services were integrated with other preventive services from the outset, especially maternal and child health.

- From the beginning, the family planning program participated in and/or sponsored an active program of research for policy planning, learning, and innovation.

- Program leaders sought to improve access to and acceptance of services by providing them for free or at extremely low prices.

- The program initiated a huge mass media campaign to increase knowledge, attitudes, and practices in relation to family planning in the early to mid-1970s that supplemented the community-level work done by the paramedical and volunteer cadres.

Problems and Constraints

Inevitably, the program faced many problems and constraints, some avoidable, some not. One could argue that the management constraints were part of the growing pains of a new program, and many of these were correctable, if not avoidable. Note that the following list of the problems and constraints, which includes those related to the setting and those related to the program's leadership and management, makes little effort to assess their significance.

- The country had no history of modern contraception as of 1967, and thus no experience or expertise. This inevitably had an important impact on early performance. The program's management worked to overcome this problem, but this naturally occurred only gradually.

- The principal target group was the conservative, pro-natalist, but chronically underserved rural population. This contextual problem had an important and enduring negative impact. In addition, rural areas were seriously underdeveloped relative to towns and cities, with far less access to communications, transportation, social services, and other infrastructure.

- The lack of active endorsement and support of the program by religious leaders was an important issue.

- The urban focus of the existing infrastructure, which the program had to rely on, resulted in poor rural coverage and was a major constraint to access by rural women. Even though the program tried to address the problem via efforts to expand rural services and information using traditional practitioners, paramedics, and volunteers, it was never solved.

- The almost total reliance on the pill biased the program toward younger, urban women. These women were more interested in spacing than older rural women, who wanted to stop having children entirely. Moreover, urban women had easier access to commercially available contraceptives.

- The country's increased oil revenues had a negative impact on people's perceptions of the need for limiting population growth and fertility. Ultimately, this appears to have had an impact on the support for the program from within the government as well as among the general population.

- Management lacked the authority to control the direction of the program, to coordinate it with other stakeholders, and to exert influence over Ministry of Health and other service facilities as well as other financial and human resources.

- The program's strategies, policies, and objectives were vague, and implementation planning was not done on a nationwide basis. One example was the amorphous focus on all married women of reproductive age, which precluded effective targeting and planning.

- Record keeping was poor, virtually no evaluation of program results was carried out, and thus, national leaders received little feedback regarding the program's progress (World Bank 1982).

- While the program's heavy reliance on pills was largely unavoidable, why so little effort was invested in promoting condoms and in laying the groundwork for the eventual introduction of long-acting methods is less clear. To exacerbate the problem, pill supply policies were too restrictive in that they allowed women to obtain only one cycle of pills per visit.

- On the demand side, communications efforts were poorly targeted and may have placed excessive reliance on mass media, with too little use of market research to improve communications strategies, including targeting, messages, channels, and impact assessment. In addition, the effectiveness of young and unmarried motivation cadres was unclear, and the program made too few efforts to engage in aggressive direct motivation of new acceptors and of dropouts.

- The shortage of doctors and nurses, especially in rural areas, was exacerbated by over-medicalized policies and an allocation of scarce human resources that was not cost-effective.

Conclusions

One of the most striking aspects of the list of the program's problems and weaknesses is how many of them also affected—or would affect—every other nascent family planning effort in Asia and elsewhere (Moore, Asayesh, and Montague 1974). Even more striking is that even today, 35 years later, many, if not most, of these problems continue to be weak areas in maternal and child health, reproductive health, and other public health programs. These chronic problems include weak strategies and plans, for example, to maximize access to services; vague priority setting and targeting; weak supervisory systems and questionable quality of care; weak monitoring and evaluation systems, with few data generated for decision making and few lessons learned; little use of cost-effectiveness analysis; and poor coordination within and between sectors.

On the positive side of the ledger, the program's achievements were impressive, especially given that Iran was a pioneer in designing and implementing a national family planning program from scratch. The common view in those early days of family planning was that "successful national family planning programs seem to exist primarily in small, rapidly modernizing countries which are either islands or peninsulas" (Moore, Asayesh, and Montague 1974, p. 400). This restrictive view would persist for some years. Given the widespread belief in this view, and given Iran's challenging realities, it would have been difficult to be optimistic about its chances to carry out a successful program. Putting this view aside, a fair conclusion is that during its first stage, the Iranian family planning program performed well relative to comparable first-wave countries like Egypt, Pakistan, and Turkey.

Postscript: Assessing Later Developments

Most of this narrative is focused on the first stage of Iran's family planning program, that is the shah-initiated program that operated from 1967 to 1979. However, the subsequent two stages—from 1979 to 1988 and from 1988 to the present—represent important later developments that help us understand the contributions of the shah's initiatives. This section offers a brief overview of these subsequent stages.

The Second Stage of the Family Planning Program: 1979–88
The leaders of the 1979 Islamic Revolution decided essentially to halt the extant family planning program. One reason was simply that they did not believe that population growth was a problem. Influencing this judgment were the human losses that had occurred during the eight-year war with Iraq, which began in mid-1981. The new revolutionary authorities revived Islamic law, cut back on women's rights, and in general orchestrated a shift from secular toward traditional values. Part of these changes involved suspending the high-profile official family planning program, including dropping the previous fertility control policy; abolishing the Family Planning Division of the Ministry of Health; dissolving the High Council for Coordination of Family Planning Council; ceasing the information, education, and communications program entirely; and closing clinics that specialized in family planning. However, contrary to popular belief, the suspension of the official program did not signal the end of family planning services and supplies in Iran. Family planning services continued to be provided by the Ministry of Health's MCHN facilities, by retail outlets, and by private clinics and practitioners.

Despite the explicitly pro-natalist policies of the Islamic Republic of Iran, data from this period reveal that despite a brief drop in annual family planning clients at the outset of the revolution in 1979 (from 5.2 million to 4.2 million), the number of clients had risen to 5.6 million by 1981. The number of clients continued to increase slowly to a high of more than 7 million by 1987. Several surveys conducted during this period revealed that most families were in favor of limiting the number of children they had (Mehryar and others 2000). Yet even with these increases in contraceptive use, the total fertility rate increased markedly, and with it so did population size. The 1986 census revealed that the total population had grown from 33.7 million in 1976 to nearly 50 million (Aghajanian 1994; Bulatao and Richardson 1994).

The Third Stage of the Family Planning Program: 1988 to the Present
By 1988, the national leaders came to appreciate the negative implications of the 1986 census. Also by that time, the war with Iraq was over and the leadership could again consider family planning as a national priority. Accordingly, beginning in early 1988, ministries and government departments were directed to consider what

policies and programs were needed to control population growth. Possibly learning from the shortcomings of the first stage of the family planning program, but more likely resulting from its own religious leanings and the mullah-dominated power structure, the government exerted considerable efforts to consult with and obtain the support of most members of the religious establishment. By early 1989, the government announced the national family planning policy, which was approved by parliament. Following the previous pattern, the Ministry of Health was given responsibility for the program and generous resources to provide free contraceptive services to all married couples. Another emulation of the earlier program was to establish a series of mechanisms to ensure intersectoral cooperation among the numerous ministries and agencies involved in some way with the program. There is no doubt that the current program benefited enormously from the efforts of the shah's program to spread knowledge of family planning among all segments of the population, from the thousands of people trained at that time, and from the growth of the private sector's role in contraceptive provision since 1961.

The rising contraceptive prevalence rates indicate the success of the program, rising from 49 percent in 1989 to 76 percent by 1997. Another significant achievement has been to reduce the urban-rural gap in prevalence to only 10 percent, a feat achieved in large part through the extensive deployment of local rural health workers. In tandem with the increase in prevalence rates, the population growth rate dropped from 3.9 percent in the 1980s to 2.5 percent by 1991. Similarly, the crude birth rate fell from 43 live births per 1,000 population in 1973–76 to 21 in 1996. Even though the rate of population growth has been falling, the number of people added each year remains close to historic highs, and could go even higher. Given its age structure, the population will still double eventually, even with replacement-level fertility (Aghajanian 1994; Bulatao and Richardson 1994; Mehryar and others 2000).

Notes

1. The figure of 2,450 clinics was based on 1972 population figures. The estimate was calculated on the assumption of a rural population of 18 million and a target ratio of 1 clinic per 10,000 population, which comes to 1,800 clinics. For the urban population of 13 million, the ratio was estimated at 1 clinic per 20,000 population, or 650 clinics (Friesen and Moore 1972).
2. Prevalence numbers have proven particularly difficult to reconstruct with any degree of confidence because they vary a great deal depending on the source. Bulatao and Richardson (1994) is the source for the more conservative numbers shown in this section, which are based primarily on service statistics.
3. While reading such an unusually critical project assessment by a major donor is stimulating, it is only fair to point out that the Bank has had many unsatisfactory experiences in a number of countries of the kind recorded here. Moreover, the Bank was relatively new to family planning programming and, even though Bank staff members had judged this a "risky" project from the outset, they chose to go ahead with it anyway. This makes one wonder whether the Bank's approach to project formulation and management was at least partly to blame for some of the problems noted.

References

Aghajanian, Akbar. 1994. "Family Planning and Contraceptive Use in Iran, 1967–1992." *International Family Planning Perspectives* 20 (2): 66–69.

Ajami, I. 1976. "Differential Fertility in Peasant Communities: A Study of Six Iranian villages." *Population Studies* 30 (3): 453–563.

Assar, M., and Z. Jaksic. 1975. "A Health Services Development Project in Iran." In *Health by the People*, ed. K. W. Newell, 112–27. Geneva: World Health Organization.

Berelson, Bernard. 1978. "Programs and Prospects for Fertility Reduction: What? Where?" Working Paper, Center for Policy Studies, Population Council, New York.

Bulatao, Rodolfo A., and Gail Richardson. 1994. "Fertility and Family Planning in Iran." Discussion Paper Series 13, World Bank, Washington, DC.

Economic and Social Commission for Asia and the Pacific. 1974. "Family Planning Practice and Its Socio-Demographic and Communication Correlates." In *Husband-Wife Communication and Practice of Family Planning*, 113–33. Asian Population Studies Series 16 (E/CN.11/1212). Bangkok: Economic and Social Commission for Asia and the Pacific.

———. 1977. "Health Worker Pilot Project." *Asian and Pacific Population Programme News* 6 (4): 23.

Friesen, John K. 1969. *Iran. Country Profiles Series.* New York: Population Council.

Friesen, John K., and Richard Moore. 1972. "Iran." *Country Profiles.* New York: Population Council.

Gillespie, R. W., and M. Loghmani. 1972. "The Isfahan Communications Projects." Unpublished report, Ministry of Health, Family Planning Division, Tehran.

Keeny, S. M., W. P. Mauldin, G. F. Brown, and L. M. Hellman. 1967. "Iran: Report on Population Growth and Family Planning." *Studies in Family Planning* 20 (June): 3–6.

Lieberman, S. S., Robert W. Gillespie, and M. Loghmani. 1973. "The Isfahan Communications Project." *Studies in Family Planning* IV (4): 73–100.

Mehryar, Amir H., Joel Montague, Farzaneh Roudi, and Farzaneh Tajdini. 2000. "Iranian Family Planning Program at the Threshold of the 21st Century." Paper presented at the International Union for Scientific Study of Population seminar on "Family Planning Programmes in the 21st Century," Dhaka.

Moore, Richard. 1974. "Supply and Demand Aspects of Oral Pill Delivery in Iranian Family Planning Clinics." Ph.D. dissertation, Cornell University, Ithaca, NY.

Moore, Richard, Khalil Asayesh, and Joel Montague. 1974. "Population and Family Planning in Iran." *Middle East Journal* 28 (4): 396–408.

Ronaghy, H. A. 1976. "Middle Level Health Workers Training Project in Iran." In *Village Health Workers: Proceedings of a Workshop, Shiraz, Iran, March 1976*, ed. H. A. Ronaghy, Y. Mousseau-Gershman, and A. Dorozynski, 11–13. Ottawa: International Development Research Centre.

Ronaghy, H. A., E. Najaradeh, T. A. Schwartz, S. S. Russell, S. Solter, and B. Zeighami. 1976. "The Front Line Health Worker: Selection, Training, and Performance." *American Journal of Public Health* 66 (3): 273–77.

Treadway, R. C., R. W. Gillespie, and M. Loghmani. 1976. "The Model Family Planning Project in Isfahan, Iran." *Studies in Family Planning* VII (11): 308–21.

UNFPA (United Nations Population Fund). 1973. *Annual Report.* New York: UNFPA.

Westinghouse Population Center. 1973. *Distribution of Contraceptives in the Commercial Sector of Iran.* Columbia, MD: Westinghouse Population Center.

World Bank. 1973. *Report and Recommendation of the President to the Executive Directors on a Proposed Loan to the Government of Iran for a Population Project.* Washington, DC: World Bank.

————. 1982. "Project Performance Audit Report: Iran Population Project (Loan 928-IRN)." Report, 3790, World Bank, Washington, DC.

Zatuchni, Gerald I. 1975. "Iran." *Studies in Family Planning* 6 (8): 302–4.

Zeighami, B., and E. Zeighami. 1976. "Evaluation of Iranian Village Health Workers' Efficacy." In *Village Health Workers: Proceedings of a Workshop, Shiraz, Iran, March 1976,* ed. H. A. Ronaghy, Y. Mousseau-Gershman, and A. Dorozynski, 14–20. Ottawa: International Development Research Centre.

Zeighami, E., B. Zeighami, A. E. Eftekhari, and P. Khoshnevis. 1976. "Effectiveness of the Iranian Auxiliary Midwife in IUD Insertion." *Studies in Family Planning* 7 (9): 261–63.

Zeighami, E., B. Zeighami, I. Javidian, and S. Zimmer. 1977. "The Rural Health Worker as a Family Planning Provider: A Village Trial in Iran." *Studies in Family Planning* 8 (7): 184–87.

Ziai, L. 1974. "Population Education in Iran." In *Population Education in the Asian Region: A Conference on Needs and Directions*, ed. J. Middleton, 88–92. Report of the International Conference on Population Education in the Asian Region, Tagaytay City, Philippines, January 14–21. Honolulu: East-West Center.

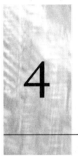

4 Tunisia: The Debut of Family Planning

GEORGE F. BROWN

Tunisia is one of the three countries of the Arab Maghreb in North Africa and is situated on the southern border of the Mediterranean. Along with Algeria and Morocco, it was colonized by France and gained independence in 1956. Its population is almost entirely Muslim and Arab, with a significant blending of Berber stock, the original inhabitants of the region. At the time of independence, Tunisia was largely rural and agricultural, with a limited industrial base and few natural resources. Habib Bourguiba was the uncontested national leader before and during the independence period, and from 1956 to 1987 was Tunisia's first president. Tunisia has charted a progressive social and economic policy and has held a relatively neutral political position since independence, retaining close ties with France as well as with its Maghreb neighbors and with the United States. Because of Bourguiba's liberal political and social policies, Tunisia's relations with other Arab countries were initially frequently strained. From independence onward, Tunisia has been a one-party state, with only weak political opposition. The Neo-Destour Party, which Bourguiba had created during the fight for independence, was the single political voice of the government.

Shortly after independence, President Bourguiba initiated a series of remarkable social changes that affected the lives of all Tunisians, especially women (Daly 1966; Gueddana 2001). He liberalized laws, codes, and regulations affecting many aspects of social life, the most notable of which included the following:

- Improving the status of women by enabling them to acquire rights as complete citizens, including giving them the right to vote and to remove the veil

- Prohibiting polygamy and giving women full legal divorce rights

- Raising the minimum age of marriage to 17 years for women and 20 years for men

- Removing barriers to the importation and sale of contraceptives and the provision of information on contraceptives

- Legalizing abortion for personal (nonmedical) reasons after the fifth child

- Limiting government family allowances to the first four children

- Encouraging literacy, especially female literacy

- Legalizing female sterilization.

All these steps, taken well before the start of the National Family Planning Program, were remarkable for the time, especially in a Muslim state. Even today, such dramatic improvements in the status of women are well ahead of all other Muslim societies. The measures were generally well received by the population, including religious leaders, reflecting the relatively progressive political and cultural nature of Tunisian society. The changes provided a promising basis for the initiation of a national family planning program.

The Beginnings

The government's first national Economic and Social Development Plan, released in 1962, pointed out that demographic growth must be decreased to achieve social and economic objectives, although the plan's 10-year perspective assumed that population growth would decrease in line with social and economic development and without government intervention (Daly 1966).

Discussions on the possibility of initiating a government family planning effort began in early 1962 between a Ford Foundation representative who had worked in Pakistan and was familiar with early family planning efforts in that country, Tunisian officials, and the Population Council (Mauldin, Berelson, and Hardy 1963). Government development planners were also concerned about rapid population growth. Box 4.1 provides a timeline of major events.

Following a visit to Tunis by the Population Council staff in 1963, the government drew up a preliminary plan for an experimental family planning program. A group of senior Tunisian officials visited several Asian countries in 1963, and another group visited the United States in 1964 to attend the Second International Conference on the Intrauterine Device and to hold discussions with various experts on population policy, family planning, and contraceptive technologies. In early 1964, a national seminar in Tunis reviewed all aspects of population and family planning; attracted favorable press and radio reports; and notably included participation by representatives of the National Women's Organization, labor unions, and the Neo-Destour Party. President Bourguiba gave a strong supportive speech, emphasizing the need to reduce population growth to achieve economic and social development (Daly 1966).

The Experimental Program, 1964–66

The operational phase of an experimental program began in 1964 with a national survey of knowledge, attitudes, and practices in relation to family planning, which demonstrated a strong demand by women with four or more children to limit their

BOX 4.1 Timeline for Population and Family Planning

1956–61: Legislation is passed to improve the status of women, including the right to vote and to remove the veil, the prohibition of polygamy, an increase in the minimum age of marriage, the provision of equal divorce rights, and the legalization of abortion after the fifth child and of female sterilization.

1962: The government's 10-year Economic and Social Development Plan urges reduced population growth rate to achieve economic and social goals.

The government and Ford Foundation officials discuss collaboration in relation to population issues.

1963: Tunisian officials visit population and family planning programs in Asia.

The government designs an experimental family planning program, emphasizing intrauterine devices.

1964: Tunisian officials visit U.S. population and family planning programs and attend the International Intrauterine Device Conference.

A national family planning conference is held.

The experimental family planning program begins.

A survey of knowledge, attitudes, and practices in relation to family planning is conducted.

Population Council technical assistance is initiated.

1965: Mobile family planning clinics are inaugurated.

The Neo-Destour Party and the National Women's Union become actively engaged.

1966: The National Family Planning Program is launched.

President Bourguiba, in a speech, expresses concern about reducing the population growth rate too rapidly.

President Bourguiba signs the United Nations Declaration on Population.

1967: Oral contraceptives are made widely available.

A postpartum program is initiated.

U.S. Agency for International Development assistance commences.

1968: The Tunisian Family Planning Association is launched.

President Bourguiba speaks in strong support of family planning.

1973: The National Office for Family Planning and Development is established.

The management of the Family Planning Program is strengthened, increasing the range of methods and improving education.

The abortion law is further liberalized, removing earlier restrictions.

family size. Knowledge and use of contraception was generally low. The survey report stated that "a large proportion of respondents say they are interested in knowing about methods of family limitation and state they would make use of them" (Morsa 1966, p. 590).

Family planning clinical work began in June 1964 with funding provided by the Ford Foundation and technical assistance by the Population Council. (The Swedish International Development Cooperation Agency had initiated an earlier maternal and child health clinical program, including contraception, in a small rural area.) The program was managed within the Ministry of Health under Dr. Amor Daly, the medical director, with no staff specifically dedicated to program management. Physicians and midwives were trained in contraceptive techniques, with an emphasis on the

Lippes loop intrauterine device (IUD). Throughout the experimental phase, a strong emphasis was given to the IUD, with a secondary focus on oral contraceptives and little attention paid to barrier methods or sterilization.

Initially, family planning was introduced in 12 clinics and hospitals in the major urban centers. By the end of the experimental period in 1966, 39 centers offered family planning and several mobile units had begun visiting outlying centers in most provinces on a weekly basis, offering primarily IUDs. The three major hospitals in Tunis had active family planning clinics and served as training centers for health workers nationwide.

Two enthusiastic medical officers in relatively rural provinces (Beja and Le Kef) organized large weekly events and gatherings of clients in villages for IUD insertions and transported some women to the district hospital for services, including sterilization. The Neo-Destour Party cells in these two provinces were active in mobilizing the local population, providing information, providing transportation for women, and citing President Bourguiba's speeches (Editors 1966). This high level of political activism and a measure of heavy-handed political pressure were clearly coercive at times, but were not generalized, and were not part of the Ministry of Health's official program. The strong measures by the Neo-Destour Party were occasionally repeated in later years. In the first year of the experimental program, Beja and Le Kef accounted for almost half of all IUD insertions. The use of mobile units to reach rural areas served as a model for an extensive national program using mobile units in later years.

Throughout Tunisia, the press and radio were the primary sources of general information about family planning and population issues. The National Women's Organization was a public advocate as well. Beyond that, information and communication efforts were extremely limited, and information provided to clients was inadequate (Povey and Brown 1968).

By the end of the experimental program, 27,817 women had visited 39 clinics and 18,523 of them had received an IUD. These results, while modest, represented a significant start, but problems quickly emerged, namely weak administration, lack of health and educational personnel, poor counseling and follow-up care, weak public information and education, and little evaluation. The heavy emphasis on IUDs undoubtedly limited individual choice, and negative rumors developed concerning this method. Follow-up visits were inadequate, and little emphasis was given to the management of side effects. These shortcomings no doubt contributed to the negative attitudes toward the IUD that emerged over time.

Almost all the limited research and evaluation focused on the clinical performance of the IUD (Brown and Sabbagh 1965; Vallin and others 1968). The studies demonstrated that the IUD was effective for more than 70 percent of women during one year of use and that the overall results were similar to international experience with IUDs at that time. Overall, the experimental phase introduced the concept of family planning and contraception to the population and to health professionals, mobilized national institutions, and set the stage for the national program to come. No significant opposition to the program emerged, and reaction to the concept of and need for family planning was generally positive.

The National Program, 1966–72

The National Family Planning Program was officially inaugurated in June 1966. Even though it was conceived as a national program, no family planning administrative structure was identifiable within the Ministry of Health. Several ministry officials had some responsibility, but all decisions were referred to Dr. Amor Daly, the medical director, who was also burdened with many other duties. All services were provided free of charge, including abortion and sterilization.

The three Tunis hospitals continued to offer services, including the provision of oral contraceptives, sterilization, and abortion. As for the rest of the country, where the health infrastructure was weak, the program relied heavily on mobile family planning teams, one for each province. Each team consisted of a gynecologist (often on contract from Eastern Europe or the then-Soviet Union), a midwife, a nurse's aide, a driver, and a clerk. Each team had a vehicle with medical equipment and a folding table for IUD insertions. The teams visited rural clinics, and sometimes schools or government offices, on a regular, usually weekly, schedule. The main purpose was IUD insertion, and many units did nothing else. Those that also distributed condoms and vaginal spermicides and dealt with gynecological complaints appeared to be more acceptable to rural communities. The teams were an expensive experiment and generally experienced a low level of demand for their services, especially in the southern rural provinces, and were clearly not cost-effective (Lapham 1970). Because of low demand and high costs, the mobile teams in some southern rural provinces were discontinued after a few months. In 1967, oral contraceptives were made available for distribution throughout the program, but health personnel were often reticent to dispense them because of their belief that women would not use them successfully. A postpartum program, which provided contraceptive information and supplies to women before and immediately after delivery, was also initiated in the major hospitals and was linked with the Population Council's International Postpartum Program (Lapham 1970; Povey and Brown 1968).

Just as the national program was beginning, a significant setback occurred in August 1966. A speech by President Bourguiba seemed to signal a change of direction when he said, "We must have children if we are not to become a nation of old people" (Povey and Brown 1968, p. 621). This was totally unexpected. Apparently he had been given inaccurate information about the national population growth rate and was led to believe that the population growth rate had dropped to 2.3 percent, whereas the correct rate was 2.8 percent. He concluded that Tunisian couples must increase procreation and protect against the example of France, with its low fertility between the world wars. While this was a temporary setback, and probably slowed down the early stages of the program, it seemed to have little long-term impact. Interestingly, at about the same time, President Bourguiba was one of 12 heads of state to sign the Declaration of Population, a statement developed at the initiative of John D. Rockefeller III and issued by United Nations Secretary General U Thant (United Nations 1967). This statement emphasized the problem of unplanned population growth throughout the world and stated that voluntary family planning is in the vital interests of both nations and families.

Despite the president's speech, the national program moved forward. Public information and education were strengthened somewhat during this period, but were mostly limited to the educational efforts of social workers and National Women's Union workers. While the political party remained active, the excessively heavy-handed efforts of the experimental period were tempered by the president's speech, which was no doubt a positive development. Mobile education teams were eventually deployed on a small scale in tandem with the mobile clinics, but had little impact. Overall, information and education were a weak part of the initial stages of the national program, in part because the health education program, originally part of the Ministry of Health, was transferred to the Ministry of Social Affairs and suffered from low budgets and inadequate coordination. Nonetheless, the public's attitude toward family planning was seen to be increasingly positive, and contraception was discussed more openly (Daly 1969; Povey and Brown 1968).

Other developments during this period included the creation of the Tunisian Family Planning Association in 1968, led by Dr. Tawhida Ben Cheikh, the first Tunisian female gynecologist, and supported by the International Planned Parenthood Federation. The association undertook advocacy and educational programs and countered some of the opposition to the relaxed abortion laws. Other national groups prominently supported the National Family Planning Program, including the Neo-Destour Party, the National Women's Union, religious leaders, and the media (Gueddana 2001).

Other donors, notably the U.S. Agency for International Development and the Swedish International Development Cooperation Agency, began to provide support to the program. In later years, the U.S. government became by far the largest supporter of the program.

Results

Lapham (1970, 1971) undertook an analysis of the results of the program from its inception in 1964 through 1969. He estimated that the crude birth rate had declined from 50 live births per 1,000 population in 1964 to 43 in 1968. Increased age at marriage was the most important factor in this decline, with the use of contraception contributing to less than one-third of the decline. As table 4.1 shows, the number of contraceptive acceptors, while small, rose consistently during 1964 to 1969, with the IUD predominating. The use of other methods also increased (as did abortions). This is notable in demonstrating the beginnings of a wide mix of contraceptive methods and a broad range of choice that continues to characterize Tunisia's Family Planning Program.

In general, the government deemed the Tunisian program to be successful during this early stage, although a number of significant weaknesses were evident, especially in relation to staffing, public information and education, administration, clinical counseling and follow-up care, and research and evaluation. Little attention was paid to the private sector, although sales of oral contraceptives by private pharmacies

TABLE 4.1 Estimated Number of Contraceptive Acceptors, 1964–69

Method	1964	1965	1966	1967	1968	1969
IUD	1,030	11,575	20,539	23,546	27,085	28,610
Oral contraceptives	0	183	140	431	2,884	4,212
Condoms	1,055	521	310	298	1,295	1,654
Other barrier methods	428	164	80	52	147	283
Female sterilization	278	604	1,263	1,855	3,200	4,481

Source: Lapham 1970.

almost certainly increased during this period. Nevertheless, the substantial increase in the minimum age of marriage promulgated by the president prior to the start of the program clearly had a substantially larger impact on the birth rate than did the Family Planning Program (Ayad and Jamai 2001).

Program Expansion: 1973 to the Present

The creation of the National Office for Family Planning and Development in 1973 marked the maturing of the program beyond family planning services and greatly strengthened its capacity (Gastineau and Sandron 2000; Gueddana 2001). For the first time, a full-time professional staff was dedicated to the program. The emphasis was broadened to include a focus on overall social well-being; an expanded training effort; a significant research effort, including economic and social research; and a broader public information and education program, along with attention paid to social policies and legislation and their impact. President Bourguiba renewed his support for family planning and inaugurated an annual prize in his name for its promotion.

Clinical family planning services and training were greatly expanded and were broadened to the private sector. Figure 4.1 shows the steady increase in contraceptive prevalence from 12 percent in 1971 to 60 percent in 1994, that is, an average increase of 2.1 percentage points per year over 23 years, well above the international average.

Figure 4.2 demonstrates the significant choice of contraceptive methods available to Tunisian women and men, resulting in an unusually wide mix of methods. The IUD, oral contraception, and female sterilization were all used extensively during 1978 to 1994, and condoms and other methods were also made available. The abortion law was further liberalized in 1973 to eliminate any restrictions. Condom use increased slightly during the period, other barrier methods were available but infrequently used, and vasectomy was never popular. Indeed, little attention was directed toward men, including the information and education program. Traditional methods remained somewhat important. By 2002, both Morocco and Tunisia had reached 60 percent of couples using a contraceptive method, but in Tunisia the increase has been faster and began somewhat sooner.

Further liberalization of laws concerning social security, abortion, and female sterilization all contributed to a dramatic increase in program outreach and depth.

FIGURE 4.1 Contraceptive Prevalence, 1971–94

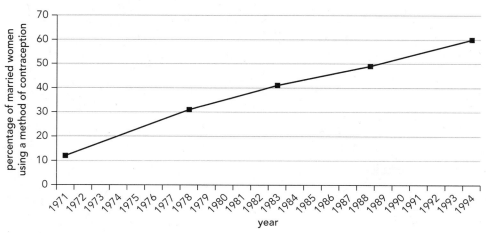

Source: National surveys.

FIGURE 4.2 Methods of Contraception Used, 1978–94

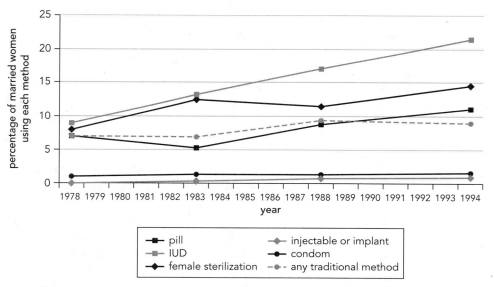

Source: National surveys.

Substantially increased financial support was provided by the U.S. Agency for International Development, the World Bank, the United Nations Population Fund, and other international donors. As Tunisia witnessed significant political and social changes in the 1980s, the National Office for Family Planning and Development continued to expand. In 1987, President Ben Ali succeeded President Bourguiba, but support for the program was maintained. By 2006, the total fertility rate had reached two births per woman, or below replacement level. This is the lowest rate of any country on the African continent and is lower than that in most other developing countries (Population Reference Bureau 2006). Thus, in 40 years, Tunisia has fully achieved its goal of reducing fertility and achieving low population growth rates.

The government's social and economic policies certainly contributed to the dramatic decline in fertility rates, especially, as noted earlier, the increase in the minimum age of marriage. Indirectly, the greatly improved status of women and the significant increase in the education of both women and men contributed substantially to the decline in fertility.

International Influence

As Tunisia's Family Planning Program was the first in the Arab world and the first on the African continent, it was presented and widely discussed at such milestone events as the First Conference on International Family Planning, held in Geneva in 1965 (Berelson and others 1966), and the First African Population Conference, held in Nigeria in 1966. Tunisia's path-breaking social policies and efforts to expand the status of women were widely noted at the early stages of the program and continue to draw international attention (Vallin and Locoh 2001).

The most obvious early influence was on neighboring Morocco. Exchanges were held among senior officials of the two countries before Morocco launched its own National Family Planning Program in 1966. In later years, technical exchanges between Tunisian officials and officials of Sub-Saharan Francophone African countries resulted in structured training seminars in contraceptive technologies being held in Tunisia for clinicians from a range of Francophone African countries.

Reflections on Tunisia's Early Population and Social Policies

The postindependence social liberalization policies and laws initiated by President Bourguiba were unique in the Muslim world, and were fundamentally important in setting the stage for the successful National Family Planning Program. No other developing country had formulated and promulgated such a comprehensive set of policies, laws, and administrative actions to improve the status of women; promote literacy; encourage a small family norm; improve economic conditions; and increase access to contraception, sterilization, and abortion. Even 40 years later, few countries enjoy such a comprehensive population policy.

Speculating what prompted President Bourguiba to undertake such a liberal population and social development policy is an interesting endeavor. During a visit to Tunisia in 1966, John D. Rockefeller III, chair of the Population Council's Board of Trustees, and Frank Notestein, the Population Council's president, met with President Bourguiba. Rockefeller complimented the president on his far-sighted population policy and asked him how he had developed his ideas. Bourguiba replied, *"J'ai de baggage dans ma tête"* ("I've got a lot of brains") (statement by President Bourguiba to John D. Rockefeller III, Spring 1966, recorded by the author).

While this enigmatic response was not revealing, a journalist wrote some years later that "when Bourguiba was a small boy, his mother died giving birth to her eighth child, and the boy never forgot either his loss or the reason for it."[1] (Geyer 2000, p. 1). Whatever the influences on him, or perhaps because of his own brilliance, Bourguiba's consistent commitment over many years to social development, women's rights, and family planning had an important effect on population policies and programs in Tunisia and beyond.

Conclusions

The experimental stage of the National Family Planning Program in 1964 and its early expansion in 1966 provided a solid base and set the stage for the more comprehensive effort that began in the 1970s. A strong population and social development policy put in place well before the experimental program in 1964 was enormously important in providing the underpinnings and preparing the public for family planning. The introduction of new contraceptive technologies, especially the IUD, was a key element. The availability of other methods, including oral contraceptives, sterilization, and abortion were also notable. The beginnings were modest and halting, and mistakes were made, but the program received strong political support at the highest levels and made creative course corrections over the years. As a result, over 40 years Tunisia's contraceptive prevalence has increased from less than 10 percent of married women of childbearing age to more than 60 percent; the total fertility rate has decreased from six births per woman to two, or below replacement level; and the population growth rate has declined from 2.8 percent to 1.1 percent (Population Reference Bureau 2006).

As the new Family Planning Program expanded steadily, important changes in society had a major impact on fertility and the acceptance of family planning, including the increase in age of marriage; a decline in mortality; and a rapid improvement in education, especially female education (Vallin and Locoh 2001). Tunisia's remarkable success and creativity in relation to both population and development policy and family planning implementation has set an important example to other countries in the region and throughout the world.

Note

1. Geyer, G. A. "Habib Bourguiba's Original Thinking Led to Tunisia's Success." UExpress Syndicate. http://www.bourguiba.com.

References

Ayad, M., and H. Jamai. 2001. "Les Déterminants de la Fécondité." In *Population et Développement en Tunisie*, ed. J. Vallin and T. Locoh, 171–202. Paris: Ceres Editions.

Berelson B., R. K. Anderson, O. Harkavy, J. Maier, W. P. Mauldin, and S. J. Segal, eds. 1966. *Family Planning and Population Programs*. Chicago: University of Chicago Press.

Brown, G. F., and G. Sabbagh. 1965. "L'Efficacité de la Contraception Intra-utérine en Milieu Tunisien." *La Tunisie Médicale* 44 (5): 318–21.

Daly, A. 1966. "Tunisia." In *Family Planning and Population Programs*, ed. B. Berelson, R. K. Anderson, O. Harkavy, J. Maier, W. P. Mauldin, and S. J. Segal, 151–62. Chicago: University of Chicago Press.

———. 1969. "Tunisia: The Liberation of Women and the Improvement of Society." In *Family Planning Programs: An International Survey,* ed. B. Berelson, 113–24. New York: Basic Books.

Editors. 1966. "Tunisia: The Role of the Political Party." *Studies in Family Planning* 1 (13): 5–6.

Gastineau, B., and F. Sandron. 2000. *La Politique de Planification Familiale en Tunisie, 1964–2000."* Paris: Ceres Editions.

Gueddana, N. 2001. "L'expérience du Programme de Planification Familiale (1956–1996)." In *Population et Développement en Tunisie,* ed. J. Vallin and T. Locoh, 202–32. Paris: Ceres Editions.

Lapham, R. J. 1970. "Family Planning and Fertility in Tunisia." *Demography* 7 (2): 241–53.

———. 1971. "Family Planning in Tunisia and Morocco: A Summary and Evaluation of the Recent Record." *Studies in Family Planning* 2 (7): 101–110.

Mauldin, W. P., B. Berelson, and J. Hardy. 1963. "Tunisia: Proposed Family Planning Program." *Studies in Family Planning* 1 (2): 3–4.

Morsa, J. 1966. "The Tunisia Survey: A Preliminary Analysis." In *Family Planning and Population Programs,* ed. B. Berelson, R. K. Anderson, O. Harkavy, J. Maier, W. P. Mauldin, and S. J. Segal, 581–94. Chicago: University of Chicago Press.

Population Reference Bureau. 2006. *World Population Data Sheet.* Washington, DC: Population Reference Bureau.

Povey, W. G., and G. F. Brown. 1968. "Tunisia's Experience in Family Planning." *Demography* 5 (2): 620–26.

United Nations. 1967. "Declaration of Population." *Studies in Family Planning* 1 (16): 1–12.

Vallin J., M. Limaim, G. Brown, and G. Sabbagh. 1968. "L'Efficacité de la Contraception Intra-utérine dans le Gouvernorat du Kef (Tunisie)." *La Tunisie Médicale* 46 (2): 121–30.

Vallin J., and T. Locoh. 2001. "Les Leçons de l'Expérience Tunisienne." In *Population et Développement en Tunisie*, ed. J. Vallin and T. Locoh, 569–82. Paris: Ceres Editions.

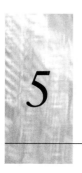

5 Morocco: First Steps in Family Planning

GEORGE F. BROWN

Morocco, part of the Arab Maghreb, is situated in the northwestern corner of Africa. In 1966, at the beginning of its family planning efforts, Morocco's population was 13 million. By 2005, it had grown to 30 million. Morocco's population is almost entirely Muslim (99 percent) and is largely Arabic speaking, with several Berber languages spoken by significant minorities in the mountainous Atlas region. Morocco, along with its neighboring Maghreb countries, Algeria and Tunisia, was colonized by the French in 1912. Spain also colonized northern Morocco. Independence was achieved in 1956. Morocco is principally an agrarian society, and at independence, literacy was low—averaging 18 percent for men and 2 percent for women in rural areas and increasing to 41 percent for men and 17 percent for women in urban areas. The age of marriage was low, especially in rural areas, averaging 15.5 years for women and 22.3 years for men.

Politically, Morocco is a monarchy with a parliament that is largely supportive of the monarchy. It is primarily a one-party state, although some limited political opposition exists, and political unrest has been significant, especially in the 1970s, when a failed attempt to overthrow the monarchy took place. The king is the spiritual and religious head of this religiously conservative country.

In 1966, the total fertility rate was a high 7.2 births per woman and mortality rates were declining, although they were still relatively high. The population growth rate in 1966 was estimated to be 3.2 percent.

Beginnings

Government concerns about high population growth initially stemmed from a 1965 analysis by the Ministry of Economic Planning that calculated the economic repercussions of rapid population growth on education, housing, employment, and other development sectors. The analysis also included population projections based on a decline in the birth rate and demonstrated the tremendous economic gains that would ensue if the growth rate were decreased to 2.5 percent by 1985 (Brown 1968;

Castadot and Laraqui 1973; Kingdom of Morocco 1965). At the same time, a World Bank mission to Morocco underlined that economic growth was being equaled or exceeded by population growth. An equally important element was the influence of neighboring Tunisia's population policies and its National Family Planning Program, which had started in 1964. Exchange visits between senior development planning and health officials of the two countries took place in 1965 (Brown 1968). Box 5.1 presents a timeline of major events.

BOX 5.1 Population and Family Planning Timeline, 1965–71

1965: The Planning Commission undertakes an analysis of population projections, their impact on certain aspects of the economy, and proposed solution with United Nations technical support.

Initial discussions take place between officials of the Moroccan and Tunisian governments on population and family planning.

The Ministry of Health obtains contraceptive supplies and commences discussions with the Ford Foundation, the Population Council, and the International Planned Parenthood Federation.

The first group of medical personnel attend training courses in Brussels and London sponsored by the International Planned Parenthood Federation.

1966: The first family planning clinics open. The Ministry of Health requests each province to set up family planning services, emphasizing intrauterine devices (IUDs).

The Ford Foundation provides the government with a grant for family planning supplies, equipment, and technical assistance.

The National Population Commission and provincial commissions are created by royal decree.

King Hassan II signs the United Nations Declaration on Population.

A national family planning seminar is held in Rabat with wide publicity.

A study on knowledge, attitudes, and practices in urban areas is conducted with assistance from the Swedish International Development Cooperation Agency.

The Population Council provides a resident technical assistance staff.

1967: A royal decree abrogates colonial-era law prohibiting contraceptives.

Family planning services expand to each province.

A study on knowledge, attitudes, and practices in rural areas is conducted, also with assistance from the Swedish International Development Cooperation Agency.

1968: The National Population Commission holds its first meeting.

The Five-Year Development Plan (1968–72) emphasizes the importance of reducing population growth rates and includes a strong national family planning program, with the goal of reducing the birth rate by 10 percent and inserting 500,000 IUDs over five years.

Program evaluation begins.

Training of family planning health assistants is initiated.

The distribution of oral contraceptives through health centers starts.

1969: The first full-time medical director of family planning is appointed and efforts to invigorate the program are undertaken.

A subsidized commercial condom sales program through tobacco outlets begins in Casablanca.

The emphasis on oral contraceptives is strengthened.

The U.S. Agency for International Development commences financial and technical support to the Family Planning Program.

1970: The Ministry of Economic Planning urges rapid strengthening of the program and engagement by all physicians.

Princess Lalla Fatima Zohra, president of the Moroccan Women's Association, presides at a public meeting on family planning in Rabat.

The family planning health assistants program is abandoned, and education responsibilities are given to all health personnel.

The commercial condom distribution through tobacco outlets is abandoned because of a lack of demand.

The minister of finance announces expansion of the Family Planning Program at a meeting of the Organisation for Economic Co-operation and Development in Paris. The government increases family planning budget commitments.

1971: The French Family Planning Movement organizes a national seminar.

The Moroccan Family Planning Association is created, chaired by Princess Lalla Fatima Zohra. The International Planned Parenthood Federation provides assistance.

Evaluation reveals that only 20 percent of the national plan's target is achieved, with IUD and pill acceptors combined, and that fewer than 1 percent of women of reproductive age are being reached.

Contacts with Ford Foundation and Population Council staff members working in Tunisia led to an initial grant from the foundation and technical support from the council in 1966, and a group of Moroccan physicians went to Europe for training in contraception with support from the International Planned Parenthood Federation. In the same year, the Ministry of Health launched the first family planning services and held a national seminar on the subject. At that meeting, the minister of health made some important pronouncements (Castadot and Laraqui 1973) and underlined the substantial health gains that would result from birth spacing, and the minister of development affirmed the need for a national effort to respond to high fertility and to related public health needs and to reduce population growth to achieve economic and social advancement and improve women's health (Castadot and Laraqui 1973). Also in 1966, King Hassan II was one of 12 heads of state to sign the United Nations Declaration on Population (United Nations 1967).

In addition, a 1966 royal decree created the High Commission on Population and provincial commissions. Even though these commissions rarely met, their creation reflected awareness of the need to involve high levels of society and government. As a more immediately practical action, a colonial-era law preventing the sale of contraceptives was abrogated in 1967 (Brown 1968; Castadot and Laraqui 1973).

The First National Family Planning Survey

To determine knowledge, attitudes, and practices in relation to family planning, the government undertook an urban survey in 1966 and a rural survey in 1967, as well as a smaller survey in a region near Rabat. Support was provided by the Swedish International Development Cooperation Agency. These surveys revealed generally favorable attitudes about family planning, particularly among women with three or more children, but knowledge and practices in relation to family planning were extremely limited. While most women with three or more children indicated that they did not want more children, many expressed reluctance to try a family planning method, citing religious, cultural, and marital concerns, as well as a lack of information and negative rumors about contraceptives (Kingdom of Morocco 1970; Lapham 1970). Overall, government officials were encouraged by the level of interest among Moroccan couples and their willingness to offer their views on matters that had hitherto been considered too sensitive even for interviewers to raise. The challenge of raising knowledge levels and making family planning methods available were daunting, but were deemed to be surmountable.

The Initial Family Planning Program, 1966–70

The Ministry of Health was made responsible for the National Family Planning Program, which was initiated in 1966. The program was integrated into the existing public health service system under the ministry's Division of Technical Services, and therefore did not receive any dedicated leadership or strong administrative management. Ministry officials believed that full integration of family planning within overall health services was essential to maximize available resources without duplication and to ensure sound medical procedures. Services were established in urban health centers in most of the 20 provinces and in several large cities. Casablanca, the largest city, established multiple centers. By 1968, 110 such centers were offering family planning services as part of their overall public health operations. A limited number of rural centers were established in a few provinces (Brown 1968).

Initially, the program was almost entirely based on the Lippes loop intrauterine device (IUD). At the outset, the minister of health stated that he would not have initiated the Family Planning Program without the availability of the IUD, as he believed that only this long-acting method would be suitable and effectively used by Moroccan women (Larbi Chraibi, personal communication with George Brown, 1966). Oral contraceptives were added a year after the initial program was under way, but only at a modest level, with one cycle of pills dispensed by a physician at the initial clinic visit and clients directed to purchase subsequent cycles at pharmacies. Initially, many physicians (most of them French or other Europeans) were opposed to oral contraceptives, fearing side effects and the presumed difficulty of Moroccan women to take them consistently. Oral contraceptives were commercially available in pharmacies, but no effort was made to collaborate with pharmacies to stimulate sales or to lower prices. In 1968, clinics began to offer clients three cycles of pills. Condoms and vaginal spermicides were available in some centers, but were not actively promoted. Female sterilization was rarely performed, vasectomy was not available, and abortion was illegal and therefore not recorded.

In 1966, the structure of health services in Morocco was weak, with limited rural health services and with expatriate health personnel from France and Eastern Europe accounting for the large majority of the staff for public health management and services. Over a period of years, as more Moroccan health personnel were trained, the situation gradually improved, but initially this was a significant limitation. Many of the European physicians had not been trained in family planning, and were often even more conservative and unwilling to provide contraceptive services than Moroccan physicians. Similarly, the departments of Health Education and Statistics within the Ministry of Health were weak, and research was extremely limited. The family planning education effort was limited to clinic-based communication to clients, with little or no publicity in the press or other media. Indeed, the program was almost invisible publicly, reflecting a conservative and tentative approach to the subject. The newly established medical school was closely tied to the French university system, and the first dean of medicine was opposed to introducing family planning into the curriculum. No clinical research was undertaken until 1969, when alternative IUDs were tested on a limited, experimental basis.

The early IUD acceptors over the first two years of the program were, on average, 30.8 years old with 5.3 children. Thus, the clients served were largely women who had reached the end of their desired childbearing, but who had a substantial number of years of potential childbearing ahead of them. No special effort was made to reach out to younger women, and services were available only for married women (Brown 1968).

Family Planning Education and Information

Ministry of Health officials soon recognized that inadequate education of clients, and of the population at large, was a major weakness of the program. In 1968, the ministry initiated a special program to train 35 health assistants from among those who had recently graduated from nursing school. The intensive 14-week course included both theoretical and practical training. The health assistants were then assigned in teams to regional health centers in five major cities, where they provided contraceptive information to prospective clients in maternal and child health clinics. However, the health assistant program had significant problems: the assistants were young; the assistants were chosen arbitrarily and did not volunteer; the clients were mostly women, but half the health assistants were men; and the health personnel and supervisors the assistants were subsequently assigned to were poorly trained themselves (Garnier 1969). The health assistant program was abandoned after a year, and the assistants were reabsorbed into the cadres of the Ministry of Health. In 1969, seminars were held for teachers in nursing schools and family planning was integrated into the schools' curricula. The more difficult task of training the bulk of health personnel remained to be tackled.

Beyond this modest information and education effort, the ministry produced pamphlets and wall charts for use in health clinics and a film. In the first three years of the program, no public statements or support were forthcoming from senior levels of government, which seemed to inhibit any serious public discussion of family planning. Even though King Hassan II signed the United Nations Declaration on Population in 1966, he made no mention of family planning or population in any of his speeches in the country. Most high-level government officials followed his example, and the press was largely silent. This began to change in May 1970, when Princess

Lalla Fatima Zohra, president of the National Union of Moroccan Women, presided at a public meeting on family planning in Rabat, and in early 1971, when a seminar sponsored by the French Family Planning Movement was held in Rabat and was highly publicized in the Moroccan press (Lapham 1971).

The Moroccan Family Planning Association was established in 1971 with assistance from the International Planned Parenthood Federation. Its aim was to educate and inform the public by distributing materials on family planning, and it succeeded in speaking publicly on family planning while the government remained weak or silent. The National Union of Moroccan Women also helped to inform women by publishing articles on family planning in its weekly news magazine and by organizing meetings (Castadot and Laraqui 1973).

Structural Changes

A positive senior administrative change was made in 1969 with the creation of a new position: a dedicated senior officer who would be in charge of the overall program. Dr. Abdelkader Laraqui was named secretary-general and national director of the Family Planning Program. He was not initially given any significant staff support, but the decision to create this position was a recognition that more effort was needed to energize the program. Initially, Laraqui's office issued directives to provincial medical officers to improve family planning efforts, but had limited capacity or resources to implement them. Some regional directors were more enthusiastic than others, so the result was a highly uneven program effort (Lapham 1971).

Service statistics became more structured and systematic under the Ministry of Health's Department of Statistics, and a small amount of evaluative research was initiated, but more comprehensive research and evaluation efforts remained to be developed.

Commercial Sales of Contraceptives

Oral contraceptives had been commercially available from the onset of the program, but were relatively expensive and were probably initially purchased in small numbers by middle-class urban women and foreigners. Sales gradually expanded as the program matured and more women received introductory cycles of pills from the public health clinics. Prices also declined somewhat, but the Family Planning Program made no effort to collaborate directly with the pharmacies or to seek price reductions. Estimates indicate that sales of oral contraceptives in pharmacies increased from 10,000 cycles per month in 1966 to 53,000 cycles per month in 1970 (Lapham 1971).

In 1969, the government initiated a pioneering social marketing effort to introduce subsidized sales of condoms through the National Tobacco Board, a quasi-autonomous public enterprise that held the monopoly for tobacco sales throughout the country. This initiative was informed by early social marketing efforts with condoms in India. The Ministry of Health provided the National Tobacco Board with more than 1 million condoms for sale at a low price (US$0.04 for three condoms) through the board's 633 outlets in Casablanca. While the senior executives of the National Tobacco Board were willing to undertake distribution, they made no effort to publicize the program, instruct retailers, or provide point-of-sale information, and the Ministry of Health made no effort to support or encourage informational efforts. As a result, only 100,800 condoms were sold during the first year, and the program was abandoned (Castadot and Laraqui 1973). Clearly this program suffered from the same problem as the family planning effort as a whole: a lack of information and a reticence to go public with new initiatives in an area perceived to be sensitive. Another 20 years passed before a renewed and successful social marketing program for condoms was put into place.

Population and Development Plan, 1968–72

In 1968, the Ministry of Economic Planning issued its Five-Year Plan (1968–72), and set out some highly ambitious goals for demographic change and family planning. As noted in the plan (Kingdom of Morocco 1968, as cited and translated by Castadot and Laraqui 1973, p. 5), "The Moroccan population is growing very quickly. One can envision the long-term consequences of this growth—further unemployment, overpopulation of the cities—if it is not remedied by adequate measures. It is vital to bring into play with greatest speed a demographic policy composed of the following items:

- Implementation of a family planning policy
- Creation of new job opportunities
- Creation of an urban renewal plan to include slum rehabilitation
- Creation of a temporary emigration policy."

The demographic policy envisaged a gradual decrease in the birth rate from 50 to 45 per 1,000 population by 1972 and to 35 by 1985. It also envisaged raising the minimum age of marriage to 18 years for women and 21 years for men and introducing legal reforms in relation to family assistance. (These reforms had not been implemented by 1972.) To attain these demographic objectives, the plan called for strengthening the Family Planning Program as well as a program of public education, with highly ambitious targets: inserting 500,000 IUDs during the plan period and making oral and other contraceptives widely available. A corps of 600 male and female motivators was to be recruited, and substantial funding was proposed to undertake these tasks.

The appearance of these objectives in the plan did not translate into action; little explicit program implementation was undertaken, at least initially; and the Ministry of Health did not receive a significant increase of government financial resources. At this time, the U.S. Agency for International Development initiated its first grant to the ministry in support of the new plan, and thereafter steadily increased its assistance and soon became the most important international donor (Hajji and others 2003).

Clearly the plan's goals were completely unrealistic, especially the IUD targets, which were more than 10 times the annual number of insertions achieved during the program's early years. The plan also reinforced the almost total emphasis on the IUD over other contraceptives. Nevertheless, the Five-Year Plan unequivocally set forward a strong rationale for decreasing population growth and expanding family planning efforts. The plan's failure to translate recommendations into practical implementation emerged as a pattern that was repeated in succeeding years.

Results

The first five years of the program (1966–70) achieved a slow but steady increase in contraceptive use. As table 5.1 shows, the total number of acceptors increased to 25,067 in 1970, and the early emphasis on the IUD shifted such that by 1970, more acceptors were using oral contraceptives. Indeed, as the table does not include commercial sales of oral contraceptives, it therefore underestimates the use of this method. Other methods, including sterilization and condom use, had low levels of use (Lapham 1971).

The program failed by far to reach the optimistic objectives set forth in the 1968–72 Five-Year Plan. Lapham (1971) estimated that by 1970, the program had reached only 0.9 percent of women of reproductive age, which was far too few women to have any impact on the birth rate.

The low levels of IUD use reflected poor follow-up and a large number of dropouts from the program, estimated at 60 percent in 1972 (Robbins and others 1976). Women did not receive adequate information about side effects, and expulsions of IUDs resulted in pregnancies as well as negative rumors, further discrediting the method. It became evident that most women preferred oral contraceptives, even though they had to purchase them in pharmacies. By 1972, more than 19,000 oral contraceptive acceptors were registered, compared with only 5,300 IUD acceptors. Thus, the pattern of preference for oral contraceptives was established early in the program, despite the government's heavy emphasis on IUDs.

Administratively, the program was introduced into all 20 provinces, with at least some of the health personnel trained. Several provincial medical directors were active and organized significant training and services, especially in the major cities. Other

TABLE 5.1 Estimated Number of Contraceptive Acceptors, 1966–70

Method	1966	1967	1968	1969	1970
IUDs (first insertions)	6,427	5,036	6,520	10,987	9,763
Oral contraceptives[a]	—	—	—	9,257	14,275
Condoms[a]	—	—	—	1,060	1,029
Total	6,427	5,036	6,520	21,304	25,067

Source: Brown 1968, 1969; Lapham 1971.

Note: — = not available.

a. Public sector only.

provincial heads were much slower and more conservative. Thus, the program was highly uneven in terms of the availability of services and the number of acceptors. With a few exceptions, services were weak or nonexistent in rural areas. As noted earlier, information and education were virtually nonexistent throughout the country and efforts to field health assistants and a trial condom social marketing program were abandoned. The beginnings of a central family planning management structure had been created, but no strong administrative or statistical structure had been created. The training of health personnel and health sciences students in family planning had just begun.

Overall, the results of the first four years were modest, but nevertheless significant considering the deeply conservative and religious culture of the country, yet still too small to have any impact on fertility. Of special note was the Ministry of Economic Planning, which consistently emphasized population growth and family planning as a key component of the development planning process. The services offered by the Ministry of Health were limited, yet showed some modest progress, and the number of family planning acceptors gradually increased, which is notable given the absence of any organized information program.

Program Developments, 1971–Present

The program expanded significantly in the latter part of the 1970s and in the 1980s because of greater commitment by the government and much higher levels of external support, especially from the U.S. Agency for International Development. This greater program effort was stimulated by a U.S. Agency for International Development consultant report (Robbins and others 1976) that highlighted the program's achievements and deficiencies. The report noted that the modest level of new contraceptive acceptors was exceeded by women entering reproductive age and that the program was still not achieving any significant impact on fertility, and recommended a much stronger level of commitment by the government.

The program began to take off in the 1980s with the establishment of strong central and provincial administrative structures, much more complete coverage of services, expanded training of health personnel, and far more public information and education. The steady increase of recently graduated Moroccan health professionals and the resultant displacement of expatriate physicians provided an important impetus to the program. A comprehensive system of home visits by community health workers known as the Systematic Motivational Home Visits Program was pilot tested in one province in 1977 and expanded nationwide in 1980. This was the first comprehensive effort to reach rural populations. In addition, a strong effort was made to encourage commercial sales of oral contraceptives through pharmacies, and a successful condom social marketing program was initiated in 1989. Efforts to broaden the method mix were largely unsuccessful despite attempts to introduce injectables and implants and renewed efforts to expand IUD use.

As figure 5.1 shows, by 2004, contraceptive use had reached 63 percent among married women of childbearing age. The method mix (figure 5.2) has increasingly been skewed toward oral contraceptives, which in 2004 were used by 40.1 percent

FIGURE 5.1 Contraceptive Prevalence, 1974–2004

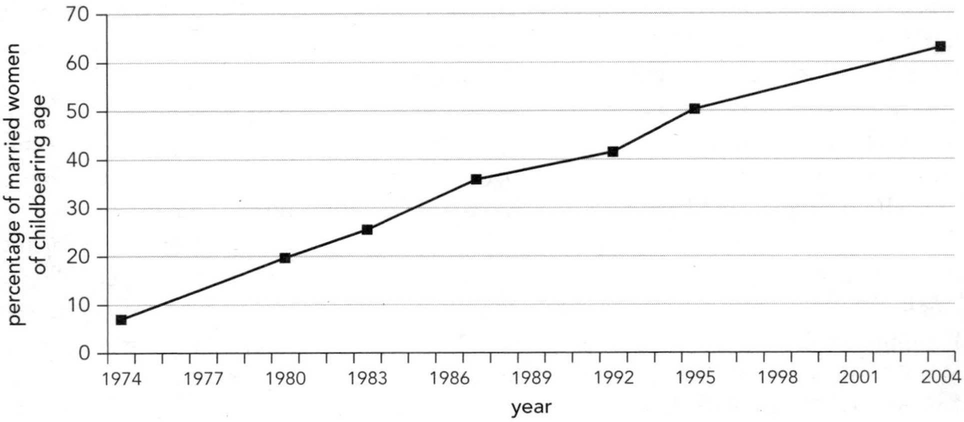

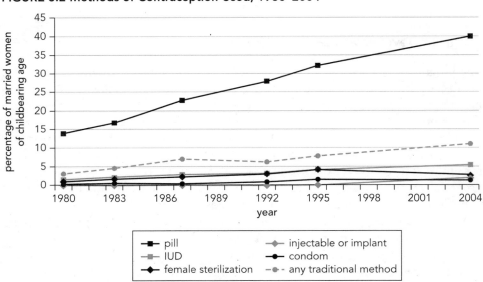

Source: Ross, Stover, and Adelaja 2005, table A.1.

FIGURE 5.2 Methods of Contraception Used, 1980–2004

Source: Ross, Stover, and Adelaja 2005, table A.1.

of married women of childbearing age, with IUDs used by only 5.4 percent. Other methods, including periodic abstinence, female sterilization, injectables, and condoms had much lower levels of use (ORC Macro 2005).

At the same time, the quality of services steadily improved. Following the International Conference on Population and Development in Cairo in 1994, the Ministry of Health broadened its reproductive health program to include family planning; maternal and child health; and sexually transmitted infections, including HIV/AIDS. Political support for the program shifted from a focus on stemming rapid population growth to emphasizing improvement of the quality of life and responding to the reproductive health needs of the population.

By 2006, the total fertility rate had dropped to 2.5 births per woman, a remarkable decrease from 7.2 in 1966; the mortality rate had also decreased substantially; life expectancy had reached 70; and the population growth rate had dropped from 3.2 percent in 1966 to 1.6 percent (Population Reference Bureau 2006).

Major changes in socioeconomic status undoubtedly played a large role in Morocco's fertility decline. From 1966 to 2006, many improvements occurred in relation to economic and social development, including increased age at marriage; higher levels of education, especially for girls; increased per capita income; decreased mortality; and urbanization. These factors all contributed to a more favorable climate for family planning and fertility decline. One analysis of the proximate determinants of fertility concluded that increased age at marriage accounted for 44 percent of Morocco's fertility decline, with 55 percent due to contraceptive use (Ayad 1999).

Conclusion

The early stages of Morocco's national population and Family Planning Program, while promising, were slow and cautious. Yet these early efforts were sustained and provided the underpinnings of a highly successful program to bring contraception to the population, satisfy women's reproductive health needs, and reduce the population growth rate. The Ministry of Economic Planning was an early supporter of government efforts to reduce fertility in order to achieve economic development. The lack of public statements and support by national leaders and the absence of public education and information contributed to the slow initial family planning effort, but at the same time allowed the program to take its first steps without undue political opposition. The early decision by the Ministry of Health to integrate family planning into basic health services resulted in a slow and uneven start-up process, but perhaps avoided excessive zeal or too many mistakes by health providers. Experimental initiatives on family planning education and commercial condom sales were deemed failures, yet both areas were renewed with vigor in later years. The shift in emphasis toward reproductive health after the Cairo conference was successfully achieved, and the original demographic rationale for the program has been dropped in favor of the goal of seeking improved reproductive health and well-being of the population.

Why have most Moroccan women decided to use oral contraceptives, in essence rejecting the government's initial enthusiasm for the IUD? Avoidance of an intrusive gynecological procedure and the side effects of the IUD were certainly prominent features, and misinformation and negative rumors probably played a part early on, building on poor client information and inadequate follow-up services and resulting in high dropout rates. The part played by the IUD in the early years should not, however, be minimized, as leading government officials believed that the IUD was essential in initiating the National Family Planning Program.

Comparing Morocco's early efforts with those of neighboring Tunisia's National Family Planning Program, which started two years earlier (see chapter 4), is instructive. Unlike Morocco, Tunisia enjoyed strong and sustained public support from the president, who had enacted many laws to improve the status of women and to encourage lower fertility. The Tunisian program was less integrated into basic health services, and expanded more quickly during its early stages, but it also suffered from excessive persuasion by the local political party, which at times was coercive in nature and resulted in some backlash. The more cautious, low-key program initiation in Morocco avoided these excesses and ultimately prevailed in a more conservative society. Both countries have succeeded to a remarkable degree in relation to fertility reduction, with Morocco being a few years behind Tunisia.

References

Ayad, M. 1999. *La fécondité au Maroc: niveaux et déterminants de 1980 a 1995*. Demographic and Health Surveys. Calverton, MD: ORC Macro.

Brown, George F. 1968. "Moroccan Family Planning Program: Progress and Problems." *Demography* 5 (2): 627–31.

———. 1969. "Le Programme de Planification Familiale au Maroc." *Revue Tunisienne de Sciences Sociales* 17–18: 283–90.

Castadot, R., and A. Laraqui. 1973. "Morocco." Country Profiles Series. New York: Population Council.

Garnier, J.-C. 1969. "Morocco: Training and Utilization of Family Planning Field Workers." *Studies in Family Planning* 1 (47): 1–5.

Hajji, N., S. Wright, G. Escudero, M. Abdou-Oukil, and M. B. Ouchrif. 2003. *Morocco Reproductive Health and Child Health Programs: 30 Years of Collaboration, USAID and Ministry of Health of Morocco, 1971–2000*. Chapel Hill, NC: University of North Carolina, Carolina Population Center.

Kingdom of Morocco. 1965. *Projections de Population, Répercussions sur Certains Aspects de l'Economie du Pays et Solutions Proposées*. Rabat: Royal Cabinet, General Delegation for National Promotion and Planning.

———. 1968. *Plan Quadriennal, 1968–72*. Rabat: Ministry of Economic Planning.

———. 1970. *Enquête d'Opinion sur la Planification Familiale, Milieu Urbain*. Rabat: Ministry of Health, Secretariat of Planning of the Prime Minister's Office.

Lapham, R. 1970. "Morocco: Family Planning Attitudes, Knowledge, and Practice in the Sais Plain." *Studies in Family Planning* 1 (58): 32.

———. 1971. "Family Planning in Tunisia and Morocco: A Summary and Evaluation of the Recent Record." *Studies in Family Planning* 2 (4): 101–10.

ORC Macro. 2005. *Enquête sur la Population et la Sante Familiale, 2003–04*. Calverton, MD: ORC Macro.

Population Reference Bureau. 2006. *2006 World Population Data Sheet*. Washington, DC: Population Reference Bureau.

Robbins, J. C., R. P. Bernard, D. Mutchler, and L. S. Zabin. 1976. "Report of the Evaluating Team of the Morocco Family Planning Program." AID/pha/C-1100 Ltr. POP/FPS 1/2/76. Washington, DC: American Public Health Association and U.S. Agency for International Development.

Ross, J. A., J. Stover, and D. Adelaja. 2005. *Profiles for Family Planning and Reproductive Health Programs: 116 Countries*, 2nd ed. Glastonbury, CT: Futures Group.

United Nations. 1967. "Declaration of Population." *Studies in Family Planning* 1 (16): 1–12.

II Europe and Central Asia

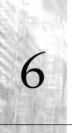

6 Emergence of the Family Planning Program in Turkey

AYŞE AKIN

Turkey, a Middle Eastern country covering some 770,000 square kilometers, lies in both Asia and Europe. It has more than 70 million people, nearly all of them (98 percent) Muslim. Between 1927 and 2000, population growth was rapid and the population grew fivefold, though the rate of growth varied from a low of 1.06 percent per year in 1940–45 to a high of 2.85 percent per year in 1955–60. By 1990–2000, however, the rate was 1.83 percent per year. A comparison of population pyramids for 1955 and 2000 shows a remarkable shift in structure from one reflecting rapid growth at the base to one in which each cohort below the age of 15 is smaller than the one above. Indeed, the 2000 pyramid is similar in shape to those of many developed countries. During the same period, average household size declined from 5.7 to 4.5, a 21 percent reduction. Not surprisingly, the proportion of the population living in urban areas rose steeply between 1950 and 2000, from 25 to 65 percent of the total population. Literacy rose for both sexes. In 1935, it was 30 percent for males and 10 percent for females, but according to the 2000 census, by that time it had reached a remarkable 94 percent for males and 81 percent for females. Thus, profound demographic and social changes have taken place in Turkey in recent years.

As of the early 1920s, Turkey had been devastated by many years of war. At that time, the population was only around 13 million, and mortality during the wars of 1911–22 had been heavy. Therefore, the national population policy was designed to increase the population as quickly as possible. That policy prohibited the importation of contraceptives, made abortion illegal, prohibited advertising and education concerning contraceptive methods and materials, and provided financial incentives for large families and was in place for many years (Tokgöz and Akın 1983).

In the 1920s and 1930s, the population growth rate was about 2 percent or less per year, but in the mid-1950s, it suddenly jumped to approximately 3 percent per year (Metiner 1969). This was after World War II, when malaria was eradicated and antibiotics and improved government child-health services all rapidly decreased mortality. In addition, the return of many men from the armed forces led to a baby boom, as in many other countries at that time (Fişek 1983; Metiner 1969).

Consequently, significant demographic changes occurred during 1945 to 1960. In 1958 to 1962, population growth was about 3.0 to 3.2 percent per year and those aged 15 years and younger accounted for 41.5 percent of the total population, the crude birth rate was about 45 live births per 1,000 population per year, and the crude death rate had fallen to about 13 deaths per 1,000 population. In addition, a serious and rapid increase in illegal abortions had occurred. All these factors had significant implications for the population in the future, leading the government to aim at a reduction in population increase from 3.2 percent to 2.0 percent per year (Cerit 1989; Üner 1984; Üner and Fişek 1961).

The Pro-Natalist Population Policy, 1923–65

As mentioned earlier, because of the heavy human losses sustained during World War I and the War of Independence, along with the generally high level of infant mortality, the government believed that population growth should be increased to meet the country's defense needs and to address the shortage of agricultural manpower. Before the declaration of the republic in 1923, Kemal Atatürk addressed the third opening of the Turkish Grand National Assembly and stated, "Our objective in the field of national health and social assistance is to protect and strengthen the general health conditions, decrease the death rate, eradicate communicable diseases, increase the population and, thus, be able to raise a dynamic generation" (Altıok 1978, pp. 53–54).

Atatürk repeated his desire to increase the population several times thereafter, so that eventually the concept was adopted as state policy, as indicated in his opening speech to the Grand National Assembly in 1924. During the ensuing years, a number of laws that had direct or indirect implications for population growth were enacted (Box 6.1). For example, in 1926, the minimum marriage age was reduced to 18 for men and to 17 for women, and in 1938 was further reduced to 17 for men and 15 for women. Several other laws were also explicitly aimed at promoting fertility. The laws on Local Administrations and on Municipalities, passed in 1929 and 1930, respectively, imposed several obligations on local administrations to implement the population increase policy by improving public health, establishing free maternity hospitals, and distributing medicines to the poor for free or at low cost. The 1930 Law on General Hygiene was the most explicit in relation to the pro-natalist position. It imposed obligations on the Ministry of Health to encourage births and to grant monetary awards or medals to women who had six or more children and prohibited the importation and sale of contraceptives (Altıok 1978; Fişek 1963, 1964b, 1986b; Fişek and Shorter 1968).

Abortion had always been a sensitive issue in Turkey. During the pro-natalist period, a number of laws attempted to prevent abortions. The Turkish Penal Code, passed in 1926 and adapted from the Italian Penal Code, considered induced abortion to be a crime. An amendment to this law was introduced in 1936 that increased the penalties for induced abortion and penalized any action that attempted to avoid conception. In another amendment as late as 1953, the penalties for abortion were again increased; however, several studies documented that the practice of abortion

BOX 6.1 Timeline of Major Events

1923:	Pro-natalist population policy is established; major legislative changes support rapid population growth.
1950s:	Maternal mortality is high because of illegally induced abortions.
1958:	A turning point occurs, and efforts to reverse the pro-natalist population policy start. The Ministry of Health forms an advisory panel to evaluate the health aspects of excessive fertility.
1959:	Survey information shows high rural infant mortality and maternal mortality; 53 percent of maternal deaths are estimated to be caused by abortion.
1960:	Military revolution takes place. Dr. Nusret Fişek becomes undersecretary of health. Advocacy activities to change the pro-natalist population policy increase.
1961:	Preparation of the new Population Planning Law begins with wide participation by the Ministry of Health, nongovernmental organizations, and individuals.
1963:	A Population Council team assesses the national situation and assists with a national survey that shows popular interest in contraception and in government help in providing it.
1964:	The first director of the new Family Planning Unit in the Ministry of Health is appointed.
1965:	Parliament passes the first anti-natalist Population Planning Law.
1965–66:	Hacettepe University establishes the Public Health Department and the Institute of Population Studies.
	Various ministries, including the ministries of Education and Defense, introduce family planning in their educational programs.
	The first 10 pilot clinics open.
1967–68:	Mobile teams reach rural families, providing them with information and services.
1979:	Activities to strengthen the earlier anti-natal Population Planning Law begin.
1983:	The Second Population Planning Law is passed, authorizing trained nonphysicians to insert intrauterine devices, legalizing induced abortion up to 10 weeks on request, allowing trained general practitioners to terminate pregnancies, legalizing surgical sterilization for men and women on request, and establishing intersectoral collaboration to provide family planning services throughout the country.
1983–2000:	Contraceptive use among married couples rises to 71 percent, abortion incidence declines, maternal deaths from unsafe abortions decline sharply, and the total fertility rate falls to 2.2 births per woman.

continued to be widespread, irrespective of the laws (Fişek 1967a, 1972; Kişnişçi and Akın 1978). Approximately one out of five pregnancies was aborted, an extremely high rate, and abortion was one of the leading causes of maternal deaths (Altıok 1978; Fişek 1963, 1964b, 1986a; Özbay and Shorter 1970).

In addition, a number of laws either granted tax exemptions for children or allocated resources based on the number of children a person had and also gave priority for land distribution to families with many children (1938), gave public sector employees modest child support payments (1944), and provided income tax reductions based on the number of children (1949). A number of laws encouraged immigration from abroad, granting legal or financial advantages to immigrants. During this period, all political parties adopted the government's pro-natalist position as reflected not only in the explicitly or implicitly pro-natalist laws passed, but in party programs and mass media materials. Opinions did not start to change until 1958.

The Move toward an Anti-Natalist Policy, 1965

Changing the pro-natalist population policy was not an easy process. It took time and involved efforts by many individuals, nongovernmental organizations (NGOs), and sectors of society. The first articles attacking population growth were written by Professor Haluk Cillov in the daily newspaper *Milliyet* and by Fakir Baykurt in the daily newspaper *Cumhuriyet*. Cillov argued that the population was growing too fast and having a major impact on cities and stressed the need to control population growth (Fişek 1963, 1964b). Also, in 1958, obstetricians and gynecologists such as Dr. Ziya Durmuş, Dr. Necdet Erenus, Professor Naşit Erez, and Dr. Zekai Tahir Burak launched an initiative to change the population policy and legalize methods of contraception. Burak was a prominent specialist and head of a large maternity hospital in Ankara, and he had noticed that many women were admitted in serious condition because of self-induced abortions and that most of them died. He documented these hospital cases to demonstrate the magnitude of adverse outcomes on women's health resulting from unwanted pregnancies and unsafe abortions. He then sent a letter to the Ministry of Health stating that maternal mortality had increased because of unsafe abortions, that measures should therefore be taken to prevent such deaths, and that contraception should be legalized.

Following Burak's letter, the Ministry of Health set up a committee to investigate issues connected with abortion, to determine the associated medical problems, and to discuss countermeasures. In its report, the committee pointed out that despite the strict provisions in the Turkish Penal Code, abortion was practiced on a large scale and the vast majority of cases were not subjected to judicial action. The report suggested that members of the medical profession were performing some of these abortions for personal profit, but that most abortions were being carried out in places that lacked medical facilities, resulting in serious medical problems and deaths. The committee's report, while acknowledging the law against abortion and accepting that it should remain illegal, indicated that abortion should be permitted under certain conditions of medical necessity. Furthermore, the committee argued that contraception should be allowed so that women would not have to bear unwanted children and that the law should be changed so that women could have the advantage of contraceptive methods and devices in the manner of other countries. Although the report did not mention any change in policy, it was important as the first official document suggesting measures to legalize family planning (Altıok 1978; Fişek 1963, 1964b, 1967a; Holzhausen 1987; State Planning Organization 1993; Üner and Fişek 1961).

Also in 1958, the Ministry of Health formed an advisory panel of university professors and well-known specialists to carry out an independent evaluation of the health aspects of excessive fertility and to recommend solutions. This panel recommended removing the existing legal barriers to contraception and making contraceptives available; however, the panel was against making abortion legal unless a medical indication existed. The panel submitted those recommendations to the Ministry of Justice for its opinion and support. Unfortunately, the Ministry of Justice did not approve the recommendations (Fişek 1964b; Levine and Üner 1978).

In 1959, a survey was carried out in 137 villages, which showed that the rural infant mortality rate was around 165 deaths per 1,000 births and estimated the maternal mortality ratio at 280 deaths per 100,000 births. Furthermore, the survey estimated that 53 percent of maternal deaths were caused by abortions. This study was also important in two other respects. First, it established the connection between abortion and maternal mortality, reinforcing the views of the Ministry of Health committee on the wide extent of abortion. Second, it was important because Professor Nusret Fişek, who directed the survey, became undersecretary of the Ministry of Health after the 1960 revolution and served in that position for six years (Altıok 1978; Fişek 1963, 1964b; State Planning Organization 1993).

A revolution led by the military took place on May 27, 1960, after which planning was instituted in all areas and a number of reforms, including regulatory and legislative changes, were implemented. A new constitution was drafted that emphasized planning and created the State Planning Organization under the Prime Minister's Office. At this time, population planning became a serious objective (Anderson 1970) and Fişek played a vital role. He was already known as a pioneer in many fields of public health, and his leadership was invaluable in preparations for the new anti-natalist Population Planning Law. He pressed the issue at both national and international platforms and communicated closely with Burak and other opinion leaders, including some in NGOs. Fişek spearheaded efforts in relation to legal changes, and later drafted the 1965 law (Anderson 1970; *Official Gazette* 1965).

After the 1960 military intervention and the establishment of the State Planning Organization, discussions began between the Ministry of Health and the State Planning Organization. Their representatives unanimously agreed that a change in the traditional population policy was necessary, and an anti-natalist position was taken in both the First Five-Year Development Plan and the Population Planning Law that was prepared for parliament. Even before that, liberalization of the old policy had been enacted by allowing limited contraceptive imports. The First Five-Year Development Plan discussed the problems caused by the high rate of population growth, arguing that it was undermining gross national product growth and that population growth had to be brought under control. The plan advocated repealing the anticonception laws, creating a family planning program, and providing family planning education to the public. The government accepted the proposals (Altıok 1978; Fişek 1964b, 1967b; State Planning Organization 1993).

In the process of changing the policy, advocacy activities were extremely important. For instance, in December 1960, Fişek organized a large forum on birth control at the Ministry of Health's Institute of Hygiene and participants included well-known physicians, religious leaders, sociologists, and demographers. The issue of birth control was discussed extensively, with representatives from each discipline stating their own perspectives and opinions. The results of this forum were discussed in the media for some time, thereby keeping the issue on the agenda. Many articles appeared in the newspapers discussing the need for an anti-natalist population policy. At the same time, the Ankara Gynecological Association organized several large annual seminars on family planning that were closely followed by the press.

A principal reason for changing the policy was the large numbers of abortions each year. Although the exact number was not determined, it was believed that the number of illegally induced abortions approached half a million each year, with around 10,000 deaths per year as a result of complications (Fişek 1967a; Metiner 1969). A second factor was the increasing mechanization of agriculture. This had led to rapid urbanization and had created a situation whereby half the people in the largest cities were living in newly established squatter settlements. The cities had neither sufficient accommodations nor jobs to support large families.

Preparations for the new law began in 1961 and involved close collaboration between Ministry of Health officials, NGOs, and individuals who had the foresight to understand the problems. The Turkish Family Planning Association and the Ankara Gynecological Association were extremely active in terms of advocacy, giving numerous lectures and holding national meetings. Changing the pro-natalist policy gradually gained support in the medical community and in the country at large, and policy makers began to be convinced. However, much more was needed in the way of evidence and support.

In early 1963, the government requested the Population Council to send a team of experts to analyze demographic factors, conduct a field survey to determine the feasibility of a nationwide family planning program, and provide recommendations for operational guidelines and costs. This led to agreement on a formal project between the government and the Population Council (Anderson 1970; Metiner 1969). The Population Council helped field a nationally representative knowledge, attitude, and practice survey that interviewed more than 5,000 people in nearly 300 villages and cities. This was the first survey of its type in Turkey. It revealed valuable information and later helped the national program. The survey report showed that an overwhelming number of women in rural areas desired a family planning program operated by the government. A full 60 percent wanted only two to four children, and most couples older than 30 and married for 10 years did not want any more children at all. Some 67 percent of villagers and 87 percent of city residents said they wished to know more about contraception (Berelson 1964; Metiner 1966, 1969).

Thus, even in 1963, when producing or marketing contraceptives was still prohibited, the data seemed to show that the small family norm was well established, that a majority of husbands and wives approved of contraception, and that about two-thirds were interested in learning more. At the same time, knowledge of contraceptive methods was limited: 43 percent of husbands and wives said they did not know of any specific way to avoid conception. This national survey and several smaller studies clearly demonstrated a favorable attitude toward family planning among Turkish families.

In 1964, before the Population Planning Law was ratified, the Ministry of Health established a family planning organization. Dr. Turgut Metiner, an experienced gynecologist who had received some of his training in the United States, was appointed as director. During this time, the Ministry of Health also supported several seminars and group discussions and instituted the preparatory phase for detailed planning for a nationwide effort.

Also in 1964, Turkish personnel were trained in various aspects of family planning in the United States, and a Population Council resident representative arrived to assist in planning, initiate local training, and help with implementation of the program. Provisions were made for additional advisers, both resident and short term, when needed to work with opinion leaders, NGOs, and communities.

All these developments helped reverse the climate of opinion.

The Population Planning Law and Its Outcomes, 1965–67

The new Population Planning Law was intended to provide the legal framework for funding and implementing a nationwide family planning program. This law was passed by the Assembly and the Senate and was signed by the president in April 1965. The law stated that the purpose of population planning was to allow individuals to have as many children as they wished and that preventive measures (contraception) to avoid pregnancy would be allowed. The Ministry of Health was given the responsibility of implementing the program, training health personnel in contraceptive administration, and providing education to the public. The law also stated the strict medical conditions under which abortion or sterilization would be allowed and the penalties for violations.

The parliamentary debate on the bill was interesting in that it revealed some of the underlying ideologies of the participants concerning population. It also revealed their profound lack of information about population dynamics. Only the Ministry of Health seemed to have a demographic framework for understanding the issues involved. This was not surprising, as discussions of population processes were relatively new in Turkey and technical knowledge was not widespread. The debate was also unusual in that an "outsider," Fişek, spoke twice in parliament to defend the bill and to provide technical details. The lack of information on population growth on the part of members of parliament and the fact that they were being pushed to reverse a 40-year-old policy accounted for some of the incoherence of the debate.

Several smaller issues emerged, one of which was symbolic: what to call the program. In the original draft of the First Five-Year Development Plan, the State Planning Organization had initially indicated that the name of the program should be the Family Planning Program. The government changed this to the Population Planning Program, the feeling being that this was more neutral and did not imply an invasion of family intimacy. Following considerable debate in parliament, the official implementation agency within the Ministry of Health was named the General Directorate of Population Planning. However, in all substantive discussions of the topic since that time, everyone has referred to the family planning program.

More meaningful debate concerned the methods to be used to reduce fertility. While most of those who supported the bill argued for allowing contraceptives, only two persons argued for making abortion more legal. Later, in 1967, a regulation was issued that enumerated the medical conditions required for abortion and sterilization, but aside from these, the 1965 population policy did not change until the 1980s (Altıok 1978).

Support and Opposition

Support for the 1965 law came from the majority of the people as well as from various sectors of society. Opposition came not from rural women, but from certain more educated groups who were, however, ill-informed. These included business people in Istanbul and Izmir, who mistakenly believed that if the country had a bigger population, they would have a bigger market. Another opposition group felt that Turkey must have a large population in order to have a big army and a powerful voice in international affairs. Others believed that if Turkey's economy improved, then the birth rate would automatically decrease. In addition, some gynecologists were opposed to the family planning program, concerned that in some way it would threaten their practices. From time to time, adverse propaganda of a purely medical nature appeared suggesting that either the oral contraceptive or the intrauterine device (IUD) were harmful. In general, opposition was avoided to the extent that no serious religious objections emerged. The Turkish population was also relatively homogeneous with a single language, which avoided ethnic competition and fears of one group growing faster than others.

Early Implementation Measures

During the program's early days, numerous steps were taken that seemed promising in relation to reaching the targets set in the First Five-Year Development Plan. The Ministry of Education planned to emphasize human reproduction in biology courses in middle and high schools starting in the 1965–66 school year and to incorporate the social, economic, and political implications of rapid growth in social studies courses. Two educational programs were envisaged for armed forces personnel, one for married personnel and the other for all enlisted men just before their release from active duty. Both the Ministry of Education and the Ministry of Defense were assigned functions under the new law, and in addition, the Ministry of Health planned closely coordinated information programs through the ministries of Rural Affairs and Agriculture. Other information, education, and communication programs were directed to many groups, such as couples with many children, unmarried people, men's and women's associations, labor unions, staff members of large industries, university students, and government employees.

The Scientific Committee, consisting of university faculty and ministry staff members, was established at the Ministry of Health to advise the High Medical Council. Subsequently, 10 pilot clinics were opened in various parts of the country, and after six months of observation, the committee licensed two types of oral contraceptives for sale and allowed the use of the Lippes loop IUD. Since then, other contraceptives have been licensed, but only after they have been examined by the Committee on Contraceptive Medicine, have been analyzed in the government laboratory, and have received the approval of the Scientific Committee.

For the deployment of actual services and for efficiency, the plan was to use existing facilities and personnel of the Ministry of Health (Fişek 1964b; Metiner 1966; Ross 1966) and to have a small central organization to train public health services personnel. This organization was established as an independent department of the

Ministry of Health under the direct supervision of the undersecretary. To overcome the shortage of clinical services workers, especially in the rural areas where 80 percent of the population lived at that time, a plan was instituted to attract 200 medical graduates, both men and women, and train them in gynecological assessment and IUD insertion. This was the basis for 200 mobile teams. Public services offered the IUD for free and other methods at cost. The target of the program was to provide services to 5 percent of all women of childbearing age each year, and the hope was that the cumulative effects of such an approach would greatly improve the health of mothers and children.

The Family Planning Association, with its 20 branches, assisted with educational work and operated several clinics. Another smaller but valuable organization was the University Women's Association of Ankara, whose members volunteered their services by visiting villages, suburban communities, and factories to provide information and to instruct mothers where to go for services.

Mobile Teams

Among the various ways to inform the public and to implement services, a key approach was the use of mobile teams. In this way, contraceptives, especially the IUD, were brought to villagers' doorsteps and to large squatter communities in the main cities. The mobile teams worked in pairs, one providing education and information and the other providing medical services. The education team included female and male educators who visited the village first, then the medical team arrived to follow up with clinical services. The mobile teams achieved remarkable successes in 1967 and 1968, finding a groundswell of interest among village women. Indeed, one of the early characteristics of family planning provision was the enthusiastic cooperation of village people whenever anyone visited to discuss or offer services. During the 1960s in Turkey, as in other countries, most married couples wanted to learn and do something about family planning.

Budget and Donors

The total budget for family planning was divided into three parts according to source. First was the Ministry of Health's annual budget for family planning authorized by parliament. Second was a grant referred to as counterpart funds, jointly agreed on by the Ministry of Finance and the U.S. Agency for International Development, that covered support for provincial family planning directors and field workers; travel expenses; incentive payments; research; program evaluation; and publication of information, education, and communication materials. The third source was grants from foreign foundations. The Swedish International Development Cooperation Agency contributed mainly for oral contraceptives; the Population Council provided assistance for consultants, vehicle maintenance, contraceptives, advanced calculators, educational materials, fellowships, and salary supplements; and the Ford Foundation helped with population research. Technical assistance came primarily from the Population Council's resident advisers and to a lesser extent from the U.S. Agency for International Development and the Ford Foundation. Turkey also received assistance from the World Health Organization for training programs, and the Family Planning Association received funds from the International Planned Parenthood Federation.

Research

The leading research institution was at Hacettepe University, which established the Institute of Population Studies in 1966 supported by a grant from the Ford Foundation. Training for the first group of students began in 1967 with a two-year program for a master's degree in population dynamics. The institute also undertook detailed surveys of population and family dynamics and engaged students for research projects in the university's Medical School. The institute published a quarterly bulletin describing family planning efforts and Turkey's population problems. In 1968, it conducted a nationwide study using a knowledge, attitude, and practice questionnaire comparable to that employed by the pioneering 1963 survey. It also fielded later demographic and health surveys in collaboration with the Ministry of Health and supported by Macro International.

Also at Hacettepe University, the Public Health Department (formerly the Community Medicine Department) was established in 1965. As part of medical education, it emphasized the preventive aspects of community medicine, including reproductive and family health. Later, this department helped the Ministry of Health extensively with family planning work, especially by means of its health service research activities, as well as through its national training programs in family planning. In 1978, the department became a World Health Organization Collaborating Center for family planning and reproductive health and continues in this role today.

Outcomes

Over time it became clear that contraceptive practices would lag behind attitudes and knowledge. By 1978, contraceptive use had risen to only 50 percent of couples, two-thirds of whom relied on traditional methods with their high failure rates (table 6.1). This has to be understood in the context of the decades of pro-natalism, the official policy before 1965, and the subsequent slow start of the national program. Before 1965, knowledge of such modern contraceptive devices as oral contraceptives, the IUD, and foam tablets was limited among the public, and even among most physicians. The only contraceptive available on the market was the condom, and the only reason the condom could be freely sold was that it qualified as a prophylactic against venereal disease. The first IUD was inserted only in 1964, and vaginal creams and foam tablets became available only in 1967 (Fişek and Shorter 1968). The overall availability of contraceptive methods was narrower than in some other countries.

However, the program also had a number of positive features that were most welcome to the leadership, especially considering the radical reversal of the well-entrenched pro-natalism that had been required in both law and practice. These positive features included the following:

- The timely assessment, with documentation, of the demographic and health realities that had suddenly changed after 1945–50, namely, the high population

TABLE 6.1 Contraceptive Use, Selected Years
percentage of married or cohabiting women aged 15–49 using contraception

Method	1963	1978	1983	1988	1993	1998	2003
Any method	22.0	50.0	61.5	63.4	62.6	63.9	71.0
IUD	0.0	4.0	8.9	17.1	18.8	19.8	20.2
Pill	1.0	8.0	9.0	7.6	4.9	4.4	4.7
Condom	4.3	4.0	4.9	8.9	6.6	8.2	10.8
Surgical sterilization (female)	0.0	0.0	0.1	2.2	2.9	4.2	5.8
Coitus interruptus	10.4	22.0	31.1	31.0	26.2	24.4	26.4
Other	12.0	12.1	8.6	10.2	3.2	2.8	4.1
Total effective-method users	5.3	18.0	27.2	32.3	34.5	37.7	42.5
Total ineffective-method users	22.4	32.0	34.2	31.0	28.1	25.5	28.5
Unmet need for contraception[a]	—	—	—	—	12.0	10.0	6.0
Abortions per 100 pregnancies	7.6	16.8	19.0	23.6	18.0	14.5	11.3

Source: National surveys by the Ministry of Health and Hacettepe University.

Note: — = not available.

a. Couples who do not want children for at least two years, who can conceive, and who are not using any method of contraception.

growth, maternal and infant mortality, abortion rate, and unmet need for contraception. The 1963 national survey was critical, as were later surveys.

- The leadership by a small number of committed, influential people, as stressed earlier.

- The strong advocacy activities, especially by the Turkish Family Planning Association and the Ankara Gynecological Association, to draw in people outside the government.

- The military government's positive stance toward family planning.

- The presence of farsighted people at the Ministry of Health.

- The preparation of infrastructure to deliver services even before the Population Planning Law was in force, including the training of health personnel and the formation of mobile teams.

- The effective collaboration with international agencies in relation to technical and financial support.

Notwithstanding the reversal of pro-natalism, the passage of new laws, and the creation of the national action program, success was incomplete, and in due course, a reappraisal seemed to be warranted.

Later Developments, 1980–83

While the profound changes described earlier amounted to a historic revolution for family planning, much was yet to come. Legal developments are considered first.

Modification of the First Population Planning Law

Clearly, the 1965 Population Planning Law was followed by substantial progress in family planning services and in the provision of information about contraceptive methods to the public. However, a review of program implementation in 1980 indicated that services still did not fully meet the needs of the public (Fişek 1983; Özbay 1975). Traditional methods were also the most frequently used means of contraception. It was not until 1993 that modern methods accounted for more than half of contraceptive methods used (figure 6.1).

The reliance primarily on traditional methods, despite people's increased knowledge, was unfortunate, as they were often ineffective and hindered the spread of modern methods. Another serious problem was that even though induced abortions were banned, the number increased annually. Abortion was used almost as a regular method of birth control by women in the higher socioeconomic strata of society, who obtained services from medical specialists at a high cost, whereas low-income women often had to resort to self-induced abortion, which usually led to serious injury or death. Estimates indicate that there were 300,000 induced abortions and 50,000 self-induced abortions in 1981 (Akın 1992). This indicated that despite the law, a significant service gap existed. Therefore, work started to modify the 1965 law to expand service delivery and to make services more available and equitable. Two strategies were followed during the preparatory phase (Akın 1999, 2001): one based on scientific studies and a second devoted to advocacy.

Scientific Approach

Several local and national epidemiological investigations were conducted, as well as several operation research studies, to demonstrate the adverse effects of illegally induced abortion. These undertakings included the following:

FIGURE 6.1 Contraceptive Prevalence, 1978–2003

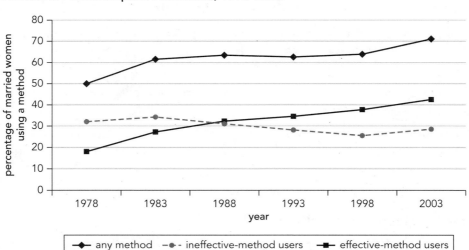

Source: National population and health surveys by the ministries of Health and Social Affairs and Hacettepe University.

- Analyses of the national surveys, by Hacettepe University's Institute of Population Studies and the Ministry of Health which were conducted every five years following the 1963 survey, established the unsatisfactory trends in fertility regulation

- Specific community-based studies on induced abortion

- Three key studies by Hacettepe University's Public Health Department, noted earlier,

  o demonstrated that trained nonphysicians can insert IUDs as successfully as physicians, leading to 201 nurse-midwives being trained and followed for one year in the field (1979)

  o provided evidence on the costs of illegal abortion for the health care system based on a World Health Organization multicenter study (1979–81)

  o introduced a safe and simple technique (manual vacuum extraction) for pregnancy termination, following which 35 general practitioners were trained in the technique and were followed for one year, demonstrating that trained general practitioners can terminate early pregnancy successfully using manual vacuum extraction (1981).

The results of these studies were used for advocacy purposes and served as a basis for specific aspects of the new law (Akın 1992).

Advocacy Activities

During the preparatory phase for modifying the Population Planning Law in 1980, another military government came into power whose leaders looked favorably upon population matters. Advocacy activities included the following:

- The results of the aforementioned studies were well disseminated and publicized at several meetings organized by the Ministry of Health, NGOs, and universities.

- The media produced programs and articles on population issues with the support of the president. Numerous items appeared in scientific journals, magazines, and newspapers.

- At the parliamentary level, the military government organized workshops on health care reform, where the results of the studies were presented to relevant government authorities.

Based on the persuasive results of the research and the supportive political atmosphere, preparations for the new law were initiated by the General Directorate for Maternal and Child Health and Family Planning (previously the General Directorate of Family Planning) (Population Planning Advisory Board 1994). The new Population Planning Law was passed in May 1983. It included the following innovations (*Official Gazette* 1983):

- Authorizing trained nonphysicians to insert IUDs

- Legalizing induced abortion up to 10 weeks into a pregnancy on request

- Licensing trained general practitioners to terminate pregnancies

- Legalizing surgical sterilization for men and women on request

- Strengthening intersectoral collaboration to provide family planning services throughout the country.

Within a few years after the new Population Planning Law came into force, the following beneficial consequences occurred:

- Maternal deaths caused by unsafe abortions had almost disappeared.

- Hospital beds were seldom occupied by patients with complications of induced abortions.

- The burdens of induced abortion on the health care system had decreased.

- The costs of induced abortions for individuals had decreased.

- The prevalence of induced abortions increased initially, but started to decrease after 1990 and continues to do so (table 6.1). The incidence of abortion per 100 women aged 15–49 fell to a negligible level (table 6.2), because contraception resulted in fewer pregnancies and because more pregnancies were wanted.

- IUD prevalence doubled between 1983 and 1988.

- In 1993, for the first time, the prevalence of effective contraceptives exceeded the prevalence of traditional methods (table 6.1, figure 6.1).

- The Population Planning Advisory Board was established within the Ministry of Health to advance family planning activities by means of intersectoral collaboration (Aytaç 1992; State Planning Organization 1994).

By 1988–2003, major changes had occurred (table 6.3). By 2003, the total fertility rate was down to 2.2 births per woman and 71 percent of couples were using contraception. Furthermore, the balance between traditional and modern methods of contraception had shifted steadily, among the general population, illiterate women, and women with at least a secondary school education.

TABLE 6.2 Induced Abortion Rates for One Year Prior to Surveys, Selected Years

Year	Number of induced abortions per year per		
	100 pregnancies	100 women aged 15–49	100 live births
1983 demographic and health survey	19.0	2.8	15.4
1988 demographic and health survey	23.6	5.5	35.1
1993 demographic and health survey	18.0	3.1	26.0
1998 demographic and health survey	14.5	2.5	20.9
2003 demographic and health survey	11.3	0.4	13.9

Source: National demographic and health surveys.

TABLE 6.3 Selected Demographic Indicators, Selected Years

Indicator	1988	1993	1998	2003
General Population				
Crude death rate (per 1,000 population)	—	22.9	23.4	19.7
Total fertility rate (births per woman)	3.4	2.7	2.6	2.2
General fertility rate (per 1,000 women aged 15–49)	—	95.0	94.0	79.0
Contraceptive use, any method (percentage of married women)	63.4	62.6	63.9	71.0
No use of any method of contraception (percentage of married women)	36.6	37.4	36.1	29.0
Modern method of contraception (percentage of married women)	31.0	34.5	37.7	42.5
Traditional method of contraception (percentage of married women)	32.3	28.1	26.1	28.5
Illiterate Women (percentage of married women)				
Modern method of contraception	—	25.0	28.1	29.9
Traditional method of contraception	—	24.0	22.5	26.9
Women with at least a Secondary School Education (percentage of married women)				
Modern method of contraception	—	48.0	52.8	50.8
Traditional method of contraception	—	38.7	22.5	26.5

Source: National surveys by the Ministry of Health and Hacettepe University.

Note: — = not available.

Lessons Learned and Conclusions

Turkey's experience with changing its population policy, both the historic 1965 reversal and the 1980 modification, demonstrated the importance of the following effective ways to realize legal changes:

- Vigorous, committed leadership

- Support from scientific evidence based on empirical research

- Advocacy through multiple channels (meetings, publications, and the media)

- Intersectoral collaboration, both within the government and with the private sector

- International collaboration and support.

A vital lesson came from the legalization of abortion, which had a great effect in preventing abortion-related complications and maternal deaths. **Three trends were mutually supporting: safer abortions, a decline in the maternal mortality ratio, and greater use of modern contraceptive methods.** Figure 6.2 shows the concurrent changes in the search for contraception and mortality. In legalization of abortion, evidence from national studies and from operations research was helpful in convincing both decision makers and opponents. International support through

FIGURE 6.2 Prevalence of Modern Methods of Contraception and the Maternal Mortality Ratio, 1963–2003

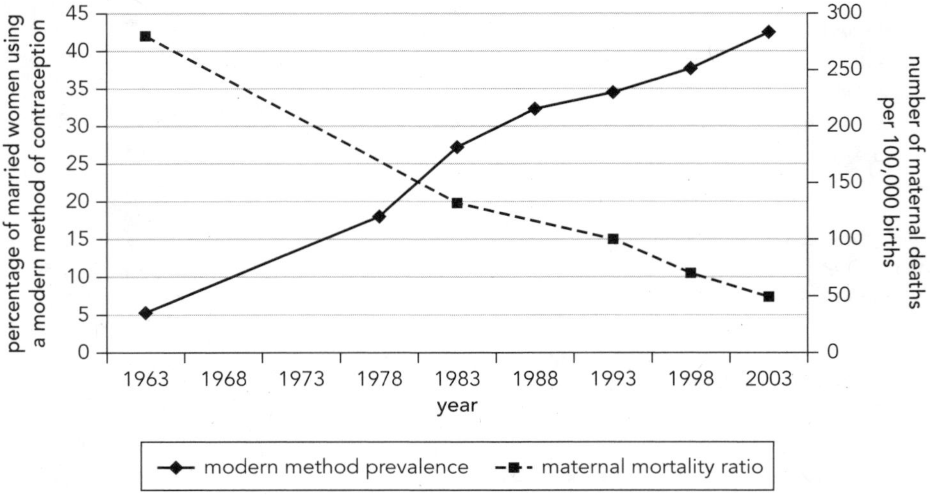

Source: Prevalence: national surveys; maternal mortality ratio: Akın and Dogan 2000; World Health Organization, Ministry of Health, and State Planning Organization estimates; AVSC; IPAS; JHPIEGO.

collaboration with agencies such as the World Health Organization, the Association for Voluntary and Safe Contraception, International Population Assistance Services, and the Johns Hopkins Program for International Education in Reproductive Health was also extremely valuable.

Even though Turkey has made marked progress in family planning, continued efforts are required to further decrease unmet need for the prevention of unwanted pregnancies. Furthermore, the social status of women has to be improved, and female empowerment should be enhanced as a deliberate public policy to help prevent early marriages, early births, and unwanted pregnancies and to minimize maternal deaths related to high-risk pregnancies. Leaders at all levels must give priority to these issues and work to ensure the success of family planning nationwide.

Future needs include undertaking systematic reviews of policies, regulations, and service facilities to provide sustainable access to high-quality family planning and reproductive health services; establishing a national management information system; enlarging the scope of scientific and operations research; expanding and strengthening training for family planning and reproductive heath; adding trainers throughout the country; engaging in efforts to improve contraceptive technologies and provide them to the public; and maintaining international cooperation and collaboration.

References

Akın, Ayşe. 1992. "The Present and Future of Family Planning in Turkey." In *Planning for the Future of Family Planning in Turkey: Proceedings of the Abant/Bolu Meeting*, 40–55. Ankara: Ministry of Health.

———. 1999. "Cultural and Psychosocial Factors Affecting Contraceptive Use and Abortion in Two Provinces of Turkey." In *Abortion in the Developing World,* ed. A. I. Mundigo and C. Indriso, 191–211. World Health Organization.

———. 2001. "Implementing the ICPD Programme of Action: The Turkish Experience." In *Sexual and Reproductive Health: Recent Advances, Future Directions,* 2 vols., ed. Chander P. Puri and Paul F. A. Van Look, vol. I, 57–69. New Delhi: New Age International.

Akın, Ayşe, and M. Dogan. 2000. *Survey on Causes of Maternal Mortality from Hospital Records in Turkey.* Ankara: Ministry of Health.

Altıok, Esen. 1978. "The Development of a Population Policy and Its Implementation." In *Population Policy Formation and Implementation in Turkey,* ed. Ned Levine and Sunday Üner, 53–74. Ankara: Hacettepe University Publications.

Anderson, Lewis Ş. 1970. *Turkey.* Country Profiles Series. New York: Population Council.

Aytaç, U. 1992. "Family Planning Work of the Ministry of Health." In *Planning for the Future of Family Planning in Turkey: Proceedings of the Abant/Bolu Meeting,* 13–25. Ankara: Ministry of Health.

Berelson, Bernard. 1964. "Turkey: National Survey on Population." *Studies in Family Planning* 1 (5): 1–5.

Cerit, S. 1989. *Türkiye'de Nüfus Doğurganlık ve Ölümlülük.* Ankara: Yeniçağ Basın-Yayın.

Fişek, Nusret H. 1963. "Türkiye'de Nüfus Planlaması Çalışmaları." Reprinted in 1998 in *Kitaplaşmamış Yazıları-II içinde- Ana Çocuk Sağlığı, Nüfus Sorunları ve Aile Planlaması,* ed. R. Derleyen Dirican, 171–72. Ankara: Türk Tabipleri Birliği Publications.

———. 1964a. "Nüfus Planlamasında Hükumetlerin Sorumluluğu." Reprinted in 1998 in *Kitaplaşmamış Yazıları-II içinde- Ana Çocuk Sağlığı, Nüfus Sorunları ve Aile Planlaması,* ed. R. Derleyen Dirican, 173–76. Ankara: Türk Tabipleri Birliği Publications.

———. 1964b. "Türkiye'de Nüfus Sorunlarının Ele Alınış Tarzı ve Planlar." Reprinted in 1998 in *Kitaplaşmamış Yazıları-II içinde- Ana Çocuk Sağlığı, Nüfus Sorunları ve Aile Planlaması,* ed. R. Derleyen Dirican, 161–70. Ankara: Türk Tabipleri Birliği Publications.

———. 1967a. "Çocuk Düşürmenin Sosyal Yönü." Reprinted in 1998 in *Kitaplaşmamış Yazıları-II içinde- Ana Çocuk Sağlığı, Nüfus Sorunları ve Aile Planlaması,* ed. R. Derleyen Dirican, 151–60. Ankara: Türk Tabipleri Birliği Publications.

———. 1967b. "Türkiye'de Nüfus Planlaması." Reprinted in 1998 in *Kitaplaşmamış Yazıları-II içinde- Ana Çocuk Sağlığı, Nüfus Sorunları ve Aile Planlaması,* ed. R. Derleyen Dirican, 177–81. Ankara: Türk Tabipleri Birliği Publications.

———. 1972. "Türkiye'de Doğurganlık, Çocuk Düşürme ve Gebeliği Önleyici Yöntem Kullanma Arasındaki İlişkiler." Reprinted in 1998 in *Kitaplaşmamış Yazıları-II içinde- Ana Çocuk Sağlığı, Nüfus Sorunları ve Aile Planlaması,* ed. R. Derleyen Dirican, 195–203. Ankara: Türk Tabipleri Birliği Publications.

———. 1983. "Dünyada ve Türkiye'de Nüfus Sorunu." In *Hekimler İçin Aile Planlaması El Kitabı,* ed. Ayşe Akın, 1–21. Ankara: Tanıt Press.

———. 1986a. "Aşırı Doğurganlık ve Sağlık." Reprinted in 1998 in *Kitaplaşmamış Yazıları-II içinde- Ana Çocuk Sağlığı, Nüfus Sorunları ve Aile Planlaması,* ed. R. Derleyen Dirican, 127–28. Ankara: Türk Tabipleri Birliği Publications.

———. 1986b. "Türkiye'de Aile Planlaması Program Stratejisi." Reprinted in 1998 in *Kitaplaşmamış Yazıları-II içinde- Ana Çocuk Sağlığı, Nüfus Sorunları ve Aile Planlaması,* ed. R. Derleyen Dirican, 182–87. Ankara: Türk Tabipleri Birliği Publications.

Fişek, Nusret H. and Frederic C. Shorter. 1968. "Fertility Control in Turkey." *Demography* 5 (2): 578–89.

Holzhausen, W. 1987. "The Population Problem in Turkey (as Seen from the Perspective of a Foreign Donor)." *Nüfusbilim Dergisi (Turkish Journal of Population Studies)* 9: 63–73.

Kişnişçi, H., and A. Akın. 1978. "Türkiye'de Düşüklerle ilgili Epidemiyolojik Bir Araştırma." In *Türkiye'de Nüfusun Yapısı ve Nüfus Sorunları—1973 Araştırması*, 113–32. Ankara: Hacettepe University Publications.

Levine, N., and S. Üner. 1978. *Population Policy Formation and Implementation in Turkey*. Ankara: Hacettepe University Publications.

Metiner Turgut. 1966. "Implications of the Conference: Turkey." In *Family Planning and Population Programs: A Review of World Developments*, ed. Bernard Berelson, R. K. Anderson, O. Harkavy, J. Maier, W. P. Mauldin, and S. J. Segal, 807–8. Chicago: University of Chicago Press.

———. 1969. "Turkey: Answering the Demands of the People." In *Population: Challenging World Crisis*, ed. Bernard Berelson, 100–10. Voice of America Forum Lectures. Washington, DC: Government Printing Office.

Official Gazette. 1965. *557 Sayılı Nüfus Planlaması Hakkında Kanun*. Ankara: General Directorate of Publications. April 10.

———. 1983. *2827 Sayılı Nüfus Planlaması Hakkında Kanun; Tüzük ve Yönetmelikler*. Ankara: General Directorate of Publications. May 27.

Özbay, Ferhunde. 1975. "Türkiye'de 1963, 1968 ve 1973 Yıllarında Aile Planlaması Uygulamalarında ve Doğurganlıktaki Değişmeler." Paper presented at the Second Conference on Turkish Demography, Çeşme-Izmir, Turkey.

Özbay, Ferhunde, and Frederic C. Shorter. 1970. "Turkey: Changes in Birth Control Practices, 1963 to 1968." *Studies in Family Planning* 1 (51): 1–7.

Population Planning Advisory Board. 1994. *Nüfus Planlaması Danışma Kurulu Çalışmaları, 1993–1994*. Ankara: Ministry of Health.

Ross, John. 1966. "Recent Events in Population Control." *Studies in Family Planning* 1 (9): 1–5.

State Planning Organization. 1993. *Turkey: National Report to the 1994 International Conference on Population and Development*. Ankara: State Planning Organization.

———. 1994. *Nüfus ve Nüfusun Yapısı*. Ankara: Government of Turkey.

Tokgöz, T., and Ayşe Akın. 1983. "Türkiye'de Aile Planlaması Çalışmaları." In *Hekimler İçin Aile Planlaması El Kitabı içinde*, ed. A. Akın, 22–29. Ankara: Tanıt Matbaası.

Üner, Sunday. 1984. *Türkiye Nüfusu: Boyutlar Sorunlar Yorumlar*. Ankara: Semih Offset Press.

Üner, R., and Nusret H. Fişek. 1961. *Türkiye'de Doğum Kontrolünün Uygulanması Üzerinde İncelemeler*. Ankara: Ministry of Health and Social Affairs.

III Latin America and the Caribbean

7 Family Planning in Chile: A Tale of the Unexpected

HERNÁN SANHUEZA

The notion that success in family planning in Latin America was a fanciful dream persisted for many years. High birth rates and the negative attitudes of many government leaders were believed to be immutable characteristics of Latin America; the opposition of the Catholic Church was considered insurmountable. Certainly, obstacles were present: early surveys revealed extremely low knowledge and use of family planning and, at least in theory, ideals of a large family size still persisted as late as the 1950s. Then came the unexpected. Almost immediately after women were given an opportunity to access family planning in the early 1960s, most of the myths and perceived obstacles were quickly proved wrong: Catholicism played almost no role in individuals' decisions about family planning, and the influence of policy makers was limited and varied significantly from the ideas and needs of most Latin Americans.

For most of its history, Latin America's struggle for development has been a vicious cycle of booms and busts and success stories have been few, but against this often grim backdrop, family planning as it relates to Chile is indeed one of the success stories. Box 7.1 provides a timeline of major events.

The Setting

Since the 1950s, Chilean public health officials and policy makers had been concerned about the country's high levels of maternal and infant mortality and morbidity. One of the motivating factors behind the creation of the National Health Service (NHS) in 1952 was the perceived need to improve coverage of the entire population with a suitable health system that would provide, among other things, good obstetric care. However, a decade later, maternal mortality remained high at 280 maternal deaths per 100,000 live births (Avendaño 1975), and by the beginning of the 1960s, it had become evident that the levels of induced abortion, which was then illegal and remains so today, continued to be high. Clearly, improving the coverage and quality of deliveries was insufficient, and the root causes of abortion needed to be dealt with

BOX 7.1 Timeline of Family Planning Activities

1950s:	Concerns about the effects of abortion and unwanted pregnancies on maternal mortality and morbidity lead to research on the epidemiology of abortion and reproductive behavior.
Late 1950s and early 1960s:	Introduction of new contraceptive technologies—intrauterine devices and oral contraceptives—occurs. A national version of the intrauterine device is developed, tested, and offered to the public.
1961–62:	First International Planned Parenthood Federation (IPPF) visit to Chile. The Chilean Committee for the Protection of the Family is formed.
1963:	The IPPF provides financial aid and international contacts to those working in family planning. Other international agencies and foundations follow suit.
1964:	The National Health Service adopts the first family planning policy.
1965:	The Chilean Association for the Protection of the Family is organized, joins the IPPF, and provides technical advice and material aid to the family planning program.
1966:	The National Health Services refines its family planning objectives and expands the program with contributions from international agencies.
1967:	The Eighth International Family Planning Conference takes place in Santiago sponsored by the Chilean Association for the Protection of the Family. President Eduardo Frei opens the conference.
1968:	The Vatican reaffirms its position opposing artificial contraception by issuing the *Encyclica Humanae Vitae*. Groups and individuals opposing family planning become more vocal and begin forming international alliances. The attitudes and behavior of the population, however, do not change substantially.
1970:	A socialist government is elected. The family planning program continues its expansion under President Salvador Allende.
1973:	A military coup takes place and General Augusto Pinochet takes over. Despite the disruption in people's lives, the family planning program continues, albeit affected by budgetary cuts to the National Health Service.
1989:	Under Pinochet, Article 19 of the Health Code is amended to further restrict access to abortion.
1990–present:	A democratic government is restored, resulting in increased freedom of expression and community participation. All administrations elected after the dictatorship continue support to family planning.
	The feminist movement becomes more vocal about gender analysis (the understanding of the societal differences in roles, needs, and opportunities between men and women) and interaction between providers and clients, contributing positively to the program.
2001–6:	After repeated legal challenges, the National Regulatory Agency allows emergency contraception (levonorgestrel pills) to be sold with a prescription. In 2004, emergency contraception is included in the norms for care of women who have suffered sexual violence, and in 2006, it is included in the fertility regulation norms of the Ministry of Health to be provided free of charge in public clinics.

by helping women prevent unwanted pregnancies. Another concern was infant mortality, which had remained more or less static with rates of more than 100 deaths per 1,000 live births since the mid-1950s (Avendaño 1975).

Ancient historical records indicate that humans have always sought means to control their fertility. A renewed interest in improving contraceptive technology had begun around the world by the end of the 1950s, as dealing with the health consequences of illegally induced abortions and unwanted fertility was virtually a universal phenomenon at that time. In Chile, the specific contraceptive that gained the attention of some physicians was the intrauterine device (IUD) made of silk suture that Dr. Ernst Graefenberg had developed in Germany in 1929. Dr. Jaime Zipper developed a Chilean version of the IUD using nylon thread in the shape of a ring. After testing its effectiveness and safety, physicians began offering the contraceptive at the Barros Luco Hospital in Santiago. Women immediately accepted the new technology. Soon afterward, an expanding number of physicians started offering IUD insertions at other service points, first in Santiago and then in other areas of the country.

In the early 1960s, the development and subsequent availability of oral contraceptives provided an enormous impetus to the nascent family planning efforts. Because of their characteristics, oral contraceptives proved to be a good complement to the IUD. As they were provided in pharmacies without the need for a prescription, and as they did not require the participation of a physician, they became extremely popular, especially among young women. Since that time, 80 to 90 percent of contraceptive users in Chile have opted for IUDs or pills.

At the beginning of the 1960s, Chile became an early adopter of family planning in Latin America given the confluence of several factors at that time, some of which also contributed to the rapid expansion of family planning in the country. First, the interest and expertise in public health that had existed for several years resulted in the formation of a cadre of trained professionals in that discipline. By that time, the country's schools of public health had developed a record of competence and were providing training to Chilean physicians and those of many other Latin American countries. Because of this public health tradition, Chile, by Latin American standards, had relatively good systems of health surveillance and statistics that allowed the public health system to identify and keep track of major health issues. Chile has also had regular census data since 1835, with censuses carried out every 10 years or so, which have provided sufficiently reliable denominator data.

Second, by that time, Chile already had an established national health system with wide coverage that provided health services for free or at a nominal cost in hospitals and other service points to blue-collar workers and their families. Furthermore, the National Health Service (NHS) covered well over 50 percent of the population.

Third, health professionals recognized the enormous need for preventing unwanted pregnancies as manifested by the high incidence of induced abortion that was taking a heavy toll in terms of maternal mortality and morbidity. By 1964–65, estimates indicated that about two out of every five maternal deaths were due to induced abortion (Avendaño 1975), and maternal mortality was estimated at 29 deaths per 10,000 live births (Cabrera and others 1975).

Fourth, a number of specialized organizations of the United Nations were based in Chile at the time, including the Latin American Demographic Center. This proximity helped Chilean organizations and individuals to interact with international agencies and to have access to specialized expertise.

Finally, a crucial component in securing access to family planning by the population was the existence of *matronas,* a specialized group of nurse-midwives. These were university-trained professionals who provided women with obstetric care, similar to the nurse practitioners in the United States today, but specializing in obstetrics. Nurse-midwives were much closer to women in need of contraception than physicians, not only because they were women themselves, but because they were more numerous and better distributed across the country than obstetricians and gynecologists. The NHS made the wise decision of allowing nurse-midwives to insert IUDs and provide other types of contraceptives starting in 1974. This expanded coverage and resolved bottlenecks that would have precluded broad access to contraception.

At the beginning of the 1960s, rapid population growth was not perceived as a problem in Chile. The common notion was that at prevailing rates of growth, the country would be able to provide for its citizens for the foreseeable future. The same feelings and beliefs existed in other Latin American countries. Although surveys carried out in five Latin American capitals during the mid-1960s showed that rapid population growth was beginning to emerge as an issue meriting consideration by decision makers, they also showed that even if 56 percent of the leaders interviewed declared that they were concerned about rapid population growth, only 25 percent thought this was a problem in their own country (Stycos 1970). Curiously, the situation then in relation to population growth was similar to people's perception with regard to HIV/AIDS in the 1980s, that is, the problem certainly affects other countries, but not ours.

By 1965, population surveys carried out by the Latin American Demographic Center had begun to show a situation of rapid population growth due to high fertility and decreasing mortality, particularly in rural areas. By that time, concern about rapid population growth and its possible negative impacts on development and on health had begun to take hold internationally, and various models had been developed to study the interaction of population variables with development using country-specific data.

History of Family Planning

In 1961, the International Planned Parenthood Federation (IPPF), through its Western Hemisphere Regional Office, contacted the Chilean health authorities to find out what was happening with regard to family planning in the country. In early 1962, an IPPF official visited Chile to establish contacts and explore the possibilities of collaboration. The series of discussions that took place during that visit involved well-known physicians and, because of the nature of the issue and of the personalities involved, they were widely publicized by the media. The meetings also provided a powerful incentive to an already motivated group of physicians, including mostly obstetricians, gynecologists, and public health specialists, to move ahead with their interest in expanding existing family planning activities. This was done with quiet, but effective, participation by the health authorities, which lent the facilities and personnel of the NHS to provide services without committing themselves officially.

The only official act by the health authorities in 1962 was the creation, by the then director general of the NHS, Dr. Gustavo Fricke, of an advisory committee to study how to reduce the incidence and the health and financial costs of abortion. He proceeded to invite the core group of physicians working in family planning at the time to constitute what was then called the Chilean Committee for the Protection of the Family. This committee, which provided the first official advice to the NHS, evolved over time, and, in 1965, constituted itself into a private not-for-profit organization, the Chilean Association for the Protection of the Family (Asociación Chilena de Protección de la Familia, APROFA), which became an IPPF affiliate. Throughout its more than 40-year history, APROFA has been providing support to Chile's family planning program.

By 1963, the IPPF had begun giving financial and material aid to Chilean organizations. This resulted in further expansion of family planning education and services.

Issues related to human sexuality and reproduction have always been sensitive and controversial. All religions have put taboos and strict limits on sexual expression and behavior, and the Catholic Church has been no exception. It is therefore noteworthy that all this was happening at a time when Chile was governed by President Jorge Alessandri and a right-wing, conservative party in this overwhelmingly Catholic country.

In 1964, a new national government was elected. The Christian Democrat President Eduardo Frei had strong ties to the Catholic Church, and so did his cabinet. Given the church's traditional opposition to artificial contraception, one might have expected a backlash in relation to family planning activities as a consequence of the elections. This did not happen. Indeed, to the contrary, the new director of the NHS carefully considered the recommendations of Fricke's advisory committee and, on the basis of those recommendations, announced the adoption of the government's first family planning policy. The purpose of the policy was to reduce the risks associated with abortion carried out under less than optimal conditions while respecting the conscience and dignity of individuals.

In 1965, under this policy, the NHS officially began providing family planning in its facilities through its mother and child health program. Around that time, other health networks that served the needs of various community groups, such as civil servants, the military, and the police, also began providing family planning to their constituencies.

This was an important year for family planning in Chile for several other reasons. APROFA, the newly formed family planning association, had started the process of affiliating itself with the IPPF and had reached agreement with the federation to plan and organize the Eighth International Family Planning Conference in Chile in 1967. Dr. Hernan Romero, chair of APROFA's Board of Directors, was appointed as executive secretary of the forthcoming conference, and this gave the association enormous visibility and leverage in the country. The preparatory activities leading to the conference resulted in the involvement of many influential organizations and individuals in both the public and the private sectors and were pivotal in determining the future characteristics of family planning in the country.

The conference, attended by more than 1,000 delegates from 87 countries, advocated two of the IPPF's main concepts, namely, that family planning is a basic human right and that a balance should be maintained between population, natural resources, and productivity as a necessary condition for human happiness, prosperity, and peace. Chile's president inaugurated the conference, thereby giving it an official seal of approval. In his speech, he mentioned that the issues raised by rapid population growth had to be studied and properly confronted. At a time when the fields of population and family planning were receiving increased attention worldwide, the conference had clear repercussions not only in Chile, but internationally.

Over the years, family planning within the mother and child health program of the NHS continued evolving, but its main focus was always trying to reduce maternal and infant mortality and promote the well-being of the family by fostering responsible parenthood and by providing the necessary means for people to decide how to go about this. Policy statements were refined and made more specific over time. For instance, a 1966 NHS circular set specific targets for the program, indicating that it aimed at reaching 100 percent of the women hospitalized for an abortion, 40 percent of the women hospitalized for delivery, and 10 percent of women of childbearing age attending its various service points. Subsequent circulars further elaborated and refined the program's objectives, but its essence did not change.

Following elections, Frei's government was succeeded in 1970 by the socialist regime of Salvador Allende. In 1973, a bloody military coup took place and was followed by the repressive and long military dictatorship of Augusto Pinochet. Each of these two latter regimes had their own ideas with respect to family planning and acted on them. For instance, during the Allende period, the Ministry of Health introduced the concept of integrated health care for women, with family planning as an integral component. Women were to receive preventive and curative health throughout their lives, starting with adolescence, and government programs had to provide such care. The Allende government also set limits to the introduction of new methods of contraception, indicating that only those approved by the U.S. Food and Drug Administration were to be used. In the case of the Pinochet government, a brief pronatalist campaign in 1978–79 hindered contraceptive use. This happened at a time of cuts in NHS personnel and resulted in a transitory increase in fertility, but by 1982, fertility had again continued to decline. Later on, in 1989, the new Abortion Act further restricted access to legal abortion.

During the 20 years that elapsed since family planning took its first steps in the 1960s until the 1980s, the NHS and other major health institutions continued to uninterruptedly provide services through various changes of government, some of which dramatically affected the lives of all Chileans. This shows a clear sign of commitment to the issue and of institutional maturity and stability. In addition, APROFA was able to adapt itself to changing political realities and to collaborate effectively with the various governments.

The Main Actors

Family planning started with the private sector as represented by a group of influential doctors concerned about some serious health issues that were resulting in high levels of maternal and infant mortality and morbidity. They received substantial help from international organizations that were observing the same realities in other countries, some of which, worried about rapid rates of population growth due to sustained high fertility and declining mortality, had begun studying the issue and collaborating with each other and with developing country institutions.

These physicians, the early pioneers, organized themselves to improve and expand their area of influence and to give continuity to the nascent movement by setting up APROFA. Some of them were professors of obstetrics and public health and started training other doctors and health personnel in family planning and related disciplines at the universities where they worked. Their professional prestige had a decisive influence over decisions made by the health authorities at the time.

The main family planning service providers during 1960 to 1980 were, and continue to be, the government through its maternal and child program, as well as other quasi-governmental health organizations, and the commercial sector, including doctors and pharmacies, where oral contraceptives are still sold without a prescription.

The partnership between APROFA, the private association affiliated with the IPPF, and the NHS was crucial as it evolved over time. APROFA was the engine that first promoted the interest and then the actions undertaken by the NHS in relation to family planning. The association also served as a link between international assistance and the government. Through a series of agreements with the NHS, APROFA provided for many years the bulk of the imported contraceptives, equipment, and other commodities the NHS used to expand programs. APROFA also helped coordinate training activities for health personnel in Chile and from other Latin American countries. In addition, APROFA provided technical assistance to the NHS in the development of service statistics and surveillance systems.

In a profoundly conservative society, according to some observers the most conservative in Latin America, and with the quiet approval of the government, APROFA was one of the first organizations to start training teachers in basic sex education. At the time, all those involved tacitly recognized that they would face criticism for bringing issues of sexuality into the classroom and that a private organization was better suited to take the brunt of such criticism.

The IPPF was the first international agency to express interest in family planning in Chile, starting in 1961, and has been collaborating with the country ever since. Other international organizations also became involved in various aspects of family planning and population programs in Chile in the mid-1960s and played an important role in their development, influencing the magnitude, speed, and shape of family planning. Their participation also created occasional controversy and suspicion in some circles and the perception that family planning was receiving special favors from donors to the detriment of other aspects of development. Some of the most important agencies included the Ford and Rockefeller foundations, the Population Council, the U.S. Agency for International Development, the United Nations Population Fund, and the Pathfinder Fund.

The IPPF provided core funding and institutional support for the operations of APROFA from its inception. It also served as a channel of funding from the U.S. Agency for International Development for contraceptive commodities and equipment. Over the years, it has provided funding and technical assistance for a variety of projects and programs, ranging from training teachers in sex education to introducing concepts and techniques of institutional sustainability.

The Ford Foundation contributed substantially to the development of population dynamics and reproductive biology. It provided important support for research and training to the Latin American Demographic Center and to the Latin American Association for the Study of Human Reproduction, both based in Santiago. It also provided fellowships to professionals for graduate studies abroad. The Rockefeller Foundation supported family planning program development and evaluation, including postpartum family planning.

A number of other international organizations also provided various types of assistance. The Population Council helped fund research in human reproduction and program activities. The Pathfinder Fund funded training courses for physicians and other health personnel. The U.S. Agency for International Development provided financial support indirectly through other organizations and directly to the NHS for infrastructure, equipment, and salaries. It also contributed resources to the Ministry of Education for training teachers in family life and sex education and donated contraceptives to the national family planning program until 1992. The United Nations Population Fund signed an agreement with the government in 1972 to support the maternal and child health care program and the program to promote family well-being, including providing health education and promoting services to facilitate planned and responsible parenthood.

The results of Chile's collaboration with the international community included sharing the lessons learned; training professionals from other countries; and undertaking research, particularly in reproductive biology, contraceptive development, and public health.

The Chilean Contribution to Family Planning Internationally

The international family planning community has duly acknowledged the contribution of some Chileans. Dr. Jaime Zipper's inputs into developing a new, improved form of IUD and promoting its use resulted in a quantum leap of progress in the field. The early introduction of this Chilean version of the IUD had long-lasting effects in Chile, where most women continue to use IUDs. Dr. Benjamin Viel, a prestigious professor of public health, contributed to the formation of numerous medical students and physicians in family planning and to the education of decision makers and the general public on the interaction between population variables and health; Drs. Juan Diaz and Anibal Faundes have a consistent and successful track record on basic and applied research and training in relation to reproductive health issues and their impact on society; and the team work of Drs. Horacio Croxatto and Soledad Diaz at the Chilean Institute of Reproductive Medicine has been at the forefront of research on the physiology of reproduction, the development and evaluation of contraceptive methods, the dynamic interaction between service provision and clients of family planning programs, and the introduction of emergency contraception.

Opposition to Family Planning

Compared with the opposition to family planning in the United States and in some other Latin American countries, the opposition in Chile was milder, more akin to what happened in European countries.

The Role of the Catholic Church

Contrary to what might have been expected, the reaction of the Catholic Church to the new family planning initiatives was not strong. Romero, the first chair of the Board of Directors of APROFA, stated that at a meeting he attended at the Saint Lucas Academy of Medicine—a Catholic, conservative, medical think tank—a deeply religious obstetrician had publicly defended the use of the IUD (Romero 1969). Participating at the meeting was Cardinal Raul Silva Henriquez. The cardinal closed the session by saying that it was the duty of many couples to regulate the sizes of their family and that no general or rigid rules could be established for choosing the methods employed. Then he went on to say that each couple should use its own judgment when making decisions.

The position of the Catholic Church in Chile on contraception only began to change and to harden after the Vatican issued the *Encyclica Humanae Vitae* (subtitled *On the Regulation of Birth*) in 1968, but even then, adamant opposition to family planning was something the church hierarchy advocated rather than the parish or village priest. Most people did not even realize that the church was opposed to contraception. A 1970 survey in western Santiago found that a small minority of women had a negative opinion of family planning, and that of these, only 8 percent opposed family planning for religious reasons (Vaessen and Sanhueza 1971). The most important reason, as is still the case, was the perception that contraception might pose a risk to their health. However, official religious opposition was somewhat of a damper among some decision makers, and some Catholic physicians began to argue that both IUDs and oral contraceptives could be abortifacients or that they caused serious complications and side effects. Nevertheless, this did not constitute a major deterrent to the health authorities to move ahead or to Catholic women to use contraception.

The 1960s were difficult years for the Catholic hierarchy in Rome. The school of liberation theology was making major inroads, particularly in Latin America, aiming at redefining the mission of the church in the areas of social justice, poverty, and human rights. To a large extent at the urging of the Latin American Episcopal Council, created in 1955, Pope John XXIII had called for the organization of the Second Vatican Council (1962–65), a series of meetings that would take place over several years to reconsider the position of the church in the modern world. In the early 1960s, the Latin American Episcopal Council was in the process of organizing a conference of Latin American bishops, which would take place in Medellín, Colombia, in 1968. The social concerns expressed by Catholic bishops in Latin America had received ample press coverage and had influenced the thinking of the continent's political leadership. However, upon the death of Pope John XXIII in 1963, the new pope, Paul VI, concerned about the socialist undertones of the Latin American church, returned the

Catholic hierarchy to a traditional, conservative stance. Paul VI's *Encyclica Humanae Vitae* rejects the use of any artificial means of contraception under any circumstance and has remained as the position of the Vatican since 1968. Following the issuance of that work, those who opposed family planning for religious reasons became more vociferous and better organized and financed, placing institutional barriers in the way of family planning and of sex education and delaying government actions in Chile and elsewhere. Despite this, the attitude of the vast majority of the population has not changed. People have continued to use modern and effective family planning methods, complemented by abortion, as they need them.

Political Opposition

Organized political groups did not voice major opposition to family planning as a matter of health and individual rights. Some sectors of the extreme left were suspicious of the motives of international organizations in providing funding for "population control." The rhetoric was that this was another expression of northern imperialism wanting to curtail population growth as a means of frustrating the revolution of the proletariat in the developing world. This position was probably strengthened by population growth alarmists, who foresaw a catastrophe of major proportions for humankind if immediate action was not taken to stop population growth. This argument did not prove to be a major obstacle in Chile, as the main expressed objective of family planning was to help individuals avoid unwanted fertility and was never seen as a tool designed to curtail population growth.

Human Rights Opposition

Some feminists and other human rights groups argued against the terminology that was used at the beginning of the family planning programs, such as birth control, arguing that it implied that some external force was at work to stop women from having children. This mild opposition subsided when the terminology was changed to fertility regulation. More important, the organized women's movement had also expressed concerns about the potential complications arising from contraceptive use, about the paternalistic approach of doctors when providing services, and about the need to include a gender perspective into the program's activities. The arguments and criticisms raised by the feminist movement initially resulted in friction with the family planning establishment, but had a positive effect in the long run by forcing programs to analyze themselves. This helped improve many aspects of service provision by, among other things, asserting clients' rights to being treated with dignity, receiving appropriate counseling, and participating in making decisions.

Program Results

Chile's population was 7.6 million in the early 1960s, with a crude birth rate of 37 live births per 1,000 population and a death rate of 12 deaths per 1,000 population. Substantial population growth had started in the early 1950s, because of sustained high fertility and declining mortality, and the rate of natural population increase reached its peak in the early 1960s at 2.5 percent per year. This was a period when Chilean women averaged more than five children and the infant mortality rate was 114 deaths per 1,000 live births (United Nations 2002).

As family planning knowledge and contraceptive use became more prevalent in the 1960s, fertility began to decline, and by the early 1990s, fertility, general mortality, and infant mortality had declined substantially. By 1990–95, the crude birth rate had fallen to 22.5 live births per 1,000 population and the death rate to 6.4 deaths per 1,000 population. Infant mortality had been reduced spectacularly to 16.9 deaths per 1,000 live births, and the rate of natural increase of the population was 1.6 percent (United Nations 2002).

All this took place during a period of expansion of family planning activities and contraceptive use, with substantial modernization of Chilean society, improvements in education levels and primary health care, better living conditions, and significant rural-urban migration that resulted in about 85 percent of the population living in cities by 1990. Many factors influenced this transition. As a result of the population's improved access to and use of effective family planning, multiparity went down, as did the number of unwanted births. The total number of births fell, and spacing between births was longer. Concurrently, maternal mortality declined from a high rate of 283 deaths per 100,000 live births in 1964 to 40 in 1990 (APROFA 1992) and to about 20 in 2000 (Ministry of Health 2006). During the 1970s and 1980s, the average age at which women had their first child remained at about 24, but the spacing between births increased from two years to three years and the total number of births declined markedly, especially among older women. The reduction in fertility was particularly noticeable among the less educated sectors of the population (National Institute of Statistics 1989).

As Chile does not have the benefit of regular national fertility surveys among representative samples of all women of childbearing age that other countries in Latin America and worldwide have had, information about family planning use has been derived from service statistics, such as the number of registered, active users at NHS facilities and at other health services. Institutions like APROFA and the Ministry of Health also attempted to obtain information about the use of oral and other contraceptives provided without medical participation by obtaining figures from pharmaceutical companies about their distributions to pharmacies. The service statistics were then related to census and vital statistics data in an attempt to draw conclusions about program effectiveness. This procedure can only describe observed trends and cannot address causality, as many other factors affecting people's attitudes and behavior were at play, some of which were previously noted.

The available information indicates rapid acceptance and use of family planning once the program started. Between 1964 and 1974, the number of active users of contraception among women of childbearing age who were beneficiaries of NHS services and of other health networks and pharmacies grew from about 59,000 to 539,000. This represented an increase in coverage of the target population from 3.5 to 22.9 percent (Cabrera and others 1975). The number of women of childbearing age who were active users of the program grew 86 percent, along with a concomitant drop of 29.8 percent in the birth rate and of 38.5 percent in infant mortality (Cabrera and others 1975).

More recent information from the Ministry of Health shows that the number of contraceptive users who are clients of the NHS (now called the National System of Health Services) grew from 600,000 in 1990 to 1.1 million in 2004, a major increase. During this period, fertility continued to decline and the total fertility rate had reached 1.9 births per woman by 2003 (Ministry of Health 2006).

The best information about contraceptive mix comes from a 1989–90 APROFA population survey that included a sample of 1,400 women of childbearing age living in both urban and rural areas, and showed contraceptive use prevalence among 56.6 percent of such women in urban areas and 53.6 percent in rural areas. About half of the women sampled were using IUDs. A higher percentage of urban women (26 percent) were using oral contraceptives than were their rural counterparts (22 percent). At the same time, female sterilization was higher among rural women (17 percent) than urban women (10 percent). Statistics from the National System of Health Services for 2001 show that among those using public health facilities, most contraceptive users (58 percent) used the IUD and about 3 percent used oral contraceptives, while female sterilization accounted for only 2.5 percent of contraceptive users (Schiappacasse and others 2003).

A 2000 national household survey looking at health and the quality of life showed that 52.5 percent of those interviewed declared they did not use contraception, but 8 out of every 10 nonusers said that the reason was that they did not need it. Among users, more than half obtained their contraceptives from public health sources, more than a quarter from private health providers, and the rest from pharmacies (Ministry of Health 2006).

Induced Abortion

As illegally induced abortion was one of the motivating factors for family planning, further comments on this topic are warranted. Abortion has always been a common practice in Chile despite being illegal, and because of this situation, obtaining specific data about the magnitude and other characteristics of abortion has been difficult. In the 1950s, the main sources of information on abortion were hospital and emergency room records, which were recognized as seriously understating the issue. Plaza and Briones (1962) conclude that abortions represented 41 percent of discharges from emergency rooms and 8 percent of total discharges from hospitals in their study. The treatment of abortion-related issues consumed about one-quarter of all obstetrical resources. In addition, hospital statistics indicated an enormous increase in hospitalizations following abortion from 8.4 per 100 live births in 1937 to 22.3 in 1960 (Armijo and Monreal 1964).

In the late 1950s and early 1960s, the first community studies in Latin America were carried out in Chile and provided a better idea of the situation in relation to abortion. Estimates indicated that about one-third of all pregnancies ended in abortion (Tabah and Samuel 1961) and that between 75 and 90 percent of these were induced. Most estimates conclude that abortions accounted for three out of five maternal deaths. Another household survey in 1962 in Santiago indicated that 26 percent of the 20- to 44-year-old women interviewed had had an abortion and that about one out of three abortions resulted in subsequent hospitalization (Armijo and Monreal 1964).

In the 1960s and through the 1980s, the original 1938 legislation on abortion (Article 19 of the Health Code) was in effect and allowed abortion only for "therapeutic reasons," yet despite its illegality, in most cases it was seldom denounced or prosecuted. Even though societal norms looked down on abortion, there was a tacit understanding that people resorted to it and that it was a personal, if unfortunate, decision. In 1989, during the Pinochet dictatorship, the language of Article 19 was replaced as follows: "No action may be executed that has as its goal the inducement of abortion." This meant that abortion became illegal under any circumstance, even to save the life of the pregnant woman. Denunciations and prosecutions of induced abortion became more frequent, but they continued to be rare overall except in a few hospitals, where they were clearly linked to the presence in those hospitals of a few overzealous physicians. Women who needed care following an abortion quickly identified those hospitals and stopped going to them.

The thinking among Chile's health community in the early 1960s was that providing easy access to safe and effective contraception would replace abortion as a method of fertility regulation. In a well-known paper, Requena (1966) describes a pattern whereby abortion will increase during the first stages of family planning programs as the motivation for small families exceeds the availability of contraception, but then gradually declines as contraception becomes more established.

Some researchers decided to study the impact of a well-designed family planning program on abortion, births to multiparous women, and infant mortality. For that purpose, they set up a research project in 1965 in San Gregorio, a working-class neighborhood in Santiago with a population of 36,000 people. The researchers undertook a baseline population survey using a random sample of 20 percent of the households to determine levels of fertility, abortion, and other basic characteristics of the population. Following this survey, a family planning program offering education, information, and services began in NHS facilities in the area. The program emphasized reaching women who had previously resorted to abortion, because of the likelihood of repeat abortions. The educational component of the program consisted mainly of talks to groups or individuals. Two years later, a second survey was carried out and showed that during 1966, the use of contraception had increased from 12.2 to 28.0 percent of women of childbearing age and that this had been accompanied by a decline in fertility of 19.4 percent and in the abortion rate of 40.2 percent (Faundes, Rodriguez-Galant, and Avendaño 1969). These were encouraging results, but doubt remained as to whether family planning programs on a larger scale would achieve similar results given real-life program conditions compared with a small, resource-rich social experiment of short duration.

Researchers have carried out many efforts to measure the influence of family planning on abortion rates, but they have proven difficult because of problems related to obtaining reliable data, and because of the number of variables involved in the decisions people make when exercising their sexuality and controlling their fertility, including timely access to reliable contraceptives and correct and consistent use of such contraceptives. Thus, while family planning can and does help people prevent unwanted pregnancies effectively, abortion remains a frequently used option. In Chile in 1987, that is, 27 years after the beginning of organized family planning, estimates indicate that abortion was still a method of fertility regulation. During that year, some estimates indicate that about 195,000 abortions occurred, of which 90 percent, or 176,000, were induced. By this estimate, 38.8 percent of pregnancies were ending in abortion, and in 6 out of 10 cases, this happened because of contraceptive failure. However, hospitalizations for complications of abortions had declined from 29.1 hospitalizations per 1,000 women of childbearing age in 1965 to 10.5 in 1987 (Requena 1991) and mortality rates from abortion had declined from 10.7 deaths per 10,000 live births in 1960 to 0.5 by 2000 (Schiappacasse and others 2003).

Conclusions

Because family planning services have traditionally been provided through the mother and child health program of the NHS and other health networks, by definition, important sectors of the population have been systematically excluded, such as teenagers and men. For any practical purpose, only women who have already become pregnant have had easy access to the program. Even some successful programs directed toward teenagers, like one started in 1981 by the Department of Obstetrics and Gynecology in northern Santiago, worked mainly with young girls who became pregnant and their friends.

Perhaps if an effective sex education and family planning program aimed at young teenagers before they became sexually active had been in place, this would have had a positive influence in reducing the large number of pregnancies and out-of-wedlock births among young women in Chile. The number of out-of-wedlock births has remained consistently high over the years, and because the number of total births has declined, the proportion of out-of-wedlock births to total births increased from 17.5 percent of total births in 1965 to about 33.0 percent by 1988 (Hudson 1994). More than half of births to women under age 20 were out of wedlock in the mid-1980s (Viel and Campos 1987). Fertility has declined less among teenagers that among the rest of the population, and by 2000, births to teenagers accounted for 16.2 percent of total births. This has been attributed to limited access by that group to sex education and services (Ministry of Health 2006).

In addition, Chile has tended to view family planning as a medical issue rather than a social issue. Most discussions have concentrated on technology and logistics; on providers and patients; and on effectiveness, side effects, and means of operation of contraceptive methods. These are no doubt important matters, but the human dimension of family planning is also important, including paying attention to the variety of circumstances people face when making decisions on matters of sexuality and reproduction and the consequences on people's lives of having the opportunity to meet their needs in these areas or of being deprived of such opportunities.

Finally, issues of gender differences and the power differential that has tradition-ally existed between men and women in terms of access to resources and decision making had not been considered until fairly recently. This is where the feminist movement has been instrumental by questioning the medical orthodoxy and empow-ering women in need of information, counseling, and services. These sometimes con-troversial and difficult issues have greatly contributed to making the dialogue more complex, and therefore closer to the reality of people's lives. In recent years, both public and private sector organizations and individuals have sought to address these issues and deal with the associated problems.

Unlike what happened in other countries, Chile never had a vertical program focused exclusively on family planning. Although the participation of several indi-viduals, mostly doctors, was crucial from the beginning, the country never had a sin-gle major leader in the field. The process was always conducted following an insti-tutional approach, and the services were integrated into existing health networks.

Family planning is not a panacea or a magic bullet able to address all the prob-lems of development or people's lives as some thought 40 years ago, but it is a useful and important tool that people need and want for the control of their reproductive lives. A good family planning program will improve the lives of those it touches directly and will buy some precious time for the nation as a whole to attack the root causes of poverty and establish the basis of development.

Family planning obviously does not operate in isolation, but within social contexts and policy frameworks that can facilitate or hinder people learning about and having access to it. It works better in societies where people have freedom of expression and decision making, where the government and the private sector invest in education and health and in better living conditions in general, and where women have access to broad participation in society. Over the past 20 years or so, Chile has made progress in this respect. Since the end of the military dictatorship in 1990, freedom of expres-sion and of political decision making have made momentous strides. Four presidents have been elected since that time, the last one a woman. Because of good financial management, Chile is currently perhaps the most solvent country in Latin America. It has demonstrated a concerted effort to fight poverty that has been showing positive results, although a wide gap between the haves and the have-nots still persists.

This is the context in which family planning is operating today. The country enjoys some of the best indicators on the continent in relation to maternal, perinatal, and infant mortality, and to a large extent this can be attributed to the continuity and success of family planning. The Chilean program is using the lessons learned from the international family planning experience and is actively incorporating concepts of quality improvement and gender analysis. The rights of individual clients to receive free and informed choice of contraceptive methods and respectful and confi-dential treatment from well-trained service providers will, without doubt, go a long way toward extending coverage to those in need. In an attempt to decrease unwanted pregnancies among teenagers, the government recently approved free distribution of emergency contraception for women starting at age 14. This decision engendered a great deal of controversy, but as of this writing, the president and her minister of health have remained firm on the subject.

References

APROFA (Asociación Chilena de Protección de la Familia). 1992. *Boletín de Asociación Chilena de Protección de la Familia* 28 (7–12): 1–2.

Armijo, R., and T. Monreal. 1964. "Epidemiologia del Aborto Provocado en Santiago." *Revista Medica de Chile* 92: 548–57.

Avendaño, O. 1975. "Desarrollo Histórico de la Planificación Familiar en Chile y en el Mundo." Draft, Asociación Chilena de Protección de la Familia, Santiago.

Cabrera, R., G. Delgado, E. Taucher, and O. Avendaño. 1975. "Evaluation of Ten Years of Family Planning in Chile." Presentation and panel discussion at the XVIth Chilean Congress of Obstetrics and Gynecology, December 1, Santiago.

Faundes, Anibal, G. Rodriguez-Galant, and O. Avendaño. 1969. "Efectos de un Programa de Planificación de la Familia sobre las Tasas de Fecundidad y Aborto de una Población Marginal de Santiago." *Revista Chilena de Obstetricia y Ginecologia* 34 (2): 67–76.

Hudson, Rex A., ed. 1994. *Chile: A Country Study*. Washington, DC: U.S. Library of Congress, Federal Research Division.

Ministry of Health. 2006. *Normas Nacionales Sobre Regulación de la Fertilidad*. Santiago: Ministry of Health.

National Institute of Statistics. 1989. *Anuario Demografía*. Santiago: National Institute of Statistics.

Plaza, S., and H. Briones. 1962. "El Aborto como Problema Asistencial." *Revista Medica de Chile* 91: 294–97.

Requena, M. 1966. "Condiciones Determinantes del Aborto Inducido." *Revista Medica de Chile* 94: 714–22.

———. 1991. "Induced Abortion: A Vulnerable Public Health Problem." *Enfoques de atención primaria* 6 (1): 11–18.

Romero, H. 1969. "Chile: The Abortion Epidemic." In *Population: Challenging World Crisis*, ed. B. Berelson, 149–60. Voice of America Forum Lectures. Washington, DC: Government Printing Office.

Schiappacasse, V., P. Vidal, L. Casas, C. Dides, and S. Diaz. 2003. *Chile: Situación de la Salud y los Derechos Sexuales y Reproductivos*. Santiago: National Service for Women.

Stycos, J. M. 1970. "Public and Private Opinion on Population and Family Planning." *Studies in Family Planning* 1 (51): 10–17.

Tabah, L., and R. Samuel. 1961. "Encuesta de Fecundidad y de Actitudes Relativas a la Formación de la Familia: Resultados Preliminaríes." *Cuadernos Medico Sociales* 2: 19–21.

United Nations. 2002. *World Population Prospects: The 2000 Revision. Highlights*. http://www.un.org/esa/population/publications/wpp2002/WPP2002-HIGHLIGHTS rev1.PDF.

Vaessen, M., and H. Sanhueza. 1971. *Resultados de una Encuesta sobre Planificación Familiar en el Área Occidental de Santiago*. Series A, no. 116. Santiago: Latin American Demographic Center.

Viel, Benjamin, and Waldo Campos. 1987. "Chilean History of Infant and Maternal Mortality, 1940–1986." *International Family Planning Perspectives* (special issue): 24–28.

8 Against the Odds: Colombia's Role in the Family Planning Revolution

ANTHONY R. MEASHAM AND GUILLERMO LOPEZ-ESCOBAR

This volume argues that the advent in many developing countries of population policies designed to reduce their population growth rates and make methods of family planning widely available constitutes one of the most extraordinary social and political change phenomena of the 20th century. To say that these changes were revolutionary is not hyperbole, and a case could be made that the events of the 1960s and 1970s rival other dramatic shifts in public policy in previous centuries, such as the public provision of safe water and sewage disposal. Within this overall context, few scholars or observers would have given much credence to the notion that Colombia, among the most conservative and religious countries in Latin America, would be the first nation on that continent to adopt an explicit population policy advocating a reduction in the population growth rate and the widespread availability of family planning methods, especially to the poor. Fortunately, the context, process, and sequence of events have been documented in a series of articles and books (see, for example, Daguer and Riccardi 2005; Echeverry 1991; Ott 1977; Perez 1976; Perez and Gomez 1974). This chapter, drawing heavily on the aforementioned works and supplemented by the authors' observations, attempts to summarize the extraordinary events that occurred in the 1960s and 1970s and draw lessons that could be applicable to similar issues currently and in the future. Box 8.1 presents a timeline of major events in relation to family planning in Colombia.

How Colombia Became a Population Policy Pioneer in Latin America

Population growth rates in Latin America were among the world's highest in the 1950s and 1960s, exceeding 3 percent per year in some countries, including Colombia. During 1951 to 1964, Colombia's annual growth rate was slightly more than 3 percent per year (Perez 1976). In 1973, Colombia was the fourth most populous country in Latin America with a population of 22.7 million.

Fertility declined well in advance of the formulation of a national population policy and the development of a national family planning program. Estimates indicated

BOX 8.1 Timeline of Major Events

1964: The Colombian Association of Medical Schools (Asociación Colombiana de Facultades de Medicina, ASCOFAME) begins population research through its Division of Population Studies, headed by Dr. Hernan Mendoza.

1965: Former President Lleras Camargo strongly advocates measures to control population growth at the Pan American Assembly on Population in Cali, Colombia.

The Association for the Welfare of the Colombian Family (Asociación Probienestar de la Familia Colombiana, PROFAMILIA), later affiliated with the International Planned Parenthood Federation, starts family planning services in the private sector.

1966: The Ford Foundation provides technical and financial assistance to ASCOFAME.

The administration of Guillermo León Valencia approves the use of U.S. counterpart funds to train public health personnel in family planning.

1967: The Lleras Restrepo government approves a contract between the Ministry of Health and ASCOFAME for family planning training.

ASCOFAME starts providing family planning services in government health facilities.

1968: The nascent family planning program receives setbacks: the Vatican issues the *Encyclical Humanae Vitae*, the pope visits Colombia, Mendoza dies suddenly, and the Ministry of Health–ASCOFAME contract expires.

1969: Family planning efforts recover, national program emerges, and population policy is approved.

The Ministry of Health sets up the Maternal and Child Health Program and begins providing family planning services.

Dr. Guillermo Lopez-Escobar succeeds Mendoza at ASCOFAME.

Large-scale external funding, mainly from the United States, is extended to ASCOFAME, the Ministry of Health, and PROFAMILIA.

The National Planning Department, which entered the population field in late 1968, presents a draft national population policy to the National Council on Economic and Social Policy.

The Lleras Restrepo government approves the national population policy, aimed, among other things, at changing the population growth rate by lowering fertility.

1970: A similar population policy statement is incorporated into the incoming Pastrana government's 1970–73 development plan.

that age-specific fertility rates for women aged 20–39 dropped by 26 percent between 1960–64 and 1965–69 (Simmons and Cardona 1973).

High rates of induced abortion (Lopez-Escobar 1978), resulting in a heavy death toll, a high level of disability, and numerous admissions to the country's hospitals, were well documented and of deep concern to members of the Colombian medical profession and others. However, as Ott (1977) points out, the usual concomitants of a push for a fertility control policy—negative impact on economic growth, population density, and inability to provide services to growing cohorts—were not, in general, salient issues in Colombia. Ott (1977) notes that Colombia exhibited multiple obstacles to the development of a population policy:

• Nationalism

• Pro-natalist cultural norms and traditions

• Marxist political movements

• Bureaucratic rigidities

- Shortage of trained health personnel

- Inadequate government infrastructure in rural areas.

In addition, the Catholic Church was extremely strong. Indeed, the Colombian church hierarchy had a formidable reputation as the most powerful and least progressive in Latin America.

How then did Colombia turn out to be a pioneer and leader in the formulation of population policy in the Latin American context? The answer appears to lie, to a large degree, in the actions of a small number of talented and committed Colombians and the often unpredictable course of the policy process (Bauer and Gergen 1968; Measham 1972; Ott 1977). Former president Alberto Lleras Camargo strongly advocated measures to control population growth in an August 1965 Pan American Assembly on Population held in Cali, Colombia. That set the stage for the major role in population policy development played by Carlos Lleras Restrepo, who was president from 1966 to 1970. Apart from Lleras Camargo (Ross 1966) and Lleras Restrepo, most of the small coterie of people responsible for the massive policy change consisted of physicians in the oft-noted Latin American tradition of physicians playing leading roles in many aspects of national life.

Three of the main characters in this complex and intriguing drama served at the Colombian Association of Medical Schools (Asociación Colombiana de Facultades de Medicina, ASCOFAME): Gabriel Velasquez Palau, the association's president; Hernan Mendoza, chief of population studies; and Mendoza's successor, Guillermo Lopez-Escobar. The other leaders were Antonio Ordonez Plaja, minister of health throughout the Lleras Restrepo administration; Fernando Tamayo and Gonzalo Echeverry of the Association for the Welfare of the Colombian Family (Asociación Probienestar de la Familia Colombiana, PROFAMILIA), the Colombian affiliate of the International Planned Parenthood Federation (IPPF); and Jorge Villareal of the Pan-American Federation of Associations of Medical Schools. All were physicians. The main institutional actors in the policy process that played out roughly in the years 1964–70 were the Office of the President, the Ministry of Health, the Colombian Catholic hierarchy, ASCOFAME, and PROFAMILIA. Other groups, notably some universities, labor unions, women's organizations, and nongovernmental organizations, also played a role.

Population Policy Development: 1964–70

The policy process is usually complex, idiosyncratic, and impossible to analyze in a rigorously scientific way (Lindblom 1968). Events are often unpredictable, the interactions of individuals are difficult to interpret, and the conclusions vary according to the observer's assumptions and the weight given to a multiplicity of factors. Nevertheless, the role of President Lleras Restrepo in Colombia's population policy narrative is hard to overestimate. Whether success would have been achieved without the weight of his office is doubtful, not to mention his training in economics and his bold and visionary style. Well before he became president, Lleras "recognized the macroeconomic implications of population growth" (Ott 1977, p. 5).

While in office, Lleras frequently alluded to the impact of rapid population growth on education, housing, and employment. In addition, he recognized the integral role of population trends in development planning. Lleras recruited and worked closely with qualified technocrats and substantially strengthened the National Planning Department, which was to play the key role in the formulation of Colombia's population policy.

At roughly the same time that Lleras was preparing to take over the presidency, the physicians mentioned earlier were laying the groundwork, analytically and operationally, for a national population policy and a national maternal and child health and family planning program. In 1964, ASCOFAME established its Division of Population Studies (DPS) and named Mendoza as director. Mendoza, "a man distinguished by his intellect, tough-mindedness, and enormous capacity to work" (Ott 1977, p. 3), organized national population seminars; sociodemographic surveys; abortion studies; and, notably, pilot family planning programs run by the 10 medical school members of ASCOFAME.

The fertility and health surveys carried out by ASCOFAME, and later by the Regional Population Center, clearly demonstrated the need and demand for family planning services (Bravo 1979; Simmons and Cardona 1973). Mendoza used this evidence to establish the existence of a population problem and the need to do something about it. ASCOFAME avoided confrontation with the church hierarchy during this period while it gathered data and organizational strength. The church, for its part, was awaiting the papal encyclical *Humanae Vitae*, which was proclaimed in 1968.

In 1965, Tamayo established PROFAMILIA, which quickly opened family planning clinics in the major cities (Tamayo 1978). Tamayo, a highly regarded obstetrician and gynecologist, soon recruited Gonzalo Echeverry, a fellow obstetrician, who became the architect of PROFAMILIA's rural family planning program and numerous other innovations. Unlike ASCOFAME's pilot family planning programs, which were embedded in maternal and child health services, PROFAMILIA focused on family planning alone and other relevant concerns and services, such as management of gynecological infections, cervical cancer screening, and infertility treatment.

PROFAMILIA's services were always of the highest quality, were well managed, and were meticulously monitored and evaluated. As a result, PROFAMILIA quickly became the most outstanding IPPF affiliate and a recognized pioneer in the delivery of community-based family planning services. The Ministry of Health was the last, though not the least, major player to join in the provision of family planning services, within its Maternal and Child Health Program, beginning in 1969. Even earlier, however, the administration of Guillermo León Valencia (1962–66) had approved the use of U.S. counterpart funds for training physicians in family planning. A contract between ASCOFAME and the Ministry of Health for ASCOFAME to provide this training was signed early during the Lleras administration. This support from the United States, and from the Ford Foundation to support ASCOFAME's population work, together with IPPF support for PROFAMILIA, was among the earliest external assistance for population and family planning work in Colombia.

Thus, by 1966, ASCOFAME was quietly laying the groundwork for a national population policy, training physicians, and supporting pilot family planning efforts by its medical school members; PROFAMILIA was brazenly offering high-quality family planning services, rightly confident of the demand for such services; and the Ministry of Health was playing a more cautious role through Ordonez, a close confidant of President Lleras who retained his cabinet post throughout the four-year administration. To what extent were the actions of these three institutions coordinated? The definitive answer to that intriguing question may never be known. What is known is that all seven physician leaders knew each other well, communicated frequently, and shared a strongly held motivation to make family planning services widely available, especially to the poor, and to have their country adopt an explicit population policy. The experience of one of the seven, Lopez-Escobar, suggests that the seven worked closely together in pursuit of their common cause. All seven physicians who played such major roles in this narrative were highly regarded, elite members of their profession, with strong reputations and extensive social networks among the Colombian elite. These attributes no doubt accounted in part for their boldness and their ability to withstand the criticism and attacks that were to come, notably from the church and the political left.

The leaders played roles that reflected their personal styles. Ordonez was a natural, statesmanlike spokesman, the voice of moderation and reason, which was ideally suited to his exposure to criticisms from both advocates and critics of the unfolding events. He possessed great political savvy and had the ear of the president. Tamayo was fiercely independent, did what he thought was right for his country, and challenged all and sundry to try to stop him. Few dared. Mendoza also possessed strong political and strategic instincts, but was more inclined to take a confrontational stance when he thought it was appropriate. This caused more than one egg to break, but Mendoza's critical role cannot be overstated. Both PROFAMILIA and ASCOFAME were convenient lightning rods to deflect criticisms aimed at Ordonez and the administration.

Tragedy and Conflict: 1968

Just as developments looked highly propitious for the adoption of a population policy and the expansion of the nascent national family planning program, a series of setbacks occurred in rapid succession. On July 29, 1968, the Vatican issued the encyclical *Humanae Vitae* banning the use of "artificial" methods of contraception; the pope visited Colombia on August 22–24, 1968; and Mendoza died suddenly of lung cancer on August 28, 1968. In addition, the key contract between ASCOFAME and the Ministry of Health had expired on July 1, 1968, and would not be renewed until a year later. These events clearly reduced the momentum toward the development of a population policy and national family planning program. Ott (1977) interprets the ensuing slowdown as reflecting two factors: the centrality of political considerations in the evolution of policy and the extent to which the gathering momentum had been substantially dependent on a single person, namely, Mendoza.

Adoption of a National Population Policy, 1969–70

Subsequent developments attest to the momentum that had been achieved up to August 1968 and to the main players' determination not to be thwarted in their aspirations. By happy coincidence, Congress approved Lleras Restrepo's proposed restructuring of the national planning apparatus in December 1968 and the National Planning Department was required "to study the population phenomenon and its economic and social repercussions in order to develop a population policy" (Ott 1977, p. 5). Analysis was undertaken, and discussions ensued between the National Planning Department, the Ministry of Health, the DPS, and the University of the Andes, resulting in a draft policy that was presented to the National Council on Economic and Social Policy in July 1969. President Lleras chaired the council's deliberations and the council approved the policy as part of the National Development Plan (1969–73). Ott (1977, p. 5) aptly summarized the main features of the policy as follows:

> The "immediate objectives" were to "obtain a better territorial distribution of the population and alter the present rate of population growth by lowering fertility." With respect to reducing the growth rate, two major approaches were set forth: (1) raise the educational level of the populace with the aim of developing attitudes that would facilitate the process of modernization, promote greater participation in society, and increase parental responsibility; and (2) make available family planning information and services that would "assure proper medical care and guarantee respect for the conscience of the solicitants." Moreover, studies on "the relationships between population and socioeconomic factors . . . were to be undertaken with the aim of formulating specific policy measures . . ." All this implied that population was no longer regarded as primarily a health matter; a policy designed to deal with the problem had officially become a component of overall development strategy.

National Family Planning Program, 1969–2005

Colombia had a well-developed national family planning program by the early 1970s that consisted of the Maternal and Child Health Program of the Ministry of Health, PROFAMILIA'S urban and rural programs, the smaller network of services coordinated by ASCOFAME, and a vibrant private sector. From 1969 onward, the Ministry of Health provided family planning services within its Maternal and Child Health Program, which was delivered in most of the nationwide network of 1,200 health centers and posts, and within a postpartum family planning program in approximately 30 regional hospitals (Rizo 1978). The postpartum family planning program had been initiated by ASCOFAME in 1968 and was transferred to the Ministry of Health in the early 1970s.

By 1974, PROFAMILIA was operating 40 urban family planning clinics, postpartum hospital programs, and community-based distribution programs in both urban and rural areas. PROFAMILIA was notable for its many innovative programs, including a successful joint program with the Coffee Growers' Association in some states. In 1974, approximately 550,000 cycles of oral contraceptives were sold monthly, with the private sector accounting for more than half of the sales. The combined programs of the Ministry of Health, PROFAMILIA, ASCOFAME, and the private sector meant that by the early 1970s, family planning services were accessible to the vast majority of the population, in sharp contrast to the situation a decade earlier. Table 8.1 provides data on new family planning acceptors, by program, for 1975.

TABLE 8.1 New Family Planning Acceptors in Clinic Programs, by Program and Method, 1975

Program	IUD		Pill		Sterilization		Other		Total	
	Number	Percent	Number	Percent	Number	Percent	Number	Percent	Number	Percent
PROFAMILIA[a]	32,553	43	28,739	38	8,998	12	5,111	7	75,401	43
Ministry of Health[b]	27,963	30	60,898	65	0	0	4,973	5	93,834	53
ASCOFAME	3,766	47	2,849	35	1,081	13	368	5	8,064	4
Total	64,282	36	92,486	52	10,079	6	10,452	6	177,299	100

Source: Echeverry, Londono, and Bailey 1977.

a. PROFAMILIA's urban community-based distribution program had about 49,000 new acceptors and the rural program had 23,604 new acceptors. Nearly all these acceptors selected the pill. These acceptors are not included in the totals.

b. The total number of new acceptors was estimated from data for January through October.

Contraceptive use grew rapidly and continuously from the 1960s on. In 1969, prevalence was estimated to be 28 percent among married women. By 1978, prevalence was estimated to have risen to 48 percent, an increase of 20 percentage points in less than a decade (John Ross, personal communication to Anthony Measham, 2006). Colombia now boasts one of the world's highest contraceptive prevalence rates, estimated at 76.9 percent in 2005 (Levine and others 2006). So rapid was the decline in fertility that the birth rate predicted for 1985 may have already been reached by 1975 (Perez 1976). Figure 8.1 shows the growth in overall contraceptive use among married women aged 15–49 and figure 8.2 illustrates the dramatic shifts

FIGURE 8.1 Prevalence of Contraceptive Use, All Methods, 1989–2005

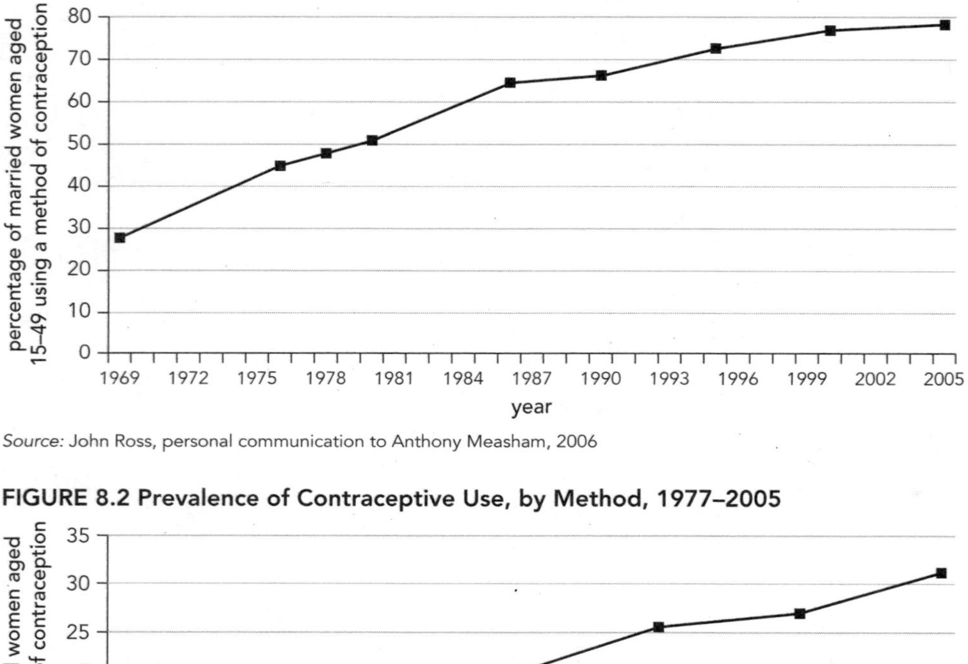

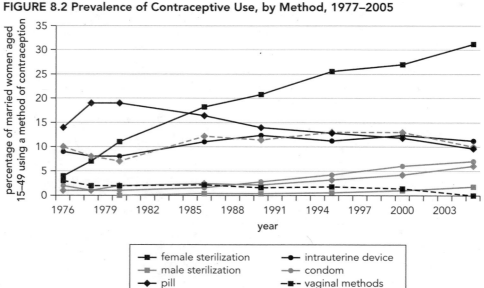

Source: John Ross, personal communication to Anthony Measham, 2006

FIGURE 8.2 Prevalence of Contraceptive Use, by Method, 1977–2005

Source: John Ross, personal communication to Anthony Measham, 2006

whereby different methods of contraception gained and lost prominence between 1977 and 2005.

Major demographic shifts occurred in Colombia between the 1950s and 1970s. The crude birth rate fell from 45 live births per 1,000 population in the 1950s to 32 in 1973 and the infant mortality rate declined from about 100 deaths per 1,000 live births in 1964 to 76 by 1973. By 1971, the crude death rate had declined to 10 deaths per 1,000 population from 15 in 1964, resulting in a population growth rate of approximately 2.2 percent per year, down from more than 3.0 percent in the 1950s (Perez 1976). In approximately two decades, these demographic shifts resulted in a quantum increase in human welfare. The extent to which the increased availability of family planning services contributed to these changes is still being debated; however, the contribution was no doubt substantial.

A Closer Look at the Context

A critical question is how, in just a few years, did Colombia manage to develop a national population policy and fertility reduction program in an inhospitable environment grounded in religious and cultural traditions? Ott (1977) provides a unique and insightful analysis of the role of ASCOFAME, undoubtedly the key institutional actor other than the government itself. Ott writes that ASCOFAME, under the leadership of Mendoza, correctly assumed that opposition to family planning and fertility reduction was tractable. In particular, the high incidence of abortion and the sizable gap between desired and actual family size suggested "a substantial unarticulated demand for family planning" (Ott 1977, p. 7). Critically, Mendoza and his colleagues recognized that the challenge they faced was essentially political: a population policy and family planning program would only be possible in the event of a nationwide change in the way family planning was viewed and, even more important, that the government was responsible for providing the necessary services.

This reasoning led ASCOFAME to conclude that enhanced public understanding of the benefits of family planning and of the essential link between population policy and economic development was critical to building political support for government action. ASCOFAME was equally astute in recognizing the political vulnerability of the church, which at that time was beset with a range of problems, including lack of consensus regarding its role in society, a shortage of priests, and low attendance at mass. The DPS therefore decided to generate support at both grassroots and policy-making levels using the following strategy and tactics:

- Undertaking research to validate the benefits of fertility control and the links between population growth and social and economic development

- Engaging in research and action programs simultaneously, for example, the pilot family planning programs in the medical schools and the hospital postpartum family planning program

- Building a base of support in the universities

- Increasing public awareness through extensive use of the mass media, speeches in the community, and a search for potential allies, for example, trade unions and women's groups

- Treating the church as a political entity

- Avoiding confrontation with opponents until the movement was strong enough to take them on and pursuing accommodation with opponents without undermining the movement's principal objectives.

While ASCOFAME's overall strategy appears brilliant with the benefit of hindsight and the knowledge that it succeeded, it was extremely risky. In particular, the extensive use of external assistance made the effort "vulnerable to accusations of U.S. influence and manipulation" (Ott 1977, p. 8). In addition, the DPS's aggressive style and willingness to engender public controversy could have damaged, even fatally, the whole enterprise, and ASCOFAME proved to be much more adept in dealing with the church than with the political left. Nevertheless, it is hard to argue with success and hard to second-guess a carefully conceived strategy that worked, and even survived the death of its principal architect long before the battle was won. Finally, recognizing the critical role played by PROFAMILIA is important, along with the fact that ASCOFAME's success would never have been accomplished without the strong support of President Lleras Restrepo and the major role played by Minister of Health Ordonez during the entire duration of that administration.

Mendoza himself aptly summarized the strategy: "The Division of Population Studies of the Colombian Association of Medical Schools believes that when someone is capable of [forcefully] and vehemently demonstrating the existence of a serious and threatening phenomenon, it is possible to create a favorable national reaction. This, in turn, leads to the possibility of reaching the goals suggested. Cultural obstacles that undoubtedly represent the most serious resistance to change can be overcome" (quoted in Ott 1977, p. 8).

Monitoring and Evaluation

The Colombian family planning program—consisting of the services provided by the Ministry of Health, PROFAMILIA, and ASCOFAME—was notable for its careful attention to monitoring and evaluation and for the making of course corrections when indicated based on the findings of service statistics and evaluative studies. A number of factors account for this enviable record. First, the DPS was the creation of the university medical schools that belonged to ASCOFAME, and hence had a strong academic tradition. Second, ASCOFAME, first under Mendoza and later under Lopez-Escobar, carried out a comprehensive research and evaluation program, much of it centered in the Evaluation Unit of the DPS.

From the late 1960s onward, ASCOFAME collated service statistics for all components of the national family planning program. ASCOFAME disseminated those findings widely and designed studies and pilot programs to test hypotheses and try out new approaches, for example, the postpartum family planning program. PROFAMILIA, too, invested heavily in research and evaluation and set up its own Evaluation Department, which undertook, for example, evaluations of its rural family planning programs and of its pioneering male and female sterilization programs (Bailey and Correa 1975; Echeverry 1975; MacCorquodale and Pullum 1974). To give two examples, when PROFAMILIA realized that its services were not reaching rural residents, it established an innovative community-based program with the Coffee Growers' Association, and when evidence showed that some urban residents in need of services were unable to reach static clinics, PROFAMILIA inaugurated an urban, community-based contraceptive delivery program.

Many other institutions added to the wealth of data and analyses of population and family planning information, including the School of Public Health at the University of Antioquia in Medellín; the 10 medical schools affiliated with ASCOFAME, notably, the University of the Valley in Cali and Los Andes, National, and Javeriana universities in Bogota; the Regional Population Center, and the Colombian Association for the Study of Population.

The Role of External Assistance

Many international agencies provided financial and technical assistance, as well as some equipment and supplies, to support the population and family planning work of several Colombian institutions. Arguably, the early support played the most critical role, that is, the financial and technical assistance provided in the mid- to late 1960s when population and family planning were still highly contentious in Colombia, and when both donors and recipients were taking risks, especially if the support emanated from North America. The situation was still volatile in the early 1970s, when a major Colombian daily newspaper extracted the Population Council's budget for Colombia and published it, saying that the total budget was for the salaries of two American technical advisers.

The Ford Foundation was one of the earliest providers of both financial and technical assistance, followed soon afterward by the IPPF, the Population Council, and the U.S. Agency for International Development (USAID). Most of the funds the Population Council provided to ASCOFAME and other entities originated from the USAID. The Bogotá office of the Ford Foundation believed in "betting on people" and made a high-return investment by betting on Mendoza. In the early 1970s, the Ford Foundation, the Population Council, the Pan American Health Organization, and the USAID each had at least one technical adviser in Colombia.

During 1973 to 1974, external agencies approved population or family planning assistance projects of one to five years duration for a total of more than US$5 million (Perez 1976). At that time, the three principal donors were the IPPF, the Pan American Health Organization, and the USAID. The IPPF funds were destined for PROFAMILIA, most of the Pan American Health Organization money went to the Ministry of Health, and the USAID funds supported big-ticket programs such as the postpartum family planning program coordinated by ASCOFAME. Other donors, in descending order of magnitude, included the University of North Carolina (mainly with USAID funds); the Pathfinder Fund; the United Nations Population Fund; World Education; General Electric TEMPO; Family Planning International Assistance; George Washington University in Washington, D.C.; the University of Chicago; World Neighbors; and the Association for Voluntary Sterilization (now EngenderHealth). Valuable support also came from the International Development Research Centre of Canada, the Family Health Foundation at Tulane University in New Orleans, and the Smithsonian Institute (with USAID funds).

How important was this assistance? Without question, the funding and technical support facilitated the formulation of a policy and the development of a high-quality family planning program. The funds—for example, those for the hospital postpartum program—allowed programs of a much larger scale than would otherwise have been possible, and probably accelerated the pace of change. In addition, the technical advisers on the ground and the multiple international contacts provided Colombian colleagues with sources of information and assistance that would otherwise have been harder to identify. However, given the sophistication of the Colombian leaders—in terms of technical capacity as well as strategy and tactics—it is hard to imagine that they would not have achieved their goals even without the external assistance.

Lessons Learned

Lindblom (1968, p. 23) has accurately described policy making as "an extremely complex analytical and political process to which there is no beginning or end, and the boundaries of which are most uncertain." Fuzzy and inchoate as it may be, the policy process usually depends critically on a small number of variables: salience of the issue, leadership, knowledge of the issue among key interest groups, political power, and government will. The sequence of events in Colombia suggests that two of these variables were most important in this case: government will, as exemplified by the determination of a bold president, Lleras Restrepo, to change policy; and first-rate leadership, notably, the contributions of Echeverry, Lopez-Escobar, Mendoza, Ordonez, and Tamayo.

Two additional points deserve emphasis. First, the idiosyncratic nature of the policy process adds a major element of uncertainty to the adoption of a new and controversial policy: it can be derailed at any time. In this case, huge obstacles were surmounted, especially the events of 1968. Whether a different outcome might have ensued in the event of unforeseen problems for the Lleras administration, a better managed campaign of opposition by the church or Congress, or a concerted effort to vilify the whole enterprise as U.S.-inspired is unknowable. Second, definitive answers are impossible to determine, as the state-of-the-art method for analyses of the policy-making process precludes scientific resolution of propositions regarding exactly why events turned out as they did.

The following three main lessons emerge from Colombia's experience:

- Political leadership and power are enormously important, as is leadership by technical experts who are strongly committed and energetic and employ shrewd strategy and tactics.

- Providing credible evidence and disseminating it widely among key interest groups is critical. In the Colombian case, ASCOFAME and other academic institutions meticulously documented the demographic situation of the country and the relationship between demographic variables and the prospects for economic and social development. Equally important, the DPS and its collaborators conducted studies and mounted demonstration programs that clearly showed the extent of demand for family planning, including the incidence of induced abortion and the gap between desired and actual fertility.

- External assistance can play an important, facilitating role in the development of population policy and national family planning programs, not least by providing financial assistance. In the case of Colombia, with an abundance of national expertise, technical assistance was less important, although it did provide important contacts with sources of information and other resources. However, the Colombian experience suggests that no substitute exists for national leadership and for nationals to carry out the bulk of the effort. External assistance may be a dangerous road to travel, as it opens up the possibility of undermining the national effort by suggesting that it is being manipulated from outside the country.

What should or could have been done differently, with the benefit of hindsight? The answer appears to be very little. The Colombian case is such an outstanding success story that imagining a better scenario is hard. Granted, Colombia was unique, even in Latin America, for its array of talented physicians and other experts, many of whom were willing to risk their careers and reputations for a cause in which they believed. Where political will is not as strong, or the boldness or sagacity of professional leaders is less evident, alternative approaches may be warranted.

Applicability of the Lessons to Other Countries or Issues

Many of the lessons learned from an examination of the Colombian case appear to be applicable to a variety of policies and programs in other countries, including policies regarding the environment, health care services, education, and undernutrition. The lessons from Colombia will most likely be most useful and readily applicable in the resolution of controversial issues of salience to a large proportion of the population. The importance of political leadership and political will are usually paramount in any democratic system, with the possible exception of federal systems, where different states and municipalities may adopt policies and programs uniquely suited to their individual needs.

The role of the individual in shaping policy making is less straightforward. One of the remarkable features of the Colombian case is the disproportionate influence exerted by a small group of individuals, most of whom belonged to the same profession. Part of the explanation for this may lie in the fact that Latin American societies in general, and Colombia in particular, have highly stratified socioeconomic structures. As a result, even in a large population, the leaders in any given profession, for example, medicine, are likely to be drawn to a substantial extent from the same, privileged background. This has several implications. First, many members of this elite group may subscribe to the notion of noblesse oblige. Second, by virtue of their socioeconomic standing, they are freer to engage in altruistic endeavors than is the case in societies with flatter structures. Third, such individuals may have more influence on the policy process than would be the case in other circumstances. Fourth, the elite in a given profession is likely to know many colleagues in a similar position, as well as many other members of their socioeconomic class, resulting in good communication, shared values, and ability to influence the outcome of events. The ability of so few individuals to have so much influence is unlikely in many other settings.

Evidence and its dissemination clearly have a strong influence on efforts to change policy and induce the development of action programs. The proponents of family planning in Colombia certainly understood this and acted on it. Particularly effective in the Colombian case were the induction of academic institutions into the policy process, the simultaneous pursuit of research and action, the heavy emphasis on evaluation and research, and the ability to translate scientific evidence into language readily understood and accessible by the lay person.

The final and perhaps most important lesson emanating from Colombia is the critical importance of a series of personal attributes and characteristics among the leaders pursuing social change. The importance of motivation and high energy is obvious. The need for patience is also evident, along with courage in the face of opposition and the sagacity to know when to be bold and when not to be. However, acute political antennae, analytical shrewdness, ability to weigh the advantages and disadvantages of various political strategies and tactics, and a willingness to change strategies and tactics as circumstances dictate seem to matter more than anything else.

References

Bailey, J., and J. Correa. 1975. "Evaluation of the PROFAMILIA Rural Family Planning Program." *Studies in Family Planning* 6 (6): 148–55.

Bauer, R. A., and K. J. Gergen. 1968. *The Study of Policy Formation*. New York: Free Press.

Bravo, G. 1979. "Socio-Economic Factors Affecting Fertility Decline in Colombia." *Population Studies* 65 (65): 116–21.

Daguer, C., and M. Riccardi. 2005. *Al derecho y al reves: La revolución de los derechos sexuales y reproductivos en Colombia*. Bogotá: Asociación Probienestar de la Familia Colombiana.

Echeverry, Gonzalo. 1975. "Development of the PROFAMILIA Rural Family Planning Program in Colombia." *Studies in Family Planning* 6 (6): 142–47.

———. 1991. *Contra Viento y Marea: Años de Planificación Familiar en Colombia*. Bogotá: Colombian Association for the Study of Population.

Echeverry, Gonzalo, J. B. Londono, and J. Bailey. 1977. "Colombia." In *Family Planning in the Developing World: A Review of Programs*, ed. W. B. Watson, 42–43. New York: Population Council.

Levine, R., A. Langer, N. Birdsall, G. Matheny, M. Wright, and A. Bayer. 2006. "Contraception." In *Disease Control Priorities in Developing Countries*, 2nd ed., ed. D. T. Jamison, J. G. Breman, Anthony R. Measham, G. Alleyne, M. Claeson, D. Evans, P. Jha, A. Mills, and P. Musgrove, 1075–90. New York: Oxford University Press.

Lindblom, C. E. 1968. *The Policy-Making Process*. Englewood Cliffs, NJ: Prentice-Hall.

Lopez-Escobar, Guillermo. 1978. *Aborto: Interrogantes, comentarios y resultados parciales de algunas investigaciones en Colombia.* Monograph 8. Bogotá: Regional Population Center.

MacCorquodale, D. W., and T. W. Pullum. 1974. "A Mathematical Model for Determining Family Planning Clinic Effectiveness." *Studies in Family Planning* 5 (7): 232–38.

Measham, Anthony R. 1972. *Family Planning in North Carolina: The Politics of a Lukewarm Issue.* Monograph 17. Chapel Hill, NC: University of North Carolina, Carolina Population Center.

Ott, E. R. 1977. "Population Policy Formation in Colombia: The Role of ASCOFAME. *Studies in Family Planning* 8 (1): 2–10.

Perez, E. 1976. *Colombia.* Country Profiles Series. New York: Population Council.

Perez, E. and F. Gomez. 1974. "Family Planning Programs: World Review." *Studies in Family Planning* 6 (8): 268–70.

Rizo, A. 1978. "Colombia 1969–1978: A Case Study in Population Dynamics. Statement, April 25, 1978." In *Population and Development: Status and Trends of Family Planning/Population Programs in Developing Countries,* vol. II, 313–30. Washington, DC: Government Printing Office.

Ross, John A. 1966. "Recent Events in Population Control." *Studies in Family Planning* 1 (9): 1–5.

Simmons, A. B., and R. Cardona. 1973. *Family Planning in Colombia: Changes in Attitude and Acceptance, 1964–69.* Ottawa: International Development Research Centre.

Tamayo, Fernando. 1978. "The Colombian Experience: A Statement to the Congress of the United States." In *Population and Development: Status and Trends of Family Planning/Population Programs in Developing Countries,* vol. II, 299–312. Washington, DC: Government Printing Office.

9 Guatemala: The Pioneering Days of the Family Planning Movement

ROBERTO SANTISO-GÁLVEZ AND JANE T. BERTRAND

This volume spotlights the most successful programs in the international family planning movement. Guatemala is not one of the internationally renowned success stories, yet it has been included in this volume precisely because the uphill battle to introduce family planning in that country—which is still being waged today—is instructive in understanding the international family planning movement. Whereas other chapters describe how political will and strong leadership were able to overcome social and cultural barriers to contraceptive use, this case study of Guatemala focuses on resistance to family planning at the highest levels, starting in the 1960s, which persisted for more than three decades and impeded the spread of family planning. Despite the establishment of a dynamic private family planning association in the mid-1960s, 40 years later, Guatemala ranks last in contraceptive use in Latin America (Population Reference Bureau 2006).

The Sociopolitical Context, Early 1960s

In the 1960s, Guatemala, whose population totaled approximately 4.8 million, faced serious sociopolitical problems. It had some of the worst socioeconomic indicators in the region: average annual per capita income was US$315, 66 percent of the population lived in rural areas, 62 percent were illiterate, 69 percent had no access to portable water, and only 21 percent had some system of human waste disposal. The birth rate was high, 44.8 births per 1,000 population, and women were having an average of 6.6 children. Youth under 15 years of age accounted for 46 percent of the population. *Machismo* and discrimination against women were pervasive. Access to health services was extremely low, and Guatemala dedicated less of its budget to the health sector than most other Latin American countries. More than half of the population was indigenous, namely, Mayans, who belonged to 23 different linguistic groups and were often illiterate, unable to speak Spanish, and culturally isolated from

The authors would like to express their appreciation to the following for providing valuable information for this chapter in the form of interviews, written accounts, and documentation: Enrique Castillo Arenales, Cynthia Burski, Johnny Long, Melida Muralles, Maria Antonieta Pineda, Oscar Rodriguez, and Ricardo López Urzúa.

137

the mainstream (Morales 1970). At the same time, conflict between the Guatemalan army and guerilla groups caused extensive societal disruption. This is the general context in which family planning began in this country, "A moment hardly appropriate to start this type of program," according to Dr. Donald MacCorquodale, the U.S. Agency for International Development (USAID) health officer during this period (personal communication from Cynthia Burski to Roberto Santiso-Gálvez 2006).

The 1960s began with considerable optimism, derived in part from the 10-Year Plan of the U.S. government's Alliance for Progress to promote development in Latin America. Various international organizations, such as the World Health Organization, the Pan American Health Organization, and the Organization of Central American States, all actively supported and participated in a plan to improve health status in the region, which gave new hope for maternal and child health in Latin America. At the same time, concern was growing about a number of population issues, including the alarming rates of illegal abortion, the need for sex education for young people, and the effects of rapid population growth on socioeconomic development. A number of researchers conducted preliminary studies on abortion, maternal mortality, contraception, sexuality, and population dynamics (for an excellent annotated bibliography of these studies, see Arias de Blois [1978]). Numerous meetings and conferences took place to analyze these different topics. The press took interest, particularly in relation to the population explosion. Radio news shows, for instance, *Guatemala Flash*, gave favorable coverage to population issues in their weekly programs, and magazines such as *La Semana* covered topics such as abortion and sex education (personal communication from Ricardo López Urzúa to the authors, 2006).

Many organizations participated in the population-related activities during the 1960s: the ministries of Health, Education, Agriculture, and Labor; universities; the National Gynecology and Obstetrics Association; workers' unions; agricultural cooperatives; and the Social Security Institute of Guatemala (*Instituto Guatemalteco de Seguro Social*, IGSS). Numerous international groups were also involved, including the United Nations Educational, Scientific, and Cultural Organization; the World Health Organization; the Latin American and Caribbean Demographic Center; the Pan American Federation of Schools of Medicine (based in Colombia); Pathfinder International; the U.S. Centers for Disease Control and Prevention; the Association for Voluntary Sterilization (JHPIEGO); and Juárez and Associates. All shared the common goal of improving the quality of life for Guatemalans by combating poverty, illiteracy, low levels of education, and poor health status. Notably, most of these groups had a favorable attitude toward family planning.

The story of the pioneering days of family planning in Guatemala during 1960 to 1970 is quite similar as in other countries in Latin America, that is, it started with a core group of dedicated pioneers who recognized the acute need for family planning, established an organization to offer services to the population, and fought assiduously to win government support for the program. Yet in contrast to many other countries where the government either championed the family planning movement itself or embraced it after private family planning associations had established the feasibility and acceptability of such a program, the Guatemalan government did not provide strong support until 2000 and then did not sustain it after a change in presidents.

Family Planning Pioneers

The beginning of family planning in Guatemala dates back to 1962, when the International Planned Parenthood Federation (IPPF) was fomenting interest in this topic in many Latin American countries. Dr. Ofelia Mendoza, IPPF technical director for the Western Hemisphere Region, had traveled to most countries in the region in the early 1960s, identifying people who recognized the need for family planning and encouraging them to establish private associations that would eventually become IPPF affiliates. Mendoza proposed that interested professionals create such associations, whose objectives would be to promote the concept of family planning among the general public and offer quality services to those in need. Box 9.1 presents a timeline of major events in relation to family planning in Guatemala.

BOX 9.1 Timeline for Family Planning

1962:	Nineteen health professionals form a preliminary board of directors for a private family planning association.
1963:	These founding members develop statutes for the private family planning association.
1964:	The Association of Family Well-Being (*Asociación Pro Bienestar de la Familia*, APROFAM) attains legal status.
1965:	APROFAM opens its first clinic in Guatemala City with a doctor, nurse, and social worker.
	IGSS opens a family planning clinic.
1967:	The USAID signs a tripartite agreement (entitled Population and Rural Health: 1969–1973) with the Ministry of Health and APROFAM. The latter is authorized to establish family planning services in 20 Ministry of Health centers.
1968:	The Vatican issues the *Encyclica Humanae Vitae*. The Catholic Church in Guatemala intensifies its opposition to APROFAM.
	Yielding to pressure from the Catholic Church, IGSS imposes tight restrictions on access to family planning services.
1969:	The government reorganizes the Ministry of Health and creates the Division of Maternal, Child, and Family Health, which includes family planning. The ministry is slow to spread information about family planning service delivery to its health centers.
1970:	The USAID amends its agreement to create the integrated Office of Information, Education, and Training within the Ministry of Health. The ministry agrees to extend family planning to 450 facilities.
	APROFAM takes responsibility for distributing contraceptives and training ministry personnel.
1973:	The agreement between the USAID and the ministry is extended to 1976.
1976:	A USAID evaluation of the activities under the tripartite agreement yields mixed results.
	An earthquake kills 25,000 people and destroys much of the Ministry of Health's infrastructure.
	The ministry dedicates its efforts to reconstructing its infrastructure. It closes the Office of Information, Education, and Training.
	The USAID signs a second agreement with the Ministry of Health and APROFAM covering the period from 1976 to 1980.
1977–78:	The activities under the tripartite agreement advance well, and coverage is extended to 492 outlets.
	Pro-natalist groups begin attacks against the intrauterine device.

(Continued)

BOX 9.1 Timeline for Family Planning (continued)

1979:	Succumbing to religious pressure, the ministry suspends the family planning program, orders all intrauterine devices to be extracted, and suspends sterilization and its collaboration with APROFAM.
	The private sector persuades the ministry to restart the family planning program, but it does so only at 144 health units and it only permits physicians to provide services.
1980–83:	The USAID and the Ministry of Health sign a new agreement effective through 1987.
	Two coups d'etat take place. The family planning program remains unaffected. President Ríos Montt, an evangelical Christian, provides some support to family planning.
1985:	Supporters of family planning succeed in getting Article 47 into the new Guatemalan constitution, which guarantees couples the right to have the number of children they desire. However, the opposition succeeds in inserting an article stating that life begins at conception with the objective of attacking contraceptives as being abortifacients.
1986:	The archbishop of Guatemala sends a letter to President Ronald Reagan asking him to suspend U.S. assistance to family planning because of allegations of mass sterilization of women without their consent. President Reagan sends a commission to Guatemala that concludes that the allegations are unfounded.
	A change at the Ministry of Health slightly favors family planning.
1992:	The USAID and the Ministry of Health sign an agreement covering the period from 1992 to 1996.
	Several members of Congress prepare the Social Development Law.
1993:	Although initially in favor of the law, President Jorge Serrano succumbs to religious pressures and does not approve it.
	A coup d'etat results in another president.
1994–96:	President Ramiro de León Carpio instructs the Guatemalan delegation to the International Conference on Population and Development to vote the Vatican position.
	The family planning program continues to operate at a reduced level.
	The media highlight the controversy about family planning.
1996–2000:	President Alvaro Arzú confronts those in favor of family planning and those opposed, decides to subject the topic to public discussion, and continues the program without strong political support.
2000–04:	President Alfonso Portillo provides political backing for family planning.
	The Social Development Law, which strongly supports reproductive health, is put into effect (2001).
	The social development and population policy guides the implementation and monitoring of family planning (2002).
	The Law of Taxes on Alcoholic Beverages earmarks funds for reproductive health (2004).
2005–06:	The funds generated by the Law of Taxes on Alcoholic Beverages and earmarked for reproductive health are not spent accordingly.
	Civil society prepares the Law for Universal and Equitable Access to Family Planning Services and Its Integration with the National Reproductive Health Program to assure funding for contraception.
	The law is approved in Congress, but is vetoed by President Oscar Berger with support from the Catholic Church and evangelical Christian groups, because of the requirement to teach topics such as sex education in schools.
2006:	The president issues his veto too late, allowing the law to become operational.
	Civil society organizes to ensure the auditing of earmarked funds to guarantee that they are used for reproductive health and the purchase of contraceptives.

In March 1962, 19 Guatemalan health professionals responded to Mendoza's call to create a private association dedicated to family planning. These founding members established a preliminary board of directors headed by Dr. Enrique Castillo Arenales (Pineda 1977). Subsequently, Castillo and Yolanda Gálvez, a nurse, attended an IPPF meeting in New York with representatives from other countries to further discuss the need for family planning in the region. Following the New York meeting, the preliminary board formed two committees, one to recruit additional members and the other to draft the statutes of the new association (Galich 1971). The process of gaining legal status for the association moved slowly until Castillo used his political connections to achieve results. The Ministry of the Interior approved the statutes in August 1964. In October, the local official newspaper *Diario de Centro América* reported that the Association of Family Well-Being (*Asociación Pro Bienestar de la Familia*, APROFAM) had gained legal status. Dr. Roberto Santiso-Gálvez was named director. In 1969, APROFAM officially became an IPPF affiliate.

APROFAM's Response to the Lack of Government Support for Family Planning

A number of developing countries described in this volume had a population policy that served as a catalyst for expanding contraceptive services in the 1960s and 1970s, such as India, Indonesia, and the Republic of Korea. Other countries such as Costa Rica did not have the benefit of such a policy, but nonetheless made significant progress. Still other countries developed a population policy that did little to advance the cause of family planning, for example, Ghana. Guatemala, by contrast, had neither a population policy nor the political will to support a family planning agenda. On several occasions, APROFAM attempted to create a national population policy in collaboration with legislators favorable to the issue, but it never got off the ground because of religious and political opposition and a lack of commitment on the part of the government. Indeed, the Social Development Law did not come into effect until 2001 and the development and population policy did not became official until 2002, and even now, some observers question the effect of this legislation on actual service delivery and contraceptive use.

From the mid-1960s, APROFAM began to fill the void in family planning leadership. It established the following objectives for the family planning program:

• Improve family health.

• Encourage family unity.

• Increase awareness and use of modern methods of fertility control.

To these ends, the program emphasized providing information and education for the population, delivering quality family planning services, and coordinating with other public and private institutions with similar objectives.

APROFAM opened its first clinic in January 1965 in the Latin American Hospital in Guatemala City, staffed by a physician, a social worker, and a nurse. The philosophy of the service providers was to provide quality services so that satisfied clients would refer their friends to the clinic. Clients could choose between the pill and the intrauterine device (IUD), originally the Margulis IUD and then the Lippes loop IUD.

From the start, the social worker did outreach work in government maternity hospitals and with women at their workplaces or at health centers. This had the intended result of creating demand, and APROFAM had to increase its clinic's hours of operation. From the time APROFAM established its clinical services, the IPPF/Western Hemisphere Region provided financial support for the outreach and information, education, and communication work. Both the IPPF and Pathfinder International donated contraceptive commodities. The method mix expanded to include vaginal creams, vaginal tablets, and condoms.

APROFAM added more physicians to the clinic's staff, and their duties included providing on-site training to other clinic personnel. Clinic staff members, including the physicians, also went to other Latin American countries for training.

The response to the family planning services increased steadily (figure 9.1), and APROFAM moved to a larger facility on Avenida Bolivar, located in a densely populated area of Guatemala City.

In the same year that APROFAM opened its first clinic in Guatemala City, IGSS also established its own family planning program. IGSS is a semi-autonomous institution, and all employers with more than four employees are obliged to register with IGSS. The employer contributes 10 percent of payroll and workers contribute 4 percent of their wages to obtain health and social services. In collaboration with APROFAM, IGSS created the Family Counseling Clinic as part of its maternity services, primarily to combat the high level of illegal abortion among the working class. APROFAM's contribution consisted of training clinic personnel and supplying

FIGURE 9.1 Number of New APROFAM Clients and Repeat Visits, 1965–70

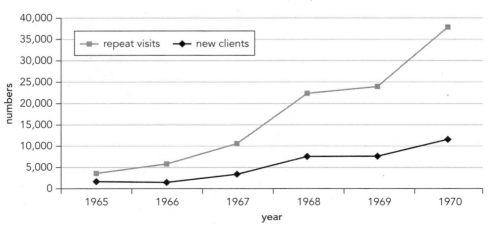

Source: APROFAM 1971.

IGSS with contraceptives. Santiso-Gálvez, then director of APROFAM, oversaw these IGSS activities.

From 1965 to 1968, the demand for family planning services at IGSS increased dramatically, and IGSS doubled its nurses and social workers and expanded its facilities. Hernán Hurtado Aguilar, then director of IGSS and a man with a strong social conscience, showed great leadership in supporting family planning delivery at IGSS during this initial period. However, in 1968, the IGSS leadership changed and the new director imposed severe limitations on family planning service delivery. To receive services, a woman had to have had an abortion, had three successive caesarian sections, or represent a high-risk case. The IGSS program was therefore drastically reduced for a number of years, although APROFAM continued to provide contraceptives.[1]

In short, APROFAM and IGSS took the lead in establishing family planning service delivery during the 1960s. In addition, APROFAM was a major player in undertaking research pertaining to family planning and reproductive health, advocating population issues among policy makers, running information and education campaigns for the general public, and training clinical personnel. APROFAM also played a critical role in developing and coordinating counterattacks when the University of San Carlos and the Catholic Church periodically threatened to bring an end to the family planning movement.

The Role of the Ministry of Health

Where was the Ministry of Health in all of this? Guatemala followed the pattern of most Latin American countries in that the IPPF affiliate was generally in the vanguard of contraceptive service delivery. Thus, the absence of the government via the Ministry of Health from the forefront of the family planning movement is not surprising. What is surprising, however, is that the government took almost 40 years to give strong support to contraceptive service delivery, in comparison with the majority of Latin American countries, which embraced family planning in the 1970s or 1980s.

The Ministry of Health first became involved in family planning in 1967, when it signed a tripartite agreement (number 520-0189) with the USAID and APROFAM to deliver family planning services. The signing occurred under the administration of President Julio César Méndez Montenegro, whose minister of health, Dr. Emilio Poitevin, launched this collaboration with great enthusiasm, promising to provide services in all existing health centers. Shortly thereafter, the ministry, yielding to political pressure from pro-natalist groups, reduced its participation from 235 health centers to 20 and from 10 mobile units in rural areas to 6. Subsequently, the mobile units ceased to function. Government support for the program was weak, staff members were inexperienced, and fears abounded about possible criticism from the Catholic Church. The tripartite agreement called for APROFAM to train Ministry of Health personnel in family planning service delivery, stock Ministry of Health facilities with contraceptives, and administer the family planning program. In this way, the Ministry of Health was able to explore the acceptability of this new service without having to fully endorse family planning (Burski 1977).

Problems with service delivery through government facilities surfaced early on. The Ministry of Health negotiated with the USAID to provide physicians with an economic incentive for each new user of the pill or IUD. The justification was that the doctors providing this service were generally underpaid and that this supplement would compensate for their extra workload. However, this economic incentive backfired. Other ministry personnel saw it as favoritism for family planning, which created further antagonism toward contraceptive service delivery. Moreover, because the ministry had delegated administration of the program to APROFAM, the latter was responsible for writing the monthly checks to the doctors participating in the program and critics complained that this system usurped the ministry's functions. The mass media publicized this controversy widely, and political opposition groups took full advantage of it to discredit the government. By 1968, the government had eliminated economic incentives, but not before they had done considerable harm to the program, to APROFAM, and to the USAID.

Despite the numerous problems in the implementation of the tripartite agreement and the poor results it produced, the USAID extended its support of the program at the end of 1969, but required the ministry to take full responsibility for the family planning program rather than delegating it to APROFAM.

In 1969, the government issued a legislative decree to reorganize the operations of the Ministry of Health. As part of this process, it established the Division of Maternal, Child, and Family Health, which included the Family Counseling Program to handle contraceptive service delivery. However, the ministry was slow to disseminate information about this new program to its personnel throughout the country. Even the euphemistic name that the Ministry of Health selected for this unit (Family Counseling) reflected its unwillingness to openly endorse family planning on the basis of its fear of attacks from religious, university, and leftist leaders.

Shortly thereafter, the government created another unit within the Division of Maternal, Child, and Family Health, the Office for Promotion, Education, and Training, which was to work closely with APROFAM to facilitate the work of the Ministry of Health in family planning. However, other units within the ministry that worked on similar types of information, education, communication, and training activities quickly grew to resent it. The new unit attempted to collaborate with other units within the Ministry of Health, but the Catholic Church continued to apply pressure by creating bad press and false information regarding family planning. For example, the immunization program agreed to develop some posters that promoted both vaccination and family planning at health centers. Rumors spread rapidly that the immunizations would sterilize children who received them, because vials were discovered that said "sterile water" in the vaccine packets. This incident carried great weight in the local press, discrediting both the immunization and the family planning programs.

The Ministry of Health program further suffered from an attempt to introduce sophisticated software for tracking service statistics and providing important feedback for decision making. Introduced by experts from the U.S. Centers for Disease

Control and Prevention in the early 1970s, local personnel never fully mastered the system, which did not meet local needs. This initiative might have fared better with closer monitoring and greater advocacy for its use within the Ministry of Health. (Years later, as technology advanced, the ministry bought a new computerized system to be used throughout its network of facilities. However, it too proved difficult to institutionalize, reflecting the challenges inherent in such systems without proper monitoring and evaluation.)

These first years of family planning service delivery within Ministry of Health facilities verged on chaos. Even the ministry was amazed that the USAID decided to extend its program of financial and technical assistance given the poor results of the first agreement. One can only surmise that this decision was based on the acute needs on the part of the Guatemalan population for all types of development assistance, coupled with the USAID's zeal to promote family planning as widely as possible in developing countries.

The USAID's Contribution

MacCorquodale arrived in 1964 to serve as health officer at the USAID Guatemala Mission. That same year, the USAID authorized its missions throughout Latin America to begin funding population and family planning programs. The mission director, Marvin Weissman, appointed MacCorquodale to begin negotiations in relation to population and family planning activities with the de facto government of Colonel Enrique Peralta Azurdia. MacCorquodale was unable to make any progress during this administration. Even though government officials received him cordially, discussions grew strained at any mention of family planning. The USAID then tried to approach other government organizations, but they too politely declined. Apparently, Guatemala was simply too Catholic. The USAID even offered support to various organizations to conduct a knowledge, attitudes, and practices survey on fertility, but no one took it up on the offer.

MacCorquodale consulted with Santiso-Gálvez, director of APROFAM, who suggested that he approach the dean of the School of Medicine at the University of San Carlos. Despite the school's strongly Marxist leanings, Santiso-Gálvez thought the dean might be interested in determining public opinion on the population issue, given the ongoing debates about rapid population growth. MacCorquodale was taken aback by the openly anti-American sentiment at the university, expressed through graffiti, posters, protests, and verbal threats from students; however, Dean Julio de León received him amiably and after hearing him out, agreed to have the university involved in a study, but warned MacCorquodale that he would be unwilling to support family planning, whatever the results of the study. MacCorquodale agreed not to engage him in that capacity.

Dr. Rolando Collado collected the data for this study, *La Familia de Guatemala,* in 1967, but had to flee the country because of death threats from anticommunist groups because of his leftist views. At about the same time, the university underwent many attacks and a number of professors were murdered by anticommunist groups, reflecting the highly volatile political climate in the country at that time. From out-side the country, Collado was able to complete the data analysis and eventually pub-lish the study's findings (Collado 1968).

MacCorquodale considered the main findings of the study to be positive and wanted to distribute them among key opinion leaders, but both the new mission director (Deane Hinton) and the new population and health officer (Dr. James King) thought that the results might play into the hands of the Marxists. MacCorquodale later commented, "*La Familia de Guatemala* never was distributed as Mr. Weissman and I would have liked. I imagine that almost all of the 2,500 copies of this study have now rotted in the warehouse and the copy that I keep in my own library is pos-sibly one of the few that still exist" (MacCorquodale 2002).

Contributions of Other Partner Agencies

In the tripartite agreement signed in 1967, the USAID also gave funding to the Uni-versity of the Valley (Universidad del Valle) to design curricular materials on sex edu-cation and human development for students from kindergarten through junior high and for the 3,000 teachers who would use these materials. Launched in 1968, this program ran through 1975 as a collaboration between the Ministry of Education and the University of the Valley. As part of the process, numerous meetings took place, both nationally and internationally. The curricular materials for both the students and the teachers ran into countless problems in the design and production stages. Finally, the Ministry of Education, which was responsible for incorporating sex edu-cation into the official curriculum, simply did not act. The materials produced for this purpose and stored in warehouses were destroyed during the 1976 earthquake, leaving many to conclude that the government had given in to pressures not to offer sex education in the schools.

Other agencies also contributed to the early days of the family planning movement in Guatemala. As part of its 10-Year Health Plan for the Americas, the Pan American Health Organization proved to be an excellent source of financial and technical assis-tance. It sponsored several regional conferences and meetings to analyze the health situation in Central America that yielded both regional and country-specific recom-mendations. One such recommendation was to incorporate family planning into ongoing maternal and child health services.

The Organization of Central American States, a division of the Organization of American States, provided scholarships and supported regional meetings about health and sex education. Dr. Juan Alwood Paredes, a Salvadoran doctor responsi-ble for the health sector within the Organization of Central American States, served as an important catalyst for these activities.

Several U.S.-based organizations contributed to strengthening family planning in Guatemala. Pathfinder International was one of the first to provide assistance in support of training, contraceptive commodities, and evaluation. A number of U.S. Centers for Disease Control and Prevention experts from the Division of Reproduc-tive Health helped design the computerized information system mentioned earlier, as well as logistics systems, and later assisted with the national contraceptive prevalence surveys (Burski 1977).

Other organizations played a key role in providing technical assistance, though after 1960–70, the period that is the main focus of this book. These included the University of Chicago for information, education, communication, and evaluation; the Population Council for operations research; Juárez and Associates for management and training; (JHPIEGO) for training and equipment for voluntary sterilization; and the Johns Hopkins Program for International Education in Reproductive Health for training in voluntary sterilization.

As concerns the importance of external aid to the establishment of family planning, despite the weak support at best, and the overt hostility at worst, from the different Guatemalan administrations over the past four decades, external aid did play a pivotal role in ensuring contraceptive access for a large portion of the population. Without the strong influx of funds, first from the IPPF for the Western Hemisphere Region and later from the USAID and its cooperating agencies, and to a lesser extent from other donors, even the dedicated pioneers would have had difficulty in sustaining the program.

Monitoring and Evaluation

During much of the 1960s and 1970s, evaluation at APROFAM consisted of tracking service statistics, for example, the number of new users and the number of repeat visits, and process indicators related to the activities conducted, such as the number of talks or meetings conducted in clinics and in the community and the number of participants at such events. One useful piece of information that APROFAM collected during the first years of service delivery was the place of residence of its clients, which guided decision making for the expansion of clinics into marginal areas. In addition, researchers conducted occasional special studies, one of which detected significant demand for pap smears. On the basis of these results, APROFAM began providing pap smears at its clinics and trained technicians in cytology (Galich 1971)[2] and was the first Guatemalan institution to carry out an information campaign for the general public about cervical cancer.

A major limitation of the monitoring and evaluation work during the 1960s and 1970s was its exclusive focus on quantitative outputs. To cite one missed opportunity, APROFAM played a critical role in training clinical personnel to deliver family planning services in its own clinics as well as in the Ministry of Health and IGSS clinics.[3] In retrospect, evaluating these training events more closely regarding course content and the subsequent performance (competence) of those trained would have been useful. As it was, APROFAM had relatively little evidence of the effectiveness of its training or information on which to base improvements in the training.

A second limitation of the monitoring and evaluation work was the difficulty in obtaining accurate counts of new users, repeat visits, dropouts, and active users. Not only did this activity consume vast amounts of staff members' time, it also yielded results of questionable accuracy because of such issues as duplication of records creating an inflated number of clients. The eventual adoption of the indicator "couple-years of protection" in the 1990s, a measure of the volume of contraception delivered by a given family planning service, largely resolved this problem.

During the early 1970s, the U.S. Centers for Disease Control and Prevention provided consultants to establish a computerized management information system. As noted earlier, this system did not prove useful, in part because of the lack of sufficient follow-up, and in part because of the low priority the Ministry of Health gave to family planning (Burski 1977). Later, in the 1980s and 1990s, APROFAM became much more engaged in operations research and other evaluation projects (together with researchers from the University of Chicago, Tulane University, and the Population Council) so that it could gain a better understanding of the dynamics of its programs. At least 15 articles documenting this work have appeared in peer-reviewed international journals. APROFAM also participated in the design, and in some cases the data collection and analysis, of all the nationally representative surveys of fertility and family planning conducted in Guatemala (1978, 1984, 1987, 1995, 1998, and 2002).

Factors that Hindered the Expansion of Family Planning in Guatemala

Several years ago, the authors of this chapter sought to establish why Guatemala lagged so far behind neighboring countries in Latin America in the acceptance of family planning. They argued that four factors stymied progress (Santiso-Gálvez and Bertrand 2004): (a) the strong influence of the Catholic Church on the government's decision making as it pertained to family planning, (b) the leftist position of the leading university, (c) the ethnic composition of the population, and (d) the civil unrest that ravaged the country from 1966 to 1996. None of these factors was unique to Guatemala, but the convergence of all four in a single country proved devastating to family planning. The first two factors in particular thwarted early efforts to develop a population policy and a strong family planning program.

The Catholic Church
In the 1960s, the vast majority of the population was Catholic. (Since then, the percentage that is evangelical Christian has risen steadily. Evangelicals tend to be equally opposed to family planning, but have not exerted the same influence over the ruling elite.) The presence of a strong Catholic Church in a given country is not by itself an impediment to family planning (consider, for example, the cases of Colombia and Mexico), but it does have a chilling effect when the church and the state join forces in their opposition to family planning. In Guatemala, officials at all levels of government were under constant pressure from the church to oppose the expansion of family planning, especially at the national level. This pervasive influence of the church dissuaded some preeminent leaders from serving on APROFAM's board of directors and caused others to resign from the board. Church leaders and government officials accused APROFAM and its board of directors of promoting abortion, which was not

the case. (Given the hostile climate for family planning, APROFAM has steered clear of any involvement in attempts to legalize abortion.) Activities only continued because a small, pioneering group of committed health professionals remained convinced of the benefits of family planning.

Soon after APROFAM opened its first family planning clinic in 1965, the Catholic Church manifested its objection in a pastoral letter opposing the program and the use of artificial contraception. However, the attacks were relatively mild for several years thereafter, a period during which the Vatican was reviewing its position on contraception. Indeed, many both inside and outside the church anticipated that the church would lessen its opposition to family planning (McLaughlin 1982). During this waiting period, some members of the Episcopal Conference of Guatemala contacted Dr. Ricardo López Urzúa and Santiso-Gálvez to discuss how to improve the educational level of young people in the country. They even proposed that each church provide a school and were willing to have experts in responsible parenthood, family planning, and contraception come to teach about these subjects (as a complement to this schooling), provided their teachings would be in accordance with the church's morals and values and that the church's position toward family planning would change as anticipated. However, the publication of the *Encyclica Humanae Vitae* in July 1968, manifestly opposing "artificial contraception," brought an abrupt halt to talks of possible collaboration between the church and local nongovernmental organizations. The church's initial opposition to APROFAM and IGSS family planning programs intensified in the wake of the Vatican's ruling, and the tripartite agreement among the Ministry of Health, APROFAM, and the USAID became the target of much of this hostility (Burksi 1977).

For four decades, starting in the 1960s, the Catholic Church tried to influence every Guatemalan government to resist the adoption and expansion of family planning. The response by different administrations has ranged from neutrality toward family planning, to weak support of family planning, to overt opposition. Perhaps the most supportive was the government of Alfonso Portillo from 2000 to 2004, but the current administration of President Oscar Berger has been less favorable. At several points throughout the past 40 years, the church has threatened to close down family planning altogether, and on more than one occasion has come close to doing so. As noted earlier, having a strong Catholic Church was not the defining impediment to the expansion of family planning, but rather it was the close ties between the Catholic Church and the ruling elite on the issue of family planning.

The University of San Carlos

The University of San Carlos was and is Guatemala's leading academic institution. Dominated by leftists in positions of authority in the 1960s and 1970s, the university played a key role in obstructing the development of a strong family planning program. The debates between university leaders and those favorable to family planning date back to the 1960s. For example, in 1968, the university sponsored a conference titled "Population and Development." Members of the faculties of economics and medicine vigorously denounced population programs as imperialistic plots by the

U.S. government and as activities counterproductive to the aim of a Marxist revolution (Osorio-Paz and Lemus-Mendoza 1968). Others from within and outside Guatemala tried to defend the benefits of such programs. The organizers of the conference—members of the economics faculty—manipulated the conclusions of the meeting so that they were extremely negative toward population and family planning programs, and subsequently presented the document to the Catholic Church, which obviously shared the faculty's position against family planning, but for different reasons.

A major factor in the hostility toward "*los norteamericanos*" or "*gringos*" (that is, the United States) was the military invasion in 1954, in which the United States had supported a coup led by Colonel Carlos Castillo Armas that unseated President Jacobo Arbenz Guzmán, who the United States viewed as a communist for having expropriated the banana farms of the United Fruit Company. The overbearing power and influence of the United States throughout the Western hemisphere was a thorn in the side of many Latin American countries during this period, and revolutionary fervor often found its voice on university campuses.

The anti-American climate at San Carlos was so intense that it caused the university to make decisions that actually went against its own self-interests. For example, it rejected a donation of US$3 million from the Kellogg Foundation for laboratory equipment for medicine and dentistry because the funding came from the United States. Ironically, the dean of the School of Medicine in Costa Rica, Dr. Rodrigo Gutiérrez, a declared Marxist and the Marxist Party's presidential candidate in various elections, opted to accept this Kellogg Foundation donation. In another case, the University of San Carlos declined the offer by Ferdinand Rath of the Latin American Demographic Center to establish its Central American branch for demographic research in Guatemala. Instead, the regional center was established in Costa Rica, subsequently produced some of the best demographic research in Latin America, and trained a number of Central American demographers.

The opposition of the University of San Carlos to family planning has had negative repercussions that are still felt to this day. First, the university authorities prohibited research in the area of human reproduction: it blocked research by Dr. Howard Tatum on the copper T IUD and subsequently refused to allow studies on injectable methods and on quinacrine (used to obstruct the fallopian tubes). Second, the university did not train or permit training of its medical students in family planning, contraception, and other aspects of human reproduction. When medical students in their final year or recent graduates were sent to practice in rural areas, they did not have even the most fundamental training in contraception. Similarly, the National School of Nursing, which was run by Catholic nuns, denied this type of training to its students. Thus, the doctors and nurses graduating from these programs did not have the necessary knowledge and competencies to deliver family planning services. Moreover, they tended to have negative attitudes to family planning, which combined with the weak to nonexistent support of family planning in government facilities to further doom family planning in the public sector. Even though the university began to allow medical students to take training courses from the Johns Hopkins Program for International Education in Reproductive Health in collaboration with

APROFAM in 1992–94, the deficiencies in in-service training in family planning continue to reverberate throughout the health system.

The Country's Ethnic Composition

More than half of Guatemalans are Mayan Indians, who comprise some 23 linguistically different groups. Despite being a majority, the indigenous population has endured for decades social and economic oppression at the hands of the Spanish-speaking *ladinos* (the white and mestizo population that has controlled economic resources since the time of the *conquistadores*). The vast majority of Mayans live in poverty in rural areas, experience high rates of maternal and infant mortality, and have low rates of education and literacy. In addition, their unique view of the world (cosmovision) conflicts with some aspects of planned fertility control. The marked differences between *ladinos* and Mayans in political power, educational levels, access to the media and Western ideas, and cultural values explain the dramatic differences in contraceptive use between the Spanish-speaking *ladinos* (52.8 percent of married women were using contraception as of 2002) and their Mayan counterparts (23.8 percent). However, this was not a major issue in the 1960s, as the early programs sought to increase demand and provide services to low-income, primarily *ladino*, populations in urban areas. Yet, at the same time, the socioeconomic characteristics and cultural values of the predominant group in the country certainly did not help the introduction of family planning in the country.

The Internal Civil Conflict

The 1960s witnessed the beginning of an internal armed conflict that would expand into civil war in the 1970s, peaking in the 1980s, and lasting until the signing of the peace agreements in 1996. This conflict first developed in the eastern highlands, where the Guatemalan army allegedly repeatedly attacked guerilla forces. Soon after, the conflict shifted to the mountainous northwestern region, home to large segments of the indigenous population. Mayans who assumed any type of leadership position during *la violencia* in the 1980s took huge risks, as many "disappeared," while others managed to flee the country. In the midst of this violent and chaotic situation, the government and nongovernmental organizations, already challenged to provide health services to rural populations, found the job next to impossible. The infrastructure for social services was virtually nonexistent in many areas. Although this situation had tremendous implications for the expansion of family planning service delivery into rural areas in the 1980s and 1990s, it did not have a major influence during the early years of family planning, when programs targeted urban areas.

Lessons Learned

The lessons learned from the Guatemala experience may be of limited value for programs in other countries with a different sociocultural context and at a different historical point in relation to family planning. Nevertheless, Guatemala's experience does shed light on the introduction of family planning in countries with little government support and unfavorable sociocultural conditions.

The experience of Guatemala illustrates the difficulty of firmly establishing family planning in a country where the Catholic Church and the government join forces in their opposition to family planning. Several strategies intended to facilitate the introduction of family planning—having the IPPF affiliate administer the Ministry of Health program and paying incentives to physicians providing contraceptive services—proved problematic. The strong opposition from the leading university in the country had strongly negative repercussions that stymied contraceptive research, training of health workers, and provision of contraceptive services. The large indigenous population in Guatemala and the incipient civil unrest were other factors that hindered the introduction of family planning, especially in the 1980s and 1990s.

Against this backdrop of obstacles, several factors kept family planning alive in the early days. First, APROFAM quickly grew to become a dynamic organization that filled the void left by the Ministry of Health. Not only did it create and later expand its own clinics, it helped IGSS establish a clinic and worked with other development partners over the years to expand access to contraception. Second, even though the ruling elite opposed family planning, the demand for contraception was strong and people responded to the offer of services. Third, the USAID did not waver in its financial and technical support for family planning, despite lackluster results. Fourth, key figures in the media kept the topic of population and family planning in the public view and periodically challenged the position of the Catholic Church.

As concerns what might have been done differently, with hindsight, more effort should have been invested in understanding the sociopolitical context and in designing and implementing programs tailored to local needs. Also, nongovernmental organizations, members of Congress, family planning advocates, women's groups, international agencies, and others could have put more pressure on the Ministry of Health to take a leadership role in family planning, rather than allowing APROFAM to assume this role. Certainly the Ministry of Health should have disseminated the legislative agreement that established family planning more widely within the ministry, and it could have avoided the antagonism toward the program that was created by the financial incentives given to family planning service providers.

For other countries struggling to introduce family planning under unfavorable conditions, the following recommendations may be pertinent:

- Study and understand the sociocultural context as it relates to family planning.

- Secure a source of sustained financial and technical support.

- Integrate family planning with other health services, for example, gynecological cancer screening, sexuality, adolescence, and infertility, both to increase the acceptability of the program among the population and to increase the efficiency of service delivery.

- Encourage the ministry of health to accept its rightful responsibilities of providing quality family planning services and working with other ministries, such as the education, labor, economy, and finance ministries, to do so.

- Improve coordination among agencies working in family planning to avoid duplication and increase the program's effectiveness.

- Ensure both preservice and in-service training in contraceptive service delivery to improve the quality of family planning services.

- Monitor the performance of those trained to ensure that they are capable of providing quality services and are doing so.

- Establish an ongoing program of monitoring and evaluation that includes quantitative and qualitative methodologies, process indicators, and impact assessment.

Conclusions

The difficulties that the pioneers in family planning confronted during the 1960s foreshadowed problems that have continued to hinder progress ever since. APROFAM stepped in to fill the leadership void left by the Ministry of Health by providing contraceptive service delivery, advocacy, training, information, education, communication, and research. Yet the lack of political support, the incessant attacks by the Catholic Church, and the periodic civil unrest all took their toll, as reflected in the still low level of contraceptive prevalence in Guatemala.

Notes

1. In the 1970s, IGSS acquired laparoscopic equipment to perform sterilization. Doctors came from Costa Rica and El Salvador to train the IGSS doctors in this procedure, and APROFAM sent IGSS personnel to receive training at Johns Hopkins University and supported the maintenance of the equipment by a skilled technician. During the 1970s, female sterilization became an important contraceptive method at IGSS.
2. This training took place at the National Cancer Institute, then subsequently in the Central American School for Cytology, which was based at the Roosevelt Hospital in Guatemala City.
3. For example, from 1967 to 1970, APROFAM trained 85 doctors, 93 nurses, 164 auxiliary nurses, 475 social promoters, and 42 others.

References

APROFAM (Asociación Pro Bienestar de la Familia). 1971. *Informe Annual de APROFAM.* Guatemala City: APROFAM.

Arias de Blois, Jorge. 1978. *Demografía Guatemalteca 1960–1976: una bibliografía anotada.* Guatemala City: Universidad del Valle.

Burski, Cynthia. 1977. *Family Planning in Guatemala.* Consultant report. Guatemala City.

Collado, Rolando. 1968. *La Familia en Guatemala.* Guatemala City: University of San Carlos.

Galich, López Luis. 1971. "Informe de Actividades de APROFAM." Paper presented at the First National Conference on the Family, Infancy, and Youth, Council for Social Well-Being, Guatemala City, April.

MacCorquodale, Donald. 2002. "How Family Planning Came to Guatemala." Unpublished document, Guatemala City.

McLaughlin, Loretta. 1982. *The Pill, John Rock, and the Church: The Biography of a Revolution*. Boston: Little Brown and Company.

Morales, Annette de Fortin Zoila. 1970. "Salud Materno Infantíl en Guatemala." Graduating thesis, University of San Carlos, Guatemala City.

Osorio-Paz, Saul, and Bernardo Lemus-Mendoza. 1968. *Seminario sobre La Población y el Desarrollo Económico*. Guatemala City: University of San Carlos, Faculty of Economic Sciences.

Pineda, Maria Antonieta. 1977. *Juntas Directivas de APROFAM*. Guatemala City: Asociación Pro Bienestar de la Familia.

Population Reference Bureau. 2006. *World Population Data Sheet*. Washington, DC: Population Reference Bureau.

Santiso-Gálvez, Roberto, and Jane Bertrand. 2004. "The Delayed Contraceptive Revolution in Guatemala." *Human Organization* 63(1): 57–67.

10 Family Planning and the World Bank in Jamaica

TIMOTHY KING

In Jamaica, as in many countries, the pioneers of family planning were men and women who sought to improve the well-being of their impoverished women compatriots, and who perhaps were also conscious of the social threats of rapid population growth. When, eventually, population control became national policy, the relationship between the initial private programs and the national effort did not always evolve smoothly, as the Jamaican experience shows (see box 10.1 for a timeline of the main events in relation to family planning in Jamaica). A related question was whether the family planning program should be a vertical one, that is, with a staff directed toward a sole objective, or whether it should be integrated within the public health service. These issues were not unique to Jamaica, but in one respect Jamaica was distinctive: it was the setting for the World Bank's first loan for family planning activities. Family planning programs entailed public expenditures that were quite different from the infrastructure investments for which almost all Bank loans had been made, and the design and appraisal of a loan for family planning that did not violate the principles that governed Bank lending at the time required a series of decisions at the highest levels of the Bank. These decisions shaped World Bank population lending for several years and subjected the Bank to a good deal of external criticism (see, for example, the comments on the Bank's attempted loan to Iran discussed in chapter 3). For that reason, this chapter focuses on the process of making this loan.

Private Endeavors

Intellectual concern about increasing population pressures on the resources of a small, mountainous, densely populated island, dependent at that time on its exports of sugar and bananas, dates back at least to the 1930s. The birth rate then was not especially high by international standards—between 1936 and 1940, it averaged

I would like to record my gratitude to Elisa Liberatori Prati, the World Bank's chief archivist, and her staff members, especially Bertha F. Wilson, for their help in providing me with access to World Bank materials, including internal documents, which are released only on special request.

BOX 10.1 Timeline of Main Events

1939:	The Jamaica Birth Control League is formed.
1950:	Lenworth and Beth Jacobs begin family planning work in St. Ann's Parish.
1954:	The Jacobses establish a clinic in St. Ann.
1956:	The Jamaica Family Planning Association is created.
1962:	The association takes over the assets of the Jamaica Family Planning League.
1963:	The Five-Year Independence Plan notes the adverse economic effects of population growth.
1966:	The Family Planning Unit is set up in the Ministry of Health.
1967:	The National Family Planning Board is established.
January 1968:	Lenworth Jacobs becomes executive director of the National Family Planning Board.
April 1968:	Robert McNamara becomes president of the World Bank.
November 1968:	Jamaica requests a World Bank loan for family planning.
January 1969:	The World Bank sends a population review mission.
December 1969:	The World Bank sends an appraisal mission for the population project.
June 1970:	The World Bank Board of Executive Directors approves a loan for the population project.
August 1970:	The National Family Planning Board is given statutory legal status.
April 1974:	Family planning is integrated with health services.
March 1977:	The World Bank loan closes.

32.1 births per 1,000 population, having fallen from about 37 in 1921 (Zachariah 1973). However, mortality had fallen more quickly: the expectation of life at birth rose from about 35 years in 1920 to about 48 in 1940 (these figures are taken from Riley 2005, who discusses alternative estimates by different authors).

Curiously, the immediate stimulus to the first organizational attempt to encourage the use of family planning was a concern about pensions (Jacobs n.d.). Seeking money for old-age pensioners, two Jamaican women approached the Morton Jam Company in London for help, and were told that this would not be forthcoming unless Jamaica did something to control its population growth. In response, in 1939, they founded the Jamaica Family Planning League; received the support of several local leaders in different fields, including Norman Manley, a future chief minister; and opened a clinic in Kingston that provided counseling and other services.

Manley's recently formed People's National Party made birth control part of its platform (Rosen 1973) The opposing Jamaican Labour Party, formed a few years later by Alexander Bustamante, claimed that this was aimed at reducing the Negro population. The Jamaican Labour Party subsequently dropped this charge, and indeed, some 20 years later formed the government that first developed a state-financed family planning program. However, during the 18 years of democratic self-rule under the same two leaders, which saw smooth transfers of the premiership from Bustamante to Manley and back again following elections, neither party did anything about family planning. The view of the family planning movement as a racial conspiracy did not disappear, and was expressed vociferously by supporters of a black power movement in the 1970s.

A 1941 report by a government committee studying the problem of unemployment also proposed that family planning services and education should be made widely available (Rosen 1973). Nothing came of this, and neither did the Jamaica Family Planning League have any discernable effect on fertility rates (the clinics averaged about 15 family planning acceptors a month in the 1940s).[1] The birth rate rose after World War II, and reached 42.4 births per 1,000 population in 1960 (Zachariah 1973). By that time, the death rate had fallen to 8.9 deaths per 1,000 population. In the early 1960s, the natural rate of population increase (the birth rate minus the death rate) of more than 3 percent was reduced to less than 1 percent by outward migration, primarily to the United Kingdom. Even though the crude birth rate fell after 1960, the 1970 census showed that this was the result of selective emigration and changes in age structure, rather than a drop in fertility.

In 1950, a physician, Dr. Lenworth Jacobs, and his wife, Beth, started a program to supply contraceptives to public health clinics in their parish of St. Ann on the north coast of Jamaica. In 1954, they established a clinic there. They raised financing from a variety of sources, including some small American foundations. In 1956, this project evolved into the Jamaica Family Planning Association (JFPA), which became affiliated with the recently formed International Planned Parenthood Federation. In 1962, the JFPA took over the assets of the Jamaica Family Planning League. In 1964, the U.S. Agency for International Development (USAID) provided the JFPA with two mobile units, USAID's first donation of that type.[2] The Jacobses continued to be the dominant figures in Jamaica's voluntary family planning movement until 1982, shortly before Lenworth Jacobs' death.

Government Plans and Programs

The Jacobses were close to the leaders of both political parties and lobbied hard for an active government program. Catholics accounted for only 7 percent of the population in the 1960 census (Ebanks, Jacobs, and Goldson 1971), but they and others were vocal in their opposition to the Jacobses' activities, and politicians kept quiet. In the early 1960s, however, the results of a fertility and family planning survey showed that, among women of low socioeconomic status, desired family sizes were well below the current average and most Jamaican women knew little about family planning but would welcome the idea. These results contributed to a change in political attitudes (Ebanks, Jacobs, and Goldson 1971; Stycos 1964). The continuing anxiety about increasing population growth worsened after the United Kingdom passed the Commonwealth Immigration Act in 1962, making it much less likely that emigration would continue to reduce the problems of a growing labor force. The chief export earners, bauxite and tourism, provided only limited employment. Open unemployment, widely estimated during the 1960s to be 15 to 20 percent of the national labor force, was already perceived as a major social and political problem. It was highly evident in Kingston, largely reflecting out-migration from the densely populated, impoverished, small-scale agriculture sector, and was particularly bad among youth: the 1960 census showed that 40 percent of those aged 14–19 and 30 percent of those aged 20–24 were unemployed. The crime problem was severe, and was almost certainly related to these figures.

Following full independence in 1962, the Jamaican Labour Party produced the Five-Year Independence Plan, 1963–68, which contained a statement that the government recognized the adverse social and individual effects of rapid population growth and intended to promote information about family planning and its availability (Williams 1969). While this was a sign that political controversies about the issue had died down, it did not mean that all sensitivity had disappeared. The government declined to participate in a national population seminar at the University of the West Indies in June 1964 (Rosen 1973). As late as 1972, the prime minister asked Edward Seaga, the Jamaican Labour Party's finance minister, not to open a conference at the university organized by the JFPA for fear it would offend Catholics. The leader of the opposition, Michael Manley, then withdrew his agreement to be the conference's closing speaker (Jacobs n.d.).

In April 1964, the Victoria Jubilee Hospital (VJH), the island's largest maternity hospital, where some 20 to 25 percent of births took place, began a pilot postpartum intrauterine device (IUD) program with funding from the Population Council. The success of this project led some three months later to an announcement by the minister of health that family planning centers would be established in 14 government hospitals. The IUD was initially the only method offered. The announcement emphasized the voluntary nature of the program. Progress was slow, principally because of a shortage of doctors and other trained staff members, and only 6,000 IUDs were inserted during the first 15 months of the program (Williams 1969). Reports of side effects of bleeding and cramps experienced by some women made the IUD unpopular, and rumors even circulated that it caused cancer.

A further indication of public support for family planning came in 1965, when the Catholic Church opened a Kingston clinic that taught the rhythm method of contraception (Ebanks, Jacobs, and Goldson 1971). This was an era of reform in the church, and many people expected that its position on contraception would change. In 1966, a Family Planning Unit was set up inside the Ministry of Health "to coordinate the activities of the Family Planning effort and to give a sense of direction to this vital Programme" (Williams 1969, p. 140). In September 1967, the Family Planning Unit was replaced by the semi-autonomous National Family Planning Board (NFPB). The NFPB was a nine-member group of professional and business leaders who met every two to three months to set policy and approve budgets. Its members were nominated by the minister of health, who retained overall responsibility for it, and it built up its own administrative staff of more than 60 people. In January 1968, Lenworth Jacobs moved from the presidency of the JFPA to become the first executive director of the NFPB. In June 1968, the NFPB published a three-year program calling for an educational campaign, a 50 percent increase in the number of clinics providing family planning services, a program to make PAP smears freely available to all women, and the training of necessary staff members. It declared a target of reducing the birth rate to 25 by 1975. In August 1970, the

NFPB became a statutory body, although its relationship with the minister of health did not change significantly.

The number of health ministry clinics that offered family planning services increased rapidly from 25 in 1966 to 50 in 1967, 94 by January 1969, and 137 by January 1970. Typically, a health center offered one to four half-day sessions a month, although four Kingston clinics became full-time clinics. A clinic team comprised a doctor, a trained nurse, a midwife, and a records clerk, with the first two employed by the Ministry of Health and the latter two by parish councils. The contraceptive methods provided included condoms, pills, IUDs, and diaphragms and other vaginal methods. These were free of charge except for the pill, for which a nominal charge (US$0.12 per cycle) was levied, but was not enforced in the case of hardship. The VJH provided female sterilization. Abortions were not legal in Jamaica at that time, except to protect the life of the mother. The focus of the program was on women. This was a logical strategy in a society in which 70 percent of births took place outside marriage. Only 20 percent of the women of reproductive age sampled in the fertility survey in the 1950s were married, 44 percent were in common law relationships, and the remainder were in "visiting relationships." As of August 1969, more than 60 percent of acceptors were choosing the pill and about 14 percent were choosing the IUD, and as of August 1970, 47,000 women had become clients of the program, or nearly 12 percent of women aged 15–44 (Ebanks, Jacobs, and Goldson 1971).

As the NFPB was responsible to the minister of health, Jacobs' move to the NFPB might have been expected to strengthen cooperation between the ministry and the JFPA, especially as Beth Jacobs became the chief executive of the JFPA; however, rivalry between the JFPA and the ministry soon surfaced. Even though the family planning program was dependent on the physical facilities of the health services, it was operated independently with a separate budget, and grumbling emerged within the Ministry of Health about the excessive influence of the JFPA on the NFPB, and the JFPA learned that ministry officials had attempted to dissuade potential foreign donors from giving support directly to the JFPA (Jacobs n.d.).

Beginning in St. Ann in 1966, the JFPA had organized a program of so-called encouragement visitors, that is, contraceptive users with good local reputations, who, the hope was, would be persuasive advocates for the adoption of family planning methods and could provide information about the availability of services. The NFPB contracted to the JFPA the task of recruiting, training, deploying, and supervising 120 encouragement visitors, working in every parish, and paid US$30 a week. Viewed from the perspective of public health professionals in the Ministry of Health, these outreach workers looked ill-qualified. Their activities were poorly coordinated with the clinics, and they accounted for only a small proportion of program acceptors.[3] In 1969, the ministry withdrew financial support for the encouragement visitor program and it was suspended. The JFPA also entered into an agreement with the NFPB that it would not increase the number of its clinics beyond the two that it had been operating.

A number of foreign agencies assisted the activities of the NFPB and the JFPA and also helped the University of the West Indies with population research. The USAID provided contraceptives, equipment, and various consultant services. The Ford Foundation provided consultant assistance for record keeping and evaluation and grants for training and research. The Population Council provided IUDs and support for postpartum programs. In addition, the Pathfinder Fund, the International Planned Parenthood Federation, the Rockefeller Foundation, the Pan American Health Organization, the United Nations Population Fund, and the Church World Service were also involved. By far the largest source of foreign money, however, was distinctly unusual, and was not a donation. It was a loan of US$2 million from the World Bank to the government of Jamaica.

The World Bank and Population

The World Bank's Board of Executive Directors approved the loan on June 16, 1970. This was the World Bank's first population project. Its content was largely dictated by an attempt to retain normal Bank lending practices in a sector that differed sharply from other areas of lending. To understand this, one needs to know something of the Bank's history, its procedures and their rationale, and also why the Bank decided to enter an area of activity for which it might appear to have been ill-suited. Indeed, the approved project was something that would have been almost unimaginable some 30 months earlier.

At that time, December 1967, President Lyndon Johnson's surprising nomination of his secretary of defense, Robert McNamara, for President of the World Bank had just been approved by the World Bank's Executives Board. (By tradition the President of the World Bank) is nominated by the United States and the Managing Director of the International Monetary Fund has been a European. McNamara would leave the Pentagon in February and go to the World Bank in April. The Bank was an institution well known to specialists on economic development, and to finance ministers and central bank governors, who were its ex officio governors and who met annually at the joint meetings the Bank held with the more publicly famous International Monetary Fund. However, few others, especially in Europe and North America, would have had any conception of the nature of the organization that was to be led by a man with one of the most recognizable names on the planet.

The International Monetary Fund and the World Bank were created in July 1944 at Bretton Woods, New Hampshire, by an international conference whose aim was to design the rules and institutions needed to ensure that the postwar international economy would function much more successfully than the prewar one had done. It was obvious that the need for investment funds both for the rebuilding of war-shattered economies and for longer-term development would be huge, and that the governments with the most urgent need to borrow externally would not have the creditworthiness to do so, at least on reasonable terms. The role of the World Bank—formally the International Bank for Reconstruction and Development (IBRD)—was to borrow in capital markets under the guarantee of its shareholders, of which by far the largest was (and remains) the United States, and to re-lend the proceeds to countries that the capital markets did not perceive as creditworthy. Close scrutiny by the Bank of both its clients' economic prospects and the prospective use to be made of its loans would ensure that its money would contribute to the reconstruction or long-term development of its clients' economies and that they would therefore be able to service the loans. Loans were normally to be made to public sector entities, and at the very least required a government guarantee. (In 1956, the Bank created a subsidiary, the International Finance Corporation, that could lend to the private sector without a government guarantee.)

The Bank opened for business in 1946. Its first four operations were program loans for reconstruction in Europe, and such lending continued into the 1950s. These would subsequently be regarded as a necessary departure from the real purpose of the Bank which, as specified in its Articles of Agreement, was to finance the foreign exchange content of investment projects, with local cost financing only "in exceptional circumstances." The Bank soon began to make only project-specific loans to developing countries, principally for infrastructure and public utilities, and, to a lesser degree, for industry and agriculture. Once an investments project was completed, the loan was closed; the country had itself to provide the finance to operate it (unless it generated enough revenue on its own); consequently, the Bank did not finance operating (recurrent) costs. The Bank developed in-house expertise and a consultant network that could help governments analyze the trade-offs involved in the choice of expenditure priorities and the selection and design of individual projects. Its ability to bring a comparative perspective to its analytical work was one of its most useful features, but the Bank could only retain a critical mass of specialized experts by concentrating them at its Washington headquarters, paying fairly generous salaries, and requiring a great amount of international travel. At the time, each project was reviewed at several levels inside the Bank before the borrowing country was invited to Washington to negotiate the final loan agreement, which was then discussed by the Bank's Board of Executive Directors before final approval. All this meant that the costs associated with each project were inevitably high. The Bank had to meet all its costs from a modest spread between its borrowing and lending rates: until 1964, loans were made at a rate of 1.25 percent above the cost of IBRD borrowing, repayable over 15 to 25 years, with a three- to five-year grace period. Subsequent methods of determining the lending rate reduced this spread. This meant that there was a minimum size of loan that the Bank was prepared to consider. The US$2 million size of the Jamaica population project was close to what was considered at the time the lowest reasonable amount for a loan.

The Bank also had another reason for having a minimum size of loan. This was a Bank desire for what was described in staff discussions as "leverage." This term would probably be regarded as politically incorrect nowadays, and the chapter author felt mildly shocked by it when he joined the World Bank in 1969, but its use was by no means sotto voce (see Mason and Asher 1973, pp. 420–56, for a discussion of the implications). The Bank saw its policy recommendations in its sectoral analyses as more than advice that a prospective borrower could take or leave—the recommendations were often turned into conditions that had to be met before a particular stage in the loan process was completed. There could be conditions to be met before a borrower was invited to negotiate the project, conditions before a negotiated project was sent to the Bank's board for approval (and until fairly recently almost every project was formally presented at a board meeting), conditions before a signed loan could be made effective and disbursement could start, and later conditions before disbursements on particular components of the project could take place. Formal loan agreements have often been supplemented by side letters describing agreed expectations concerning such things as the reorganization of key institutions and the agreement of the government to provide the required local cost financing. Conditions attached to loans have meant that the supervision of an agreed loan has been much more than a monitoring of progress: it has often involved periodic renegotiation of aspects of the loan agreement that later appeared to be unworkable or to be causing an unreasonable delay in reaping the benefits of the project. The Bank felt that a minimum size of project was essential for it to be able to impose its conditions—intended to be in the borrower's interests, but often requiring politically difficult actions—on the borrower.[4]

The Bank's need to be satisfied that future economic prospects made its loans serviceable required it to develop a capacity to analyze such prospects in considerable detail and to determine how alternative policies might affect them. Country reports have usually been discussed with senior government officials, and many undoubtedly found these discussions useful. Until program lending returned in about 1980, initially as a measure to deal with the international debt crisis, Bank loans normally did not include general policy conditions, but the size of its lending program might be influenced by its views on economic strategy and management. The possibility that the Bank might consider a country's population policy in deciding the size of the lending program became an active issue when the Bank entered the field.

The Bank kept a group of economists organizationally apart from its operational staff. They provided support to operational missions, but as the Bank had an enormous need for knowledge about economic development, the group also carried out various pieces of research, although no systematic research program existed until the early 1970s. Interestingly, while most of the Bank's research activities were on topics closely related to its lending or country analysis and while population policy did not begin to interest the Bank (officially) until 1968, the Bank provided both much of the finance and some of the research assistance for a seminal study of India's population prospects in the mid-1950s (Coale and Hoover 1958).

By the late 1950s, the capacity of the poorest countries, especially in South Asia, to service additional debt on regular World Bank terms was becoming severely limited. In 1960, the International Development Association (IDA), replenished every three years by grants from the richer Bank member countries, was organized to make soft loans that carried only a 0.75 percent service charge, originally repayable over 50 years with a 10-year grace period. (Subsequently, the loan period was shortened, varying according to the income level of the country.) Membership of the IBRD and IDA is almost identical, no distinction is made between the staff of each, and only the terms of lending differentiate IBRD and IDA projects.[5] The time discounting applied to the flow of economic benefits from a project, usually calculated using market or international prices, is the same for both types of projects. IDA resources have always been tightly constrained, and therefore available only to the relatively poor World Bank member countries.

The economic condition of a country, and not the nature of a project, is what determines its eligibility to receive IDA loans. Jamaica has never been eligible for IDA loans. At the time of the population loan to Jamaica, it had one of the highest per capita incomes in Latin America and the Caribbean, and there was never any possibility that the loan could be made on anything other than normal IBRD terms. This constraint on the Bank's lending activities was widely misunderstood outside the Bank, and misplaced criticism was eventually leveled at the Bank, especially by Ray Ravenholt, the head of the USAID's population program, with respect to the terms under which the Bank made some of its population loans.

Beginning in the early 1960s, agriculture expanded significantly as an area of lending. In 1962, the Bank made its first loan for an education project. This was its first activity in a social sector, but the strong recognition that an increase in human capital was a vital necessity for rapid economic development meant that this was less of a departure from previous lending policies than might at first appear: the justification for education loans frequently pointed to identifiable needs for a trained workforce. The education lending program concentrated on vocational and technical education and training and on general secondary education. The actual project components normally included buildings, for which the Bank had well-established operational procedures.

The Bank's decision to finance family planning resulted solely from the conviction about the seriousness of the world population problems that McNamara brought to the Bank. In his first 42 months at the World Bank, McNamara made eight major speeches. Four of these were to the annual meetings of the Board of Governors, one was in Buenos Aires to the Inter-American Press Association, one was to the New York Bond Club, and two were in academic settings (McNamara 1981). In his first speech as president, he announced that the Bank would lend for population planning. Except for his speech to the Bond Club, he made population issues a major part of all these speeches; indeed, this was the only topic of his speech at Notre Dame University in May 1969. The speech to the Bond Club was intended to reassure the Bank's creditors that in seeking to emphasize that the Bank was a development agency as well as a financial institution, and to double its lending, it was not in any way doing anything that would reduce its creditworthiness. Though not focusing on population, McNamara noted that "loans in the field of family planning have perhaps the highest economic returns of all" (McNamara 1981, p. 64). By 1971, even those Bank officials most sympathetic to the message were seriously concerned that on matters of population, McNamara was starting to sound like a cracked gramophone record.

Many others, both outside and inside the Bank, shared McNamara's deep concern about population growth. Indeed, there was a consensus on the issue in what might be termed the "liberal development community," of which McNamara would shortly become the most publicly prominent member. Speculating which of the many possible sources had the greatest influence on McNamara is both useless and irrelevant, but they were clearly external to the Bank. One of the outside gurus was Barbara Ward, who had been close to the Kennedys. Another was Hollis Chenery of Harvard, who McNamara brought to the Bank in 1970 to create an internal policy staff in whom he had confidence. McNamara also read widely, and he interacted with the Ford Foundation, which had become active in the field. There were also others whose instincts were not necessarily liberal: parts of the U.S. defense community were concerned about the effects of hungry, unemployed individuals on the stability of governments, and potentially on world peace, which could damage the security and prosperity of the United States. McNamara himself had linked security concerns with development in a speech in Montreal in May 1966: "In a modernizing society, security means development. . . . Without development there can be no security. A developing nation that does not in fact develop simply cannot remain secure" (Shapley 1993, p. 381).

In their history of the World Bank, Kapur, Lewis, and Webb (1997) see McNamara's concern with population in the context of the Bank's growing concern with poverty alleviation as an explicit development objective, separate from, and not necessarily totally complementary to, overall economic growth. They describe the years 1959–60 under the title "Approaching the Poor" and the early years of McNamara's presidency as "Poverty Moves Up." In their analysis, McNamara's concern with population was his first approach to his concern with poverty and inequality, stemming at least partly from the growing focus on these issues in the United States. Once the Bank began to focus on small farmers and the direct attack on poverty, Kapur, Lewis, and Webb (1997) suggest that the emphasis on population control fell off rapidly after 1970. While this may be broadly true for the Bank as an institution, it was not true for McNamara, and he made it the focus of his next major speech in an academic setting—his address to the Massachusetts Institute of Technology in April 1977—and his population speeches began not with references to poverty, but to the accelerating rate of increase of the global population.

McNamara was, of course, the ultimate "can-do" man: if a problem existed, a solution had to be found. If it was a development problem, and the World Bank was a development agency, then the Bank had to help achieve the solution. One of the things it could do was to include analysis of the issue in economic reports to show how population growth was impeding the achievement of other objectives and to spur governments to adopt policies to control this growth. This led to the suspicion that the Bank might make population policy part of its assessment of the creditworthiness of a country, or even a condition for lending. The Bank found itself continually denying that any such link existed. Where the idea originated is not clear, although this author was once told that it might have come from a casual remark McNamara once made at a senior staff meeting. In any case, at the 1969 annual meetings, a group of Latin American countries plus the Philippines joined in a statement that said that they understood that the Bank was not making lending conditional on specific family planning programs, because any such link would be unacceptable. The statement was read again at the board meeting that approved the first population project. However, the rumors never went away: some time in the mid-1970s, a journalist, looking for muck to rake, asked this author whether such a link was World Bank policy.

Of course, the Bank could also support fertility reduction policies directly by lending for family planning programs. Then the question arises why, if the president was concerned about stressing the global as well as the developmental aspects of the problem and the major contributors to global population growth were in South Asia and Indonesia, was the first country to which the World Bank made a loan a small Caribbean island? One might have expected that the answer to this would be "this is a new topic and we are feeling our way: let's get our feet wet in a small country with an established program so that we can learn how to do it." Alternatively, the Bank might have sounded out several potential borrowers and Jamaica was the only one to respond positively. This was not the way it happened.

The Jamaica Population Project

In May 1968, a World Bank country economic mission visited Jamaica. Except for an agricultural specialist from the Food and Agriculture Organization of the United Nations, with which the Bank had a cooperative program, its six members were all drawn from the Bank's staff. Despite the absence of a specialist on population matters, the mission's report, no doubt picking up on the evident interest of the new president of the Bank, devoted roughly similar space to population control as it did to each of the key productive sectors of agriculture, mining, and tourism and considerably more than to industry. Members of the mission appear to have been the first to suggest the possibility of a family planning project.

On September 30, McNamara opened his first annual meetings with a speech that included the statement that the Bank was seeking opportunities to finance facilities required for family planning. This possibility was immediately raised with Edward Seaga, Jamaica's minister of finance, who was attending the meeting, and with other officials of his ministry. In November, the Ministry of Finance formally requested an expert to help prepare a project. Bank staff members have often been criticized for trying to persuade reluctant governments to borrow for projects, both to further their own careers and, more altruistically, to enable the Bank to stay in business, so it should be stressed that the ministry was always totally committed to its desire for a Bank population project.

The Bank felt that it first needed to review the program in some detail and agree on an action plan for at least three years. Inquiries were made of the Population Council and others concerning suitable experts. Eventually, Sam Keeny, who had extensive experience as an adviser in Taiwan, China, led the mission, which included Dr. K. Kanagaratnam, who was in charge of Singapore's extremely successful family planning program. The Pan American Health Organization provided a consultant, and the mission included two Bank staff members. The government was happy to accept such a mission, but it did ask (verbally) that publicity be minimized. This suited the Bank well, as even though its president had just very publicly committed it to lend for family planning, none of its staff members had any idea what such a project might look like.

One major question the Bank had to consider before any discussion of a possible project could take place was what could the Bank lend for? The Bank was set up to finance the foreign component of capital investment projects, including, where necessary, the remuneration of foreign experts. The major public expenditures of a family planning project are wages, salaries, and contraceptive supplies. While the emigration of doctors and nurses was a continual problem for Jamaica, there was never any suggestion that the program itself needed foreign medical personnel. Contraceptives were being provided, or at least subsidized, through external grants. Moreover, the budget of the program was modest compared with the normal size of any loan: estimates indicated that during its 1968 fiscal year (April 1968–March 1969), the NFPB would spend no more than US$360,000, although it had a budget of US$480,000.[6]

The World Bank Loan Committee thoroughly discussed the question in December 1968. The Loan Committee was the ultimate authority on loans and lending policy below the level of the president and had to clear all prospective loans before they were sent to the board. The committee's chair was the vice president in charge of all the Bank's operational work, including both its lending and its country economic work, and committee members were, for the most part, responsible for its programs in different regions of the world. An area department (from 1972 a regional vice presidency) presented a project to the board (and previously to the Loan Committee) supported by relevant project staff members. In the case of the Jamaica project, this meant that its protagonist was the Western Hemisphere Department, which argued that the normal restrictions on lending for local or operating costs should be waived in the case of family planning projects. If the Bank confined itself to financing only the capital costs of facilities, vehicles, and expatriate personnel, even financing 100 percent of the proposed project would amount to only about US$300,000 over three years. With such a small input, the Bank would have little leverage. The department also argued that operating costs during the early years of a program could be treated as an investment in view of their lasting contribution to the program and pointed to precedents in road maintenance projects. However, some Loan Committee members felt that financing local operating costs could damage the Bank's image and standing in the financial community. It was also argued that limited eligibility for Bank financing should not deter Bank assistance if it were needed, and that the ineligible parts might obtain alternative sources of finance such as grants. It was agreed to leave the question open until the report by the review mission, which would be asked not to discuss the possible scope of Bank finance with the Jamaican authorities.

The review mission traveled to Jamaica in late January, and its draft report was ready to be sent to the government of Jamaica in March. It praised the government's commitment, and felt that the climate for acceptance of family planning was favorable. It was, however, critical of a lack of focus on recruiting and on following up individual women, noting that the program was "clinic centered rather than people centered." It recommended that the responsibilities for the field program should be transferred from the NFPB to a family planning department in the Ministry of Health, which would supervise the encouragement visitors, gradually increase their number, and improve their training. The NFPB would carry out educational and media activities aimed at raising public knowledge of and support for the program, design training programs, and provide technical advice to the proposed family planning department. The NFPB would also evaluate the program's progress against local targets that it would set, monitor service statistics on a timely basis to diagnose emerging problems and identify how to deal with them, and carry out periodic sample surveys. In addition to these major recommendations, the report made a large number of individual ones, especially in annexes devoted to evaluation and training.

The report then made a number of suggestions concerning physical facilities. It proposed an extension to the VJH, which was so overcrowded that 50 percent of mothers left less than 24 hours after delivery and many had to share beds. Postpartum acceptance of family planning was consequently only 5 to 6 percent of these mothers compared with 30 to 50 percent in other programs. The cost of the proposed extension was estimated at about US$300,000. The apparently large unmet demand for hospital deliveries led the report to suggest improvements to other maternity facilities, including the establishment of small maternity homes in remote rural areas, at an estimated total cost of US$400,000. On the basis of experience with education lending, the report estimated that the foreign component of this US$700,000 program would be around 30 percent. The report also suggested the possibility of a new training school for nurses at a cost estimated by the government of US$2 million.

The ball was thus passed back to the Loan Committee. In its presentation to the Loan Committee meeting in March, the Western Hemisphere Department argued that the government was more likely to implement the recommendations of the report satisfactorily if the Bank stayed involved. To achieve adequate leverage, the Bank should be willing to finance a larger percentage of the cost of facilities than usual—perhaps 90 percent. The chair of the Loan Committee endorsed this proposal with respect to facilities related to mother and child health. Others argued that, looking beyond Jamaica, many poor countries in need of family planning programs did not have the resources to fund their local operating costs, and therefore if the Bank were to lend for family planning projects, it would be less distorting to finance these costs, rather than look for facilities. They also argued that all family planning expenditures could be defined as investments being made to produce a final output—an averted birth— rather than recurrent with respect to that output. The chair mentioned the possibility of using grant financing from Bank profits to cover the current expenditures of family planning programs.[7] The chair decided that the president's guidance was required.

As it had been McNamara who had caused the Loan Committee to face this issue, as its members were clearly divided, and as he was personally interested in population issues, referring the matter to him was an obvious thing to do. The minutes of the Loan Committee noted that at the meeting with the chair, the president had said that he was prepared to support a loan of US$500,000 for health facilities associated with the Jamaica family planning project, whose total cost was estimated at US$700,000. The minutes go on to say: "He expressed doubts about the desirability in general of using Bank loans to finance recurrent expenditures on family planning programs, and in any case felt that so far as Jamaica was concerned, there would be no justification for this approach." Subsequently, the chair and the president took up the subject again. Clearly, the issue was capital versus operating costs rather than foreign versus local expenditures. In August, the chair informed the area department that the president was prepared to finance 70 percent of a suitable project, even if foreign costs were a smaller proportion, without the need to make a special country case to finance local costs.

This was the probably the most critical decision in the early history of the World Bank's involvement with population programs. Some years later, as the Bank began to make poverty alleviation a central concern, this constraint would be relaxed, but not so completely that it could be taken for granted: an explicit case had to be made. One can readily speculate about the competing influences on the president's decision. It came just little more than a month before he was due to make two major speeches: the first, at Notre Dame University, which focused entirely on population, and the second to the New York Bond Club, which was designed to reassure the financial community that his proposed new lending would not damage the Bank's creditworthiness. It needs also to be stressed, however, that the chair of the Loan Committee— a man whose experience, judgment, and personal qualities probably made him the most respected member of the Bank staff—while no doubt presenting both sides of the issue to the president, almost certainly favored this outcome.

The Loan Committee meeting also included the first of many discussions on the methodology of quantitative project evaluation and justification. (The report had included a brief, almost back-of-the-envelope, calculation of the benefit-cost ratio of averting a birth.) At this time in the Bank's history, it did not finance health services directly, so any contribution that a project made to the health or comfort of its beneficiaries was (formally) ignored. Some five years later, the Bank specifically addressed the issue of direct lending for health in a paper discussed by the board and subsequently published (World Bank 1975). It noted that an increasing number of Bank-assisted projects had health aspects, especially those for water supply and sanitation and family planning, including specific health components of poverty-oriented projects in both rural and urban areas. The paper recommended that health impacts should be more explicitly analyzed, and that within the existing pattern of lending, project design should increasingly include interventions to improve the health status of low-income populations. Although it did not rule out eventual direct lending for health projects, which indeed arrived in 1979, it argued against introducing such projects at that time.

In April 1968, when McNamara arrived in the Bank, only one staff member could have been regarded as a population specialist. George C. Zaidan had recently arrived in the Special Studies Division of the Economics Department, fresh from writing a Harvard doctoral thesis on the cost-benefit analysis of family planning, with special reference to Egypt. A minor reorganization of the department led to the creation of a Population Studies Division, headed by E. K. Hawkins, with Hawkins and Zaidan as its founding members. This served as the first focal point for all population activities, whether representing the Bank at international meetings or handling the early moves toward lending, but technical work on lending was at that time done in specialized project departments. These were organizationally quite distinct from country departments, which were responsible for agreeing on a proposed lending program with governments.[8] The implications of a decision to lend for family planning meant that the Bank needed a population projects department. During his participation in the review mission to Jamaica, Kanagaratnam was informally invited to head such a department, and he accepted.

The choice of a physician, with a background in family planning oriented toward maternal and child health, in combination with the decision on what the Bank could lend for, clearly influenced the direction that Bank lending activities took, and the policies it recommended, at a time when family planning specialists disagreed about the merits of vertical family planning programs versus integration with health services. Kanagaratnam could not leave Singapore for several months, and so relied heavily on staff members borrowed from elsewhere, especially from the Population Studies Division. Zaidan left the Population Studies Division to become the first division chief in the new department.

The area department sent the review mission's report to the minister of finance in late April. The accompanying letter summarized the Bank's conception of a small project. It also said that further consideration could not be given to the nurses' training school until a feasibility study had been carried out. If this suggested that the training school was justified, it could be included in the education project then under preparation. A few weeks later, as part of their periodic discussions of the lending program with the government, area department representatives discussed these proposals with both the finance and health ministers, who reacted positively to the suggestion of a family planning project, although they queried the proposal to expand the number of health centers. The minister of health sharply disagreed about the proposal to transfer field operations from the NFPB to the Ministry of Health on the grounds that the NFPB had been too recently established, that he was proposing steps to improve the quality of its management, and that his own ministry was weak and did not have the capacity to handle new responsibilities. These were technical issues outside the area department's competence, and it was agreed that Kanagaratnam, though not yet formally in his new position, would visit Jamaica to discuss them.

These discussions took place in July. The Bank accepted that the NFPB would retain its field responsibilities, but stressed that it had to be strengthened and reorganized and put on a statutory basis. Eventually, this became a condition of loan effectiveness. Kanagaratnam was accompanied by a Bank architect. The location of the extension to the VJH was moved, and it was considerably expanded from 100 beds to 160 beds, effectively doubling its capacity and increasing estimated costs more than proportionately. The new extension would include a midwifery school. Together with a suggested 10 rural maternity centers and some improvement and expansion of health services, total project costs were now estimated at US$2 million. This was the core of the proposal that the Bank sent a mission to appraise in December.

During appraisal, a software component was added to complement what had hitherto been only a hardware bricks-and-mortar project. Project components that would provide borrowers with foreign consultant services were common in Bank projects, and their existence would provide the Bank with a defense against a criticism that later surfaced during the board approval process that this was merely a hospital project. There was to be a study of whether some rearrangement of the professional functions of doctors, nurses, and midwives might be cost-effective and ease staff shortages. A short-term training adviser to the NFPB was suggested, as was a study of the optimum use of family planning staff members and facilities in Kingston. The Bank appraisal team developed these recommendations, followed up by a quick visit to Jamaica in March. Some attempt was made to get these funded by grants from other agencies, such as the USAID, but this was unsuccessful and they remained in the project.

Significantly, the project did not propose any long-term, resident foreign assistance; Jamaicans could continue to run their own show. A requirement that the Bank approve the appointment of the chief executive of the newly restructured NFPB was contentious, but remained in the loan agreement. Closely related to this was another software component: an annual external review. At the board meeting to approve the project, at least one executive director felt that follow-up should have been left to the Jamaican government, as some of the topics on which the review might focus, as described by the appraisal report, required the collection of what the executive director called "bedroom statistics," an invasion of privacy made worse if carried out by a foreign agency.

Between appraisal and the board meeting, detailed questions arose concerning project preparation, but the main Washington issue was how the project would be justified to the board. A detailed analysis of the benefits of averting a birth was prepared by the present author and widely discussed in the Bank (a preliminary version was published as King 1970). For the first time in such analyses, it distinguished social benefits from those to the family concerned. No attempt was made to hide the major limitations of the analysis: there was no way to guess how much expenditures on maternity facilities would lead to family planning acceptance and the aversion of births, and ignoring the benefits to the health and comfort of the patients involved could give an unfortunate impression. Moreover, before comparing the costs and benefits of a proposed project, the analyst normally needs to be satisfied that its design is cost-effective with respect to its major objective. Nobody could pretend that the proposed expenditures were the most cost-effective way of increasing family planning acceptance. There were always likely to be limits to how much a purely postpartum program could achieve in situations where most women preferred oral contraception. The Bank did indeed get an agreement that, by November 1970, the NFPB would produce plans for the restoration of an outreach program.

The intellectual attention given to the issue was considerable, and when the project documents went to the Loan Committee, they included an annex that provided a quantitative justification for the project. It showed that despite ignoring benefits to health and well-being, the economic benefits to averting a birth were large. The committee was split on whether the annex should be included. The majority felt it provided support to what the president had been saying in his speeches. The president and the chair, however, decided that the detailed economic analysis was potentially contentious and should be omitted. Only a broad socioeconomic justification was eventually provided to the board.

Postscript

As this book is primarily concerned with the 1960s, ending the story on the high note of board approval in June 1970 is tempting. (It also marks the end of this author's involvement with the Jamaican program.) Both the Bank and the government had good reasons to be optimistic about both the family planning program and the project. Potential opposition from the Catholic Church and the far left did not appear to threaten the broad political support for the program, and the main condition on which the Bank loan was granted—that the semi-autonomy of the NFPB be confirmed in a statute—followed soon after the loan was approved and signed.

From a project perspective, this optimism proved unjustified. The project closed in March 1977 because the loan had been fully disbursed, although the investments made under the project had not yet been completed. By that time, Bank policy dictated that one to two years after project completion, its Operations Evaluation Department would carry out an audit, discuss its findings with the government, and report these to the board. The audit report was issued in June 1979, and not surprisingly, it was highly critical.

The major problem had been the implementation of the project's hardware components. The appraisal report had laid out a tentative project timetable, showing that construction of the rural maternity centers would be completed in January 1972 and the VJH extension and related work would be finished by September 1973. The rural maternity centers were delayed and, when completed, were considerably underused, and most were eventually converted into multiple-purpose health centers. Cost inflation made the loan size inadequate, and when the project closed, the VJH extension was far from finished. Indeed, it had not been completed by the time of the audit report. The audit report noted that the VJH project was commonly referred to in parliament and by senior officials as a disaster. However, the causes of the construction delays had nothing to do with population. Some, such as the impossibility of supervising construction work at the site for a year because of strikes and political instability, were clearly external to the project. Other problems were attributed to the fact that a newly formed Bank department and inexperienced implementing institutions did not draw sufficiently on accumulated World Bank or Jamaican project expertise and experience, and that project management had therefore been weak.

The audit also discussed the software components, and in so doing questioned the wisdom of integrating a vertical family planning program with health services. When the program was originally recommended by the first World Bank mission, the minister of health had rejected this suggestion, but an understanding emerged that movement toward it would gradually take place. This was reinforced when it became evident that providing the NFPB with statutory semi-autonomy had not improved its management of the vertical program. The first and only review by external experts in June 1972 was critical of its performance. Jacobs had been replaced as executive director, but remained in his old office as medical director, and the NFPB still operated in an ad hoc way, without any sort of long-term plan. In addition, greater liaison between the Ministry of Health and the NFPB, which should have been making better use of the ministry's clinics, was seriously needed. About 60 percent of the health staff had not received training in family planning.

In contrast to the Bank's expectations, the NFPB had not revived the encouragement visitor program and instead had employed a smaller number of family planning education officers and assistants. The absence of its capacity to follow up program acceptors could be seen in the high dropout rate. The early 1970s saw about 22,000 to 25,000 new acceptors of family planning each year—around 7 percent of the female population aged 15–44—but estimates indicated that the proportion of the age cohort in the program rose only from 9 percent in 1970 to 11 percent in 1974. The external review suggested that at least 200 home visitors were needed.

The review did note one considerable improvement: the postpartum program. Postpartum staff members provided information to 70 percent of postpartum cases in 1970, and estimates suggested that 30 percent of all patients referred accepted family planning. Another calculation was that 19 percent of deliveries at that time led to family planning acceptance. As this was well before any new facilities had been completed, it illustrated the relatively weak link between investment under the World Bank project and family planning acceptance.

In its response to the review, the government noted that it was already training 300 community health aides and intended to increase this number significantly. Its long-term plan eventually called for more than 2,000 of these aides. This strategy implied increasing integration of the family planning program with general health services, a move that formally took place in 1974 with the transfer of the NFPB's 143 family planning education workers to the Ministry of Health. (The NFPB continued to exist, concerned primarily with information, education, and communication activities and evaluation.)

The integration with the health services may have reflected less the World Bank's original recommendation than political necessity. In the early 1970s, charges from the black power movement that family planning was a racist plot intensified, and a single-purpose program was politically exposed. This also contributed to the government's reluctance to use foreign advice, leading to the curtailment of some of the advisory services suggested in the project. The audit report felt that integration had reduced the attention paid to family planning, as the medical staff had other priorities and the community workers were poorly trained, and it pointed to a fall-off in the number of new acceptors after 1975.[9] Although the crude birth rate had not fallen as much as the NFPB originally hoped (from 35 live births per 1,000 population in 1968 to 25 in 1975), the audit report noted that it had dropped to about 30 in 1974, but had then leveled off.

Just as it was possible to be overly optimistic in 1970, it was easy to be too pessimistic in 1979. The rationale for integration in a country with a well-established network of clinics was a strong one, especially in the political climate of 1974. In the second half of the 1970s, clinic-based family services were supplemented by a successful USAID-assisted program to expand the commercial distribution of contraceptives. Crude birth rates are a poor indicator of fertility, and year-to-year variations can be particularly misleading. Fertility fell significantly in the 1970s: the total fertility rate, which had averaged almost 5.8 births per woman in 1965–69, averaged 5.0 in 1970–74 and 4.0 in 1975–79 (United Nations Department of Economic and Social Affairs 2005).[10] This timing strongly suggests that the increased availability of family planning must have contributed to this fertility decline, even if identifying which particular piece of program effort had the greatest effect is impossible. Fertility has continued to decline. Most recent estimates suggest that the total fertility rate is now about 2.4.[11]

Could lessons have been derived from these early years of the Jamaican program or from the World Bank's attempt to assist this program and were they? In Jamaica, the success of the postpartum program led to its extension to five other hospitals in 1973–74, but understanding had increased that a postpartum program, especially where pills are the female contraceptive of choice, needs effective follow-up, and that hospital and activities should only be part of a larger set of family planning activities in which commercial distribution is also highly important. The Bank, for its part, increasingly recognized that population control was a more complex and difficult affair than its first project had implied, and its projects began to put much more emphasis on software, especially training, research and evaluation, and technical assistance. These were important components of a second population project for Jamaica, presented to the Bank's board in June 1976. This project's primary focus was on integrating family planning with maternal and child health, including the improvement of nutrition, which had become a permissible objective of direct Bank lending. The Bank would finance the introduction of an integrated scheme in one county on a trial basis, designed to be replicable islandwide if it proved successful. Roughly 20 percent of the foreign costs, almost all financed by the Bank, were for technical assistance.

For this second project, the Bank also financed only foreign capital costs. In subsequent years, the rigidities implied by the Bank's willingness to finance some types of government expenditures and not others (irrespective of the need for them to achieve project objectives) would be increasingly relaxed, especially the distinction between local and foreign costs. They did not disappear for many years, however, and this highly desirable change in the Bank's investment lending policies therefore cannot be said to have been a result of this project.[12]

Notes

1. These figures are taken from an unpublished World Bank report. Many of the statistics used in this chapter are similarly taken from unpublished World Bank reports, which, in turn, have drawn on both published and unpublished local, mostly government, sources, and I have not usually identified the report from which a particular item of information is taken or its original source.
2. Jacobs (n.d.) says that this was the USAID's first donation, but whether this was of mobile units or more generally the first for family planning activities is not clear.
3. Acceptance data showed that only 16 percent of new acceptors in 1969, and only 4 percent in 1970, identified encouragement visitors as their source of referral (Rosen 1973), but these low figures may have reflected the disruption to the encouragement visitor program.
4. The justification for exerting leverage was not so much that the wisdom of World Bank staff members was greater than that of ministers or civil servants, but that in circumstances where some ministries (usually sectoral ones) were reluctant to carry out a necessary but politically unpopular measure favored by other ministries (typically the ministry of finance), Bank conditions could increase the pressure to do the right thing.
5. Formally, the two are separate legal entities, both part of the World Bank Group. Unless otherwise specified, or obvious from the context, the term World Bank usually refers to the World Bank Group rather than to the IBRD.
6. For comparison, the JFPA's budget was US$177,000.
7. At this time, the World Bank's profits were extremely high and the Bank had no clear policy on what to do with them. In later years, the Bank decided to devote some of these to increasing the size of IDA—its soft loan funds. In some later years, during a period of high interest rates in most of the countries in which the Bank borrowed, its profitability enabled it to set interest rates below its marginal cost of borrowing. Eventually, the Bank's major shareholders decided that it should return to the practice of relating interest rates mechanically to the cost of borrowing.
8. This was to ensure that projects' technical quality would not be compromised by considerations arising from other aspects of World Bank–country relations. In an organization that prided itself on systematic and careful analysis of alternative choices among conflicting objectives, occasional disputes between project departments and country departments were both inevitable and desirable. The trouble was that the arrangement meant that nobody below the chair of the Loan Committee had the power to resolve such disputes. A 1972 reorganization placed major project departments under the jurisdiction of five regional vice presidents.

9. Data from unpublished sources differ markedly on the extent of the decline in acceptance under the official program. Robinson (1981) reports service statistics that show a smaller fall in 1976 than does the audit report and a marked rise rather than a fall in 1977.
10. A total fertility rate of 2.1 is normally considered to be replacement rate.
11. This is the estimate in the international database of the U.S. Bureau of the Census and is consistent with the United Nations data cited.
12. The author would like to thank Tatiana Proskuryakova for providing a statement of the Bank's financing policies, approved in 2004, that is quite explicit that the Bank is now prepared to finance both local and recurrent costs of its projects.

References

Coale, Ansley J., and Edgar M. Hoover. 1958. *Population Growth and Economic Development in Low-Income Countries: A Case Study of India's Prospects.* Princeton, NJ: Princeton University Press.

Ebanks, G. E., Lenworth M. Jacobs, and Sylvia Goldson. 1971. *Jamaica.* Country Profiles Series. New York: Population Council.

Jacobs, Beth. N.d. (but probably 1996). *A History of Voluntary Family Planning in Jamaica.* St. Ann's Bay, Jamaica: Jamaica Family Planning Association.

Kapur, Devesh, John P. Lewis, and Richard Webb. 1997. *The World Bank: Its First Half Century.* Washington, DC: Brookings Institution Press.

King, Timothy. 1970. "The Measurement of the Economic Benefits from Family Planning Programs and Projects." Working Paper 71, World Bank, Economics Department, Washington, DC.

Mason, Edward S., and Robert E. Asher. 1973. *The World Bank Since Bretton Woods.* Washington, DC: Brookings Institution.

McNamara, Robert S. 1981. *The McNamara Years at the World Bank.* Baltimore, MD: Johns Hopkins University Press.

Riley, James C. 2005. *Poverty and Life Expectancy: The Jamaica Paradox.* Cambridge, U.K.: Cambridge University Press.

Robinson, W. 1981. *A Cost-Benefit Analysis of the Proposed Jamaica Family Planning Project.* Washington, DC: American Public Health Association.

Rosen, Robert C. 1973. *Law and Population Growth in Jamaica.* Law and Population Programme Monograph 10. Medford, MA: Tufts University, Fletcher School of Law and Diplomacy.

Shapley, Deborah. 1993. *Promise and Power: The Life and Times of Robert McNamara.* Boston: Little Brown.

Stycos, J. M. 1964. *The Control of Human Fertility in Jamaica.* Ithaca, NY: Cornell University Press.

United Nations Department of Economic and Social Affairs. 2005. *World Population Prospects.* New York: United Nations.

Williams, L. L. 1969. "Jamaica: Crisis on a Small Island." In *Population: Changing World Crisis,* ed. Bernard Berelson, 123–32. Voice of America Forum Lectures. Washington, DC: Voice of America.

World Bank. 1975. *Health: Sector Policy Paper.* Washington, DC: World Bank.

Zachariah, K. C. 1973. "Family Planning and Fertility Trends in Jamaica." Staff Working Paper 167, World Bank, Washington, DC.

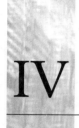

IV East Asia and the Pacific

11

The Korean Breakthrough

TAEK IL KIM AND JOHN A. ROSS

*When I meet young people, they usually ask me how many children I have. To this ques-
tion, my answer has been the same for the last 30 years: that is, "I have five children,
four sons and one daughter." But their reactions have never been the same. In the fifties,
they said "You are the most blessed man in the world." In the sixties, the response was
"You are lucky, but you should have a hard time." In the seventies, it changed to "How
come you have so many?" Nowadays, they say bluntly, "You must be crazy."*

From a 1982 field note, quoted in Kwon (1982)

In the late 1950s and early 1960s, the Republic of Korea saw its efforts to develop
being undermined by its high population growth rate. The government decided to
lower that rate through one of the first national family planning programs in the
world. As in many other countries discussed in this volume, the program relied on
increased contraceptive use, as opposed to the alternatives of increasing the marriage
age (though that occurred), relying on abortion (though that was widespread), or
exerting powerful pressures on individuals (as happened in China). To a greater
degree than in many other countries, the program used a public campaign to help
reverse traditional pro-natalist attitudes and to establish a new small family norm.
Highly specific, extensive education on contraceptives and where to obtain them
were part of the new program. To describe the Korean experience, this chapter draws
primarily on Cha (1966); Cho and Kim (1992); Cho, Kong, and Lim (1984); Han
and others (1970); Kim and Kim (1966); Kim, Ross, and Worth (1972); and Watson
(1977). Box 11.1 presents a timeline of major events.

The Setting

Five exceptional conditions set the historical context. First was the Japanese annex-
ation of the entire Korean peninsula in 1910 that continued until the end of World
War II in 1945, when the Japanese occupiers suddenly left, leaving the country in a
shambles. Second, more than a million Koreans then returned from Manchuria and
Japan, causing large absorption problems. Third, after the division of Korea at the

BOX 11.1 Timeline of Major Events

1961:   The government adopts a national family policy due to start in 1962 as part of its economic development plan.

The law prohibiting the importation and domestic production of contraceptives is abrogated.

The Planned Parenthood Federation of Korea is established as a private voluntary organization.

The slogan "Have few children and bring them up well" is adopted.

1962:   The national family planning program is started under the Ministry of Health and Social Affairs using the government's health delivery system.

Each of the country's 183 health centers sets up a family planning counseling clinic and assigns a family planning worker to the clinic.

The family planning program introduces vasectomies, condoms, and contraceptive jellies (the latter is dropped in 1963).

Training programs for family planning workers and for physicians on how to perform vasectomies are started.

1963:   The Maternal and Child Health Section is established under the Bureau of Public Health.

Two additional senior family planning workers are assigned to each of the 183 health centers.

The official 10-year family planning plan is adopted within the framework of the government's long-term economic development plan.

The prime minister sends a written order to various ministries directing them how to undertake population measures and family planning activities under their respective jurisdictions.

1964:   A family planning fieldworker is assigned to each of 1,473 township health subcenters.

A training program on inserting intrauterine devices (IUDs) is started for physicians.

The IUD is added to the national family planning program.

Family planning mobile teams are introduced to cover remote areas.

The national program adopts a family planning target system.

1965:   The family planning survey and evaluation team is established.

1968:   Family planning mothers' clubs are organized throughout the country.

The pill is introduced into the national program, initially for IUD dropouts, then for all women in 1969.

1971:   The Korean Institute for Family Planning is established

The family planning slogan "Stop at two regardless of sex" is adopted.

1972:   The program's organization is strengthened by establishing the Maternal and Child Health Bureau in the Ministry of Health and Social Affairs.

1973:   The Maternal and Child Health Law is promulgated, legalizing induced abortion under certain conditions and for medical reasons and allowing paramedics to insert IUDs.

1974:   Special urban projects are initiated in low-income areas, hospitals, and industrial sites and among army reserves.

Menstrual regulation services are added to the national program.

Tax exemptions are offered for families with up to three children.

1975:   A training program for physicians to perform female laparoscopic sterilization is launched.

The Korean Association for Voluntary Sterilization is established.

38th parallel,[1] thousands fled the Russian presence in the north and settled in the south. Meanwhile, U.S. troops were located in the south. Fourth, the most destructive of all, the north's sudden invasion of the south in June 1950 sparked the Korean War and drove fleeing populations to the southern tip of the peninsula near Pusan and destroyed much of the infrastructure. Seoul changed hands three times, and hardly a building was left standing. Fifth, the demographic structure, which had already been disrupted by the large migrations and the war's losses, was changed by a baby boom after 1953, when many soldiers returned home. Under these extreme dislocations, hard times persisted to 1961, aggravated by weak leadership at the top levels of government. Then a military coup initiated a period of profound change.

Beginnings

Even before 1961, despite the intense preference for sons and the prevailing pro-natalism, there were some indications of attitudes favoring contraceptive use. Living conditions were difficult, and especially with much of the population being refugees during the Korean War, more lenient attitudes appeared to have emerged toward pregnant women who chose abortions. In general, taking action to avoid pregnancy in the first place, and terminating it if it occurred, seemed to gain ground at that time.

Some leaders had meanwhile begun to take the first steps to promote education about contraception and even early family planning services. A mothers' association was organized, with a clinic in Seoul, and leaders of the local Methodist Church set up a number of clinics in four cities in 1957 and 1958. Faculty members at Seoul National University took an interest in family planning, and leaders of the academic community and medical profession met to develop plans for some kind of program. Simultaneously, condoms became well known because of their widespread distribution to both American and Korean soldiers and entered the black market (an old Japanese law still prohibited the importation and production of contraceptives). Visits by Koreans to other countries impressed them with the small family norm that prevailed in the West and alerted them to the international debates about explosive population growth that started in the early 1950s. All these changes began to modify the climate of opinion both inside and outside the government. As far back as 1956, the head of the Bureau of Medical Affairs in the Ministry of Health and Social Affairs made unsuccessful suggestions to start a national program in the face of opposition by the president. In 1957, without attracting the attention of higher authorities, a home demonstration program trained government workers in family planning and encouraged them to discuss it with village women. In 1959, the Maternal and Child Health Subcommittee of the Technical Advisory Committee formally discussed the need for a family planning program in the Ministry of Health and Social Affairs, though further action was not taken at that time.

The demographic situation had also become even more troubling. In addition to the mass migrations and the disrupted marriage patterns and age distributions, the baby boom that followed the end of the Korean War in 1953 had elevated the birth rate. At the same time, child mortality rates fell, and the resulting burden on an already stressed population became obvious to government planners. By 1961, the stage was set: a combination of desperate social conditions, demographic pressures, and initial responses by means of a few early services, along with modified views among prominent leaders. Into this context came a new government that opened the way to fundamental change.

A Historic Transition: 1961–62

The military revolution of May 1961 brought in a group of modern-thinking leaders who were dedicated to rebuilding the nation, both for economic development and for improved human welfare. A new feeling of freedom to debate ideas and consider departures from tradition prevailed. The government established a series of advisory panels on national renewal, one of which permitted those in public health and academia to promote ideas favorable to family planning. Work on a national population policy began, and the Ministry of Health and Social Affairs, under the strong leadership of Hee Sup Chung, was given three months to make recommendations.

Four concerns were troubling, and these had to be addressed before the government could come to the people advocating a reversal of traditional family values, namely:

- How would people respond, given the profound reliance on the large, extended family and the economic need for sons?

- What would happen to ethical and sexual mores if contraceptives were widely distributed?

- Would other government agencies accept and support the effort?

- What would fertility limitation mean for Korea's long-term development, as it would require a growing labor force. In addition, would not its international influence gain from a larger population?

In the end, the intense drive to achieve economic development overrode these concerns. The authorities decided to move ahead to lower the population growth rate, but to maintain a low profile while doing so. The new program, once created, was placed well down within the structure of the Ministry of Health and Social Affairs as an activity within the new Maternal and Child Health Section. This was judged to be a better approach than a highly visible new bureau that would hamper cooperation within the ministry and with other ministries and increase public embarrassment if the new program failed or caused a major scandal.

The new policy was quite specific: an official directive to the Ministry of Health and Social Affairs required it to do the following (Kim, Ross, and Worth 1972):

- Design a law and promulgate policies for the implementation of a family planning program.

- Abrogate the law prohibiting the importation of contraceptives, and permit the importation of all types of contraceptives.

- Promote the domestic production of contraceptives, and control their quality.

- Entrust implementation of the family planning information and education program to a special national reconstruction movement in cooperation with other government and nongovernmental agencies.

- Train family planning workers.

- Request foreign aid, and use it appropriately.

- Establish family planning clinics.

- Set up a family planning advisory council.

- Support private agencies interested in the family planning program.

The New 10-Year Plan: 1964–73

With the policy established, a concrete plan was required to decide what actions would indeed reduce fertility and by how much. In 1963, no authoritative literature existed to link massive contraceptive use to fertility declines, yet calculations were necessary to match the new population growth target in the five-year economic plan. Whereas the earlier target was to lower the growth rate from 2.9 percent per year in 1961 to 2.7 percent by 1966, the Economic Planning Board had changed this to 2.5 percent by 1966 and 2.0 percent by 1971. Thus, over 10 years the growth rate was slated to fall nearly 1 percent, a pace already achieved by Japan over the previous decade.

Calculations were then needed to specify the number of people who would adopt each contraceptive method, how long they could be expected to continue its use, and how much their fertility would decline. To achieve the goal, 45 percent of couples with wives aged 20–44 would need to be using contraception by 1971, up from only 5 percent in 1961. The government program would cover services for 32 percent of couples and private resources would do so for 13 percent. All government activities had to be tied to budget allocations, so the program needed to estimate the numbers of intrauterine device (IUD) insertions, vasectomies, and users of condoms and vaginal foam or jelly and relate these to the expected fertility rate of the couples adopting the methods. The plan took all this into account, allowing for IUD dropouts and the low effectiveness of condoms, foam, and jellies, and recognized that some couples with vasectomies would pass beyond age 45 or no longer be exposed to pregnancy by ending their marriages. It further noted that some of the 13 percent who used private resources for their family planning needs would have been motivated indirectly by the program. The results were embraced within national projections for both fertility and mortality rates and were tied to a stream of annual costs. Achieving all this in 1963 was innovative, and it anticipated extensive work in the next few years by researchers in the United States and elsewhere.

The Mechanics of the Program

With the plan in hand and its objectives clarified, the machinery of the new program had to be set up. It needed to provide good information and services to the entire population. Both information and education were necessary, as the idea of birth control was largely new to the public. The emphasis was on informing rather than persuading, as the public had to first understand the new methods and where to obtain them.

The delivery systems were different for resupply methods and clinical methods. Lay workers and mothers' clubs distributed condoms and vaginal foam and jelly (and later the pill). Private doctors were primarily responsible for the two clinical methods, the IUD and vasectomy, which they provided in their own facilities. To cover the whole country, some doctors were contracted in each area, but not every doctor, as that would dilute the number of clients per doctor. Approximately 1,075 doctors were trained and authorized to insert IUDs and 490 were trained to perform vasectomies. The doctors were paid US$1.10 per IUD insertion and US$3.30 per vasectomy. All services were free to the client, including follow-up care for side effects, and men having a vasectomy were paid about US$3 for lost work time.

The Ministry of Health and Social Affairs' own network of health centers was also central to the new program, augmented by a pivotal decision to recruit a lay family planning worker for each township. Most were female with a high school diploma, and 1,473 were selected and trained on a crash basis. They were assigned to conduct group meetings and home visits and to distribute supplies. They were also fundamental to the 1968 creation of mothers' clubs in the villages. One key to their effectiveness was their joint assignment to the health staff and to the township chief, whose job ratings were based partly on the township's progress in family planning. This arrangement strengthened support both for the new fieldworkers and for the program in general.

The administrative structure was dual, flowing both through the Ministry of Health and Social Affairs and through the Ministry of Home Affairs. The latter encompassed public officials from provincial governors down through county and township chiefs. It instructed local governments to add personnel, to match funds from the central budget, and to give due attention to the program. The Ministry of Culture and Public Information also helped by mobilizing radio, newspapers, and film networks, and later on, television.

Funding for the program came primarily from the national development budget, which reflected the firm commitment of the Economic Planning Board and its focus on reduced population growth. Additional funds came from the Ministry of Health and Social Affairs and from provincial and local budgets. Foreign donors were important, not for mainline services, but for selected functions for which government funds were not readily available, including, for example, contraceptive supplies; some of the information, education, and communications work through the Planned Parenthood Federation of Korea (PPFK); the work of the program's Evaluation Unit; most small trials and pilot projects; and the mobile teams. The donors also provided technical assistance. Annual work objectives were closely tied to the budget, as the payments to doctors covered IUDs and vasectomies and their numbers required matching budget lines. Thus, the goals for annual adoptions of contraceptives had to be covered by the budget allocations, and in turn, the budget approvals created pressures for a corresponding performance in the field. Decentralization was considerable, with both funding and goals allocated first by province, then within the province by each county, and finally by each township. The relative budget shares among areas were based partly on population characteristics and partly on the record of public response and program achievements in the preceding year.

The program's structure contained a strong private side through the planned parenthood chapter, the PPFK, a valuable arm of the national effort created in 1961 during the widespread impulse to advance family planning. The PPFK worked in close coordination with the public program to cover functions that the government could not readily handle. The PPFK handled much of the public education, partly because of the perception that it would command the trust of the people better than a government agency would. It played a key role in the creation of the mothers' clubs in 1968 at the same time as the pill was added to the program for IUD dropouts. (Initially, the pill was not made available to all women for fear that this might tempt too many away from adopting the IUD, but that restriction ended the following year.) The PPFK implemented much of the training throughout the country, administered the mobile teams and considerable foreign assistance, and conducted important studies.

Learning by Doing

At the outset of the program, no examples were available from other countries and there was no time to carry out a pilot activity given the urgent need to deal with the severe population problem. Thus, instead of being able to start with an initial design in a limited area and then gradually adapting the design nationally, the program started simultaneously across the country. Some experimental trials were initiated, but they occurred at about the same time as the national launch. Service quality was minimal at the start, but significant improvements were made in subsequent years. These benefited from rapid feedback from the field through the built-in evaluation system and from technical advice and new information from the academic groups that conducted many action-oriented trials. The leaders in this respect were the schools of public health at Seoul National University and at Yonsei University, but numerous other institutions also did important work.

Information and Education

Most of the population was reached with messages signaling something quite new in their experience: public endorsements that ran counter to the pro-natalism and large families they had always known. The country's top leaders were engaged, including the president, the prime minister, and other leading figures, who publicly endorsed and privately supported the new viewpoints.[2] This was especially true in the program's fledgling stages, when political attacks could have been tempting and antiprogram rumors needed to be headed off. The PPFK was central to the information effort, assuring a continuous flow of messages to the public. During the early years, the main channels of information were the radio, movie shorts, sound trucks, and printed materials such as posters and leaflets. On a personal level, home visits and group meetings were common throughout most rural areas. Between the 1964 and 1966 national surveys, the percentage of married women saying they knew about the new IUD rose from 11 percent to 60 percent.

Training

A massive need for training existed at the outset, and the PPFK implemented most of it in cooperation with the Ministry of Health and Social Affairs' planning staff. As a private agency, the PPFK could deal flexibly with schedules for doctors and various consultants, could handle funds more efficiently, and could work readily with foreign donors. While the PPFK ran training sessions, arranging for lecturers, texts, and facilities, the ministry retained final approval of course content, ordered workers to report for training, and oversaw the entire effort. The PPFK also handled much of the retraining needed over the years in cooperation with the ministry. This partnership arrangement worked well, with donor support for functions that the government could not readily handle.

Doctor training had to occur before the new corps of fieldworkers began to recruit clients, and doctors throughout the country were selected for early training sessions in carrying out vasectomies and inserting IUDs. While not all became part of the program—some were unsure of their skills, some were wary of client complaints, and some perceived greater income opportunities from other work—private doctors were the mainstay of the early clinical services.

A notable effort was the training of the 1,473 township workers, who averaged 1 worker for every 1,600 couples in rural areas. (In urban areas, the average was 1 worker per 2,400 couples.) The workers were selected locally and brought to a series of regional training centers in groups of 100 for initial training, followed by on-the-job experience at their county health center and by refresher training of 20 days over the next year. Other training was directed toward health personnel in the cities and at the various administrative levels. Training was a continuous part of the program over the years for doctors, the health staff, fieldworkers, and administrators.

The township lay workers were later upgraded to qualified nurses' aides, and ultimately received training as multipurpose workers for integrated rural health networks. Because the family planning program was favored in budgetary allocations, it pioneered the buildup of maternal and child health services in rural areas.

Mobile Teams

A system of mobile teams was created to serve remote areas. About 20 percent of all couples lived in the 600 townships that lacked doctors, and fieldworkers in those townships complained that they had couples wanting IUDs or vasectomies, but that they lacked access to a nearby service. In other townships, doctors were widely dispersed and inconveniently located. Quite apart from new IUD insertions, many current users needed follow-up assistance. The concept of mobile teams had been piloted earlier by the PPFK with two demonstration vans, and the decision was made to have

10 teams located in the eight largest provinces. They could not cover nearly all of the needs, but they nevertheless made an important contribution. As in other countries, the mobile teams covered four key functions:

- Providing initial and follow-up services in areas without doctors
- Providing on-the-job training to local physicians who were authorized to insert IUDs and perform vasectomies
- Helping local physicians provide clinic services to couples located far from their offices
- Carrying out public information and education programs in cooperation with local workers.

The 10 units were transferred from the Ministry of Health and Social Affairs to the PPFK in 1967, and then to direct control by the provincial governments in 1970. They were equipped to do both IUD insertions and vasectomies inside the vehicle and carried a projector for use at group meetings. Each unit included a physician, a nurse-midwife, a health educator, and a driver. Visits focused on areas without doctors and those with low achievement rates or a record of numerous side effects. Market days always drew large crowds, and the teams often coincided their visits with market days.

The work was demanding. Teams were on the road for 17–18 days a month, going to some 15 townships in 3 or 4 different counties, and often operating under rudimentary conditions and in bad weather. Nevertheless, the units performed about 5 percent of all IUD insertions each year. In four years, the units carried out more than 65,000 insertions and more than 4,000 vasectomies and trained 2,500 rural doctors. This impressive performance was attributed to vigorous administration from the top, to the use of full-time staff members, to generous salaries, to the recruitment of dedicated young doctors who had recently graduated from medical school, and to advance work with local authorities.

Evaluation and Research

The Korean program was fortunate in establishing an exceptionally rich evaluation and research operation. A special evaluation team began work in 1965 with donor support, and later with resident technical advisers. The team processed the flow of payment vouchers submitted by doctors for reimbursement that carried basic information about IUD and vasectomy adopters. The team also fielded a regular series of national knowledge, attitudes, and practices surveys; IUD follow-up surveys; and later, pill follow-up surveys. Major reports on these surveys, authored by local consultants, set out the findings, and summaries were published in international journals and presented at conferences. Leaders in the Ministry of Health and Social Affairs and the PPFK, as well as the staff of advisory panels and of interested universities and agencies, received these reports and used them to help craft periodic adjustments to the field program. Research groups at Seoul National University led by Dr. E. Hyock Kwon and at Yonsei University led by Dr. Jae Mo Yang contributed numerous studies and experiments that helped decide program modifications. By late 1967, nearly 50 reports on the Korean experience had appeared, written either locally or by interested foreign scholars.

Measures Not Taken

The Korean program was one of the strongest internationally, but it did not employ every anti-natalist measure, and it could have been stronger. As with most programs, it was based on the paradigm of reducing marital fertility through contraceptive use, which omitted alternative approaches.

First, abortion was never part of the program. Indeed, contraception eventually became so prevalent that unwanted pregnancies declined and the number of abortions also declined. However, people were familiar with abortion and many doctors provided it at relatively low cost. Even though abortion was technically illegal, prosecution was minimal. Two attempts to legalize abortion, one in 1963 and one in 1964, failed because of a lack of support by the administration and by parliament. Finally, in 1973, the Maternal and Child Health Law was passed and legalized induced abortion under certain conditions. That helped to relieve the tensions brought about by the secrecy surrounding abortion.

Second, efforts to persuade couples to marry later were not part of the program. Nevertheless, the average age of marriage rose rapidly as more women entered the labor force, as many went on to finish high school and enter college, as movement to the cities accelerated, and as women's status improved overall.

Third, incentives and disincentives were also not part of the early program. Later, starting in the late 1970s, various benefits were offered to couples who adopted sterilization at the point of having two or fewer children, and tax exemptions went to companies that provided family planning services to employees. (In addition, a law affecting women's inheritance of property was liberalized.)

Finally, the program of necessity omitted a postpartum program, as most births took place at home.[3] Also, paramedics could not insert IUDs; only doctors were authorized to do so. Female sterilization was essentially absent from the early program given the lack of clinical facilities, before the days of minilaparoscopic and laparoscopic procedures. Activity by the private sector was welcomed, and contraceptive imports were allowed in freely, but there was no social marketing at that time and the program did rather little to stimulate pharmacies or shops to sell condoms (contraceptive pills became available only in the late 1960s.)

Thus, more could have been done. However, no national program could do everything, and trying to do everything all at once could have been counterproductive, confusing management and diluting resources. In later years, the program was augmented with additional components.

Importance of Local Cultural and Historical Factors

The achievements of the Korean program occurred within a context of rapid social and economic change. Observers have cited numerous reasons for Korea's meteoric path, which transformed the society within 25 years and led to Korea becoming one of the "Asian tigers." The fast decline in the fertility rate changed the country's age distribution and released resources for family and national investments. The injection of capital in the form of foreign aid, especially by the United States, along with additional capital from donors and business sources, all helped. The intense focus on development by a new government, which had targets in every sector, certainly energized the population in the direction of change. The sense of threat from the north, the legacy of the Japanese occupation, the compression within a small peninsula, and the memory of the Korean War's devastation all contributed to the forcefulness of the push to develop. Technical assistance of all types was extensive, through economic planning at the top government levels, through skills transferred from the U.S. military to Korean soldiers and civilian employees, and through extensive overseas training, including that experienced by contract employees working in Vietnam. This was a time of opportunity for the younger generation that was entirely new.

All this took place in a context where people were already highly literate, deeply committed to education, and willing to sacrifice to advance their children's schooling. They were also ethnically homogeneous, with a single language. The status of women, which was already advanced in terms of their economic freedom and ease of travel and movement, improved as many more joined the labor force and obtained higher education. Perhaps not the least important change was that by the late 1960s, most knew that they could have children only when they wanted them.

Results

Contraceptive use rose from the historic level of less than 10 percent as shown in a 1964 national survey to about 45 percent by the mid-1970s (figure 11.1). Use ultimately reached 80 percent of couples and remained steady.

During the program's early period, the mix of contraceptive methods used responded to the program's stress on the IUD (figure 11.2). During this time, the IUD

FIGURE 11.1 Contraceptive Prevalence: Percentage of Married Women Using a Method of Contraception, 1964–97

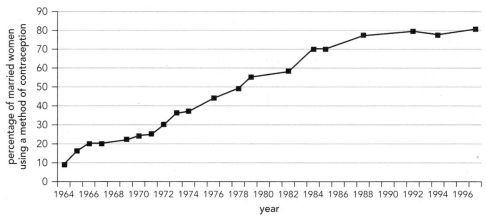

Source: Ross, Stover, and Adelaja, 2005, table A.1.

FIGURE 11.2 Contraceptive Method Mix among Married Women, 1964–79

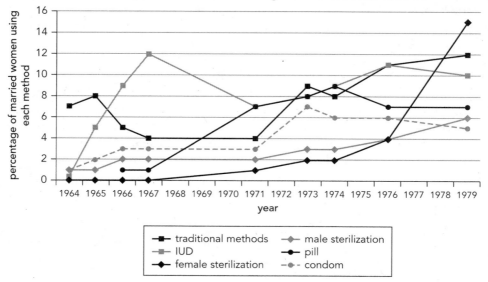

Source: Ross, Stover, and Adelaja 2005, table A.1.

gained in terms of both the percentage of couples using it and its share of the total mix. Then, in 1968, the pill was introduced for IUD dropouts and a year later for all couples, and by 1971, it had made considerable inroads on the IUD. However, it subsequently faded in importance, as in later years simpler methods of female sterilization were developed and were encouraged by the program, and sterilization then became the most prominent method of contraception.

Another way to track the rise in contraceptive use is to focus on women by duration of marriage. A 1971 survey using retrospective information showed that among women married from five to nine years in different periods, a mere 8 percent were using contraception in 1955–61, but this figure had risen to 18 percent in 1958–64, to 25 percent in 1961–67, and to 39 percent in 1964–70. Figures for women married from 10 to 14 years, who by then had as many or more children than they wanted, also showed a steep increase, from 32 percent in 1955–61 to a full 72 percent by 1964–70 (Foreit 1982).

An alternative is to track contraceptive use by number of children. Figure 11.3 shows that between 1965 and 1973, the percentage of couples who had ever used contraception increased significantly, with the increase being greater the larger the number of children. This was even notable among couples with only two children, for whom the percentage rose from 18 to 48 percent.

These changes were particularly apparent among the younger generation. Their ideal family size was declining, despite the continuing preference for sons. Indeed, among wives aged 20–29, the percentage saying that three children or more were ideal fell from more than 30 percent in 1965 to 13 percent in 1973. At the same time, the percentage saying that four children was ideal fell from 27 to 10 percent. By 1973, 40 percent of those with two children said they did not want any more.

FIGURE 11.3 Percentage of Couples Ever Using Contraception by Number of Living Children, 1965 and 1973

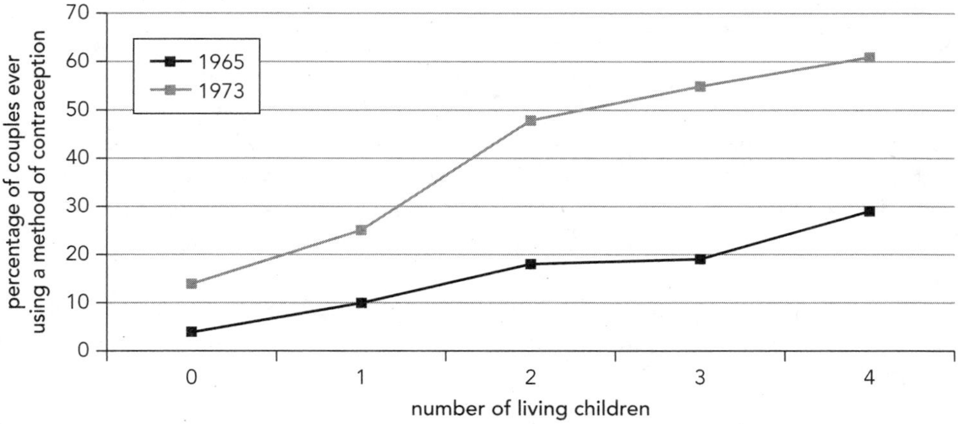

Source: Ross and Koh 1975, 26.

The program provided supplies and services to rural areas in particular, where contraceptives had been nearly unknown. Indeed, it allocated its resources and staff members disproportionately to rural areas, where education levels were lower than in urban areas. Contraceptive use by groups with a lower level of education rose faster than among groups with a higher level of education, thereby narrowing the differentials between the groups as overall use advanced. For example, from 1965 to 1973, the percentage of married women aged 30–39 with less than a primary school education who had ever used contraception rose sharply, from 20 to 53 percent, compared with a smaller rise of 54 to 72 percent for married women of the same age who had at least a middle school education. Thus, the program's stress on the most disadvantaged groups in the population helped them to gain the most. The use of abortion increased from 1965 to 1973 across the various age and family size groups. For example, the percentage of married women aged 20–29 who had ever had an abortion rose from 6 to 16 percent, and from 15 to 36 percent among those aged 30–39. Within each age group, the percentage ever having an abortion generally rose by number of living children as well. This reflected rapid social changes, as well as lags in establishing contraceptive use. The available contraceptive methods were not workable for everyone, and contraceptive failures were especially likely to end in abortion, which was fairly widely available and inexpensive. Later, the addition of the pill and female sterilization helped address these issues, and abortion rates began to come down.

Lessons Learned

The Korea experience was important, in that it occurred early on, with strong diffusion of that experience to other countries. The stream of visitors to Korea was immense, as they represented two leading cases that showed how successful programs could work. Some 150 visitors per year came from developing countries around the world, with each visitor staying for about a week and making the rounds of the field program and various university pilot projects in rural and urban areas. A flow of conference reports and publications documented the experience and results and established a permanent record for international audiences. Not all results were positive of course: a major blow was the discovery that in a mass program, IUD continuation rates were significantly below those in the early clinical trials, and that despite large numbers of adopters annually, the number using IUDs would level off as the number of terminations would increase and come to equal the number of annual new adoptions. Similarly, use of every resupply method would finally plateau. This discovery forced a revision of the annual number of users needed to meet the plan's objectives.

On the positive side, Korea, along with such early programs as those in Thailand, disproved much pessimism about the potential for change in some traditional societies. It demonstrated the following:

- The IUD, the pill, and sterilization could be acceptable to a poor, rural population.

- A reversal of cultural pro-natalism could be managed with high-level endorsement and thorough public education.

- A private family planning association could collaborate with the government and greatly strengthen the government's efforts.

- The level of fertility could come down rapidly as the outcome of a combination of program and nonprogram influences, with the program helping to stimulate the private medical sector and commercial sales.

- The use of the pill could be implemented on a mass scale and would be acceptable (even with the higher dosage pill of the late 1960s).

- A new creature of behavioral change, the national family planning program, was viable and could help modify the climate in relation to reproductive attitudes and practices. It could remove pluralistic ignorance of what others were doing, legitimating the use of the new contraceptive methods.

The Korean experience also reassured other country programs that certain field components were workable and effective. These included the widespread use of mass media, the use of field staff members who made personal contacts via home visits and group meetings, the provision of access to all contraceptive methods then available, the improvement in maternal and child health services, and the use of the private medical sector. These, however, rested on the following fundamental components:

- An ambitious program goal that was part of the long-term economic development plan

- A system of closely monitored achievement targets that was adapted over time

- A dual management system within the ministries of Health and Social Affairs and Home Affairs that was supported by a strong evaluation and research team

- The budgetary allocations from the central government along with matching funds from local governments

- The strong and continuous political commitment from the president, the prime minister, the Economic Planning Board, and the Ministry of Finance

- The active role of the PPFK in mobilizing opinion leaders and academic groups and in providing critical assistance to support the government program.

Developments after 1975

As figure 11.1 showed, contraceptive use exhibited a strong upward trend to a stable level of 80 percent. The program underwent a series of modifications in the 1980s, using incentives of various sorts to encourage sterilization and stressing the two-child family, and even the one-child family. Eventually, as the fertility rate fell well below replacement level, the government gradually reversed course to adopt a pro-natalist policy in the interests of a more advantageous age structure and a hedge against labor force needs in the long term. By that time, the effects of the program had acted in concert with the transformation of the Korean economy, resulting in vastly improved living standards and a revolution in reproductive behavior that enhanced women's health and reduced deaths among both mothers and children.

Notes

1. The Korean peninsula was divided at the 38th parallel in 1945 at the end of World War II, an action proposed by the United States and agreed to by the former Soviet Union as part of disarming the Japanese forces and ending their occupation. The Korean War (1950–53) left the division line at the demilitarized zone, which continues to the present day.
2. This support echoes current HIV/AIDS campaigns, where deep commitment by the head of state has been critical.
3. By 1972, only 13 percent of all births were at hospitals and clinics, but by 1988, 94 percent of births occurred in those settings (Cho, Seo, and Tan 1990).

References

Cha, Youn Keun. 1966. "South Korea." In *Family Planning and Population Programs: A Review of World Developments*, ed. Bernard Berelson, Richmond K. Anderson, Oscar Harkavy, John Maier, W. Parker Mauldin, and Sheldon Segal, 21–30. Chicago: University of Chicago Press.

Cho, Nam Hoon, and Hyun Oak Kim. 1992. *An Overview of the National Family Planning Program in Korea: A Summary Explanation*. Seoul: Korea Institute for Health and Social Affairs, 19–26.

Cho, Nam Hoon, Sae Kwon Kong, and Jong Kwon Lim. 1984. "Recent Changes in Contraceptive Use and Fertility in Korea." *Journal of Population and Health Studies* 4 (2): 63–79.

Cho, Nam Hoon, Moon Hee Seo, and Boon Ann Tan. 1990. "Recent Changes in the Population Control Policy and Its Future Directions in Korea." *Journal of Population, Health, and Social Welfare* 10 (2): 152–172.

Foreit, James R. 1982. "The Transition in Korean Family Planning Behavior 1935–1976: A Retrospective Cohort Analysis," *Studies in Family Planning*, 8 (9): 227–36.

Han, Dae Woo, George C. Worth, Eung Ik Kim, Thomas Bacon, and Stanley Hudson. 1970. *The Republic of Korea*. Country Profiles Series. New York: Population Council.

Kim, Taek Il, and Syng Wook Kim. 1966. "Mass Use of Intra-Uterine Contraceptive Devices in Korea." In *Family Planning and Population Programs: A Review of World Developments*, ed. Bernard Berelson, Richmond K. Anderson, Oscar Harkavy, John Maier, W. Parker Mauldin, and Sheldon Segal, 425–32. Chicago: University of Chicago Press.

Kim, Taek Il, John A. Ross, and George C. Worth. 1972. *The Korean National Family Planning Program*. New York: Population Council.

Kwon, Tai Hwan. 1982. "Exploring Sociocultural Explanations of Fertility Transition in Korea." Unpublished manuscript, Seoul.

Ross, John A., and Kap Suk Koh. 1975. "Transition to the Small Family: a Comparison of 1964–1973 Time Trends in Korea and Taiwan." In *Population Change in the Pacific Region,* ed. Yunshik Chang and Peter J. Donaldson, 121–39. Vancouver, Canada: Pacific Science Association.

Ross, John A., John Stover, and Demi Adelaja. 2005. *Profiles for Family Planning and Reproductive Health Programs: 116 Countries*, 2nd ed. Glastonbury, CT: Futures Group.

Watson, Walter B., ed. 1977. *Family Planning in the Developing World: A Review of Programs*. New York: Population Council.

12 Hong Kong: Evolution of the Family Planning Program

SUSAN FAN

Origins

The family planning movement in Hong Kong began in June 1936, when the Hong Kong Eugenics League was founded with Professor W. C. W. Nixon as president and Ellen Li as honorary secretary. In the words of Professor Gordon King, who later became chair and director of the Family Planning Association of Hong Kong (FPAHK), "The League came into being largely as the result of a visit from that wonderful pioneer of the birth-control movement, Mrs. Margaret Sanger" (FPAHK 1975, p. 4). The league was affiliated with the International Birth Control League (London and New York), the National Birth Control Association (London), and the Birth Control Clinical Research Bureau (New York). These organizations eventually became Planned Parenthood in the United States and the Family Planning Association in the United Kingdom.

The league began its work with a single clinic in the Violet Peel Maternity and Child Welfare Centre. Subsequently, it established clinics in Kowloon and in Tsan Yuk Hospital. By 1940, the league was operating five clinics staffed by several part-time female doctors and nurses. The World War II Japanese occupation ended the league's work. At that time, the estimated population of Hong Kong was 1.6 million, but the war years saw much forced deportation and starvation. By the end of the war in 1945, only about one-third of that number remained. With the liberation of Hong Kong, many people returned and a period of rapid growth ensued. By 1950, the population had risen to an estimated 2.36 million, along with housing shortages, intense overcrowding, and widespread poverty.

The need for family planning was obviously great, and in March 1950, the remaining members of the old league met to consider the challenge. They decided to change the league's name to the FPAHK, and in September 1950 made plans to reopen the

---

This chapter is adapted from Fan (2002) and is used with permission.

family planning clinic at the Violet Peel Maternity and Child Welfare Centre. From then on, the work of FPAHK continued to expand.

The International Family Planning Movement

In November 1952, the International Planned Parenthood Federation was established at an international conference in Bombay. King, as the first chair of the FPAHK, represented the association at the conference, which was attended by almost 500 delegates from 14 countries, nearly all of whom were pioneers of the family planning movement. Hong Kong, together with the Federal Republic of Germany, Holland, India, Singapore, Sweden, the United Kingdom, and the United States, were the founding members of the federation.

The Early Clinics

The FPAHK continued its work in one clinic, offering services twice a week. Because of a lack of funds, the services relied heavily on public-spirited volunteers: of the 41 workers in the clinic in 1951, 40 were volunteers. During the first year, the clinic saw 1,655 new clients. Their average age was 35, their average number of surviving children was 6.8 per family, and their average income was only US$150 per month. In the ensuing years, clinics were opened in Kowloon and then in the New Territories. Box 12.1 presents a timeline of major events.

In 1955, the FPAHK was incorporated so that it could own land and buildings. The government granted it a piece of land on Hennessy Road, Wanchai, and the Jockey Club donated US$125,000 to cover the costs of construction. This was also the year when the government provided the FPAHK with a small grant of HK$5,000 (about US$640 at that time), a big step for the association. In October 1956, Lady Grantham opened the FPAHK's first building and new headquarters. In 1960, the second center was opened in Kowloon, followed by the Yuen Long Centre in the New Territories in November 1973.

A mobile clinic operated from 1961 to 1963, visiting rural women. It offered clinical services and was used in connection with education and social work programs. Another project was the floating clinics, launched in 1966, whereby FPAHK staff members traveled with the government's two floating health clinics to visit outlying islands and villages. More clinics were opened in the resettlement areas and low-income housing developments. At the height of the FPAHK's activities, it had a total of 62 clinics distributed throughout the territory.

Community Support

The program rested upon a spirit of self-help and a sense of social responsibility, especially among the medical community, women's groups, and key leaders. Initially, volunteer doctors and nurses (and one part-time nurse) provided services. Volunteer members of the association also undertook the necessary administrative work. It was

BOX 12.1 Timeline for Family Planning Activities

1950: The Eugenics League, founded in 1936, is reorganized and renamed as the FPAHK. Birth control services are offered.

1952: The International Planned Parenthood Federation is created with Hong Kong as one of its founding members.

1955: The government begins to support the activities of the FPAHK.
Fieldwork through person-to-person motivation starts.

1956: The Subfertility Clinic opens.

1964: The International Planned Parenthood Federation starts to provide grant support.

1967: The first territory-wide survey on family planning knowledge, attitude, and practice is conducted.
Education on sexuality is introduced.

1974: The government's Medical and Health Department incorporates the FPAHK's 32 birth control clinics into its maternal and child health centers.

1975: The "Two Is Enough" campaign is launched.

1976: Minilaparotomy sterilization is introduced.

1978: The youth advisory service is created.
The first women's club opens.

1979: A pregnancy termination operation is introduced.
A premarital medical checkup service is set up.
Family planning clinics are set up in Vietnamese refugee camps.

1981: An artificial insemination service is introduced.
A study of school-age youth is carried out that later develops into the youth sexuality study.

1986: The first youth health care center is established.
The "Be a Mr. Able in Family Planning" campaign is launched.

1987: The premarital package service incorporating an educational component replaces the premarital medical checkup service.

1988: FPAHK headquarters moves to its current location in Wanchai and is officially opened in 1989.

1991: The computerized clientele management information system starts.

1992: The women's health campaign is launched.
The gynecological checkup service is introduced.

1996: The family sex education campaign is launched.

1998: The mobile clinic goes into operation.
The prepregnancy preparation service commences.
A three-year education and information project for women newly arrived from mainland China is introduced.

1999: The menopause service is introduced.
The community-level sexuality education mobile library opens.

2000: The FPAHK celebrates its 50th anniversary.

2001: The findings of the first men's health survey are released.
The Well-Men Clinic opens.

2002: Dating, marriage, and sex counseling is introduced.

2003: The Cervical Diseases Clinic opens.
The first training course on taking pap smears is introduced to support the government's territory-wide cervical screening program.

2004: The first Continuing Nursing Education Program in Sexual and Reproductive Health and the first Continuing Medical Education Program for nonspecialist doctors are held.

not until 1957 that a full-time secretary was employed to handle general correspondence and administration. In 1961, Peggy Lam joined the FPAHK as executive secretary and then as director of information, education, and communication. By this time, the FPAHK had 55 employees, a number that grew to more than 200 by 1973. It had evolved from a small, voluntary organization to a large, internationally known, and respected nongovernmental organization deeply rooted in the community.

During its early years, the FPAHK was largely funded through donations and subscriptions. In 1955, it received its first government grant of US$5,000, which was gradually increased, reaching US$1.65 million by 1974. The second largest source of income was the International Planned Parenthood Federation, and other international and local organizations also donated funds. Because of the government grant and various donations, the FPAKH was able to offer services at a low charge. Clients paid only a nominal registration fee for clinic attendance and could buy contraceptives at affordable prices.

Communication and Publicity

Traditional Chinese culture has always favored large families. In the early days of the FPAHK, many people rejected the idea of birth control, but Hong Kong ultimately came to boast one of the highest contraceptive prevalence rates in the world. Much of this change in public perception and acceptance was attributable to the association's intensive and extensive public education activities, as a result of which family planning became respectable and new attitudes were reinforced. Over the years, it used almost every available communication channel to reach the public. Printed media were the first to be used. The FPAKH produced illustrated booklets and pamphlets and distributed them free of charge. Advertisements placed in newspapers and articles also appeared from time to time. The radio was the other most common media channel before the advent of television. Announcements, talks, radio plays, songs, and interviews were broadcast on various channels and brought the association's messages into people's homes.

With the increasing popularity of movies, the screen was able to reach a large audience. A local theater produced and donated a slide show, and in 1961, the FPAHK produced its first film, *A Story of Two Families,* whose premier was attended by representatives from government departments, Kai Fong associations (neighborhood community groups), and other welfare agencies. The association continued to make and purchase films and acquired a sizable film library of more than 100 titles that it loaned to the public. Short publicity filmstrips were shown in movie theaters, and later on television.

Another means of publicity was billboard posters on the Star Ferry pier and at factories, welfare centers, housing developments, and other public places. The FPAHK also participated in numerous exhibitions and displays that it or other entities organized in various community centers. It ran a stall at the Hong Kong Products Fair from 1960 until 1974, when the Chinese Manufacturers' Association ceased to organize the exhibition.

In addition, the FPAHK held large-scale publicity events and campaigns each year. These included contests in essay writing, sewing, photography, drawing, poster design, and slogan composition and a telephone survey. Such activities promoted awareness of the FPAHK, generated interest, and encouraged participation.

Fieldwork and Home Visits

From the beginning, the FPAHK adopted the strategy of disseminating the concept of family planning through person-to-person contact. In 1955, the association's first social worker started to visit homes to motivate high-parity women to practice contraception. By 1965, the association was employing 20 fieldworkers, a number that rose to 55 by 1971. The job was not easy in those early days. Doors were slammed when the fieldworkers arrived, dogs barked at them, and they had to travel to rural districts and climb hills to visit squatter huts. Yet through their perseverance and compassion, the fieldworkers were able to overcome the suspicion, superstition, and ignorance of many women, especially those with low education and income levels.

Fieldwork was conducted in maternity homes and postnatal clinics, and in a creative step, also at the marriage and birth registries. Referral slips were sent to various social agencies so that they could refer women who needed special guidance on family planning matters to the fieldworkers, who would then visit them.

In 1974, the International Planned Parenthood Federation inaugurated a new project on community-based distribution of contraceptives, which was widely adopted by its members, including Hong Kong. Family planning information was disseminated to the rural population, and contraceptives were placed in village shops, which served as depots. Fieldworkers could sell contraceptives on the spot to women who decided to use them, and the women could get subsequent supplies from the local shops. By such means, contraception was made conveniently accessible to the rural population.

Married Life Information Service

Li, founding member and past president of the FPAHK, who contributed to the family planning movement for more than 60 years, started a marriage guidance clinic in 1959, where she served as its first counselor for several years. The service offered guidance on marital life with an emphasis on preparing young couples for marriage and sexual life. The clinic sent leaflets to couples registered at the marriage registry to encourage them to come for advice, and a growing number of couples responded, receiving help for solving marital problems and for adopting contraception. In 1966, Li became the first woman in Hong Kong to be appointed as a legislative councilor, and she promptly took the opportunity to champion the cause of family planning in the territory's legislature, calling for the formulation of a population policy and changes to existing regulations that discriminated against women.

From Family Life Education to Sexuality Education, 1967–75

In 1967, with a grant from the American Friends Service Committee, the FPAHK took on the task of developing what it termed family life education (FLE) materials. In those days, "sex" was such a taboo word that the term sex education was rarely used openly. Instead, the relatively innocuous title of FLE was widely adopted. Early work focused on finding and collecting resource materials and adapting or translating overseas literature for local use.

One of the main achievements was the drafting of a syllabus on FLE for use in primary schools, and secondary schools were also included by 1975. With the employment of an FLE officer in 1970, the association greatly expanded its scope of work in this area. Talks on the physical and psychological changes of puberty, family relationships, human reproduction and sexuality, and teenage relationships such as dating and courtship were given in primary and secondary schools, colleges, universities, and schools for physically and mentally challenged young people.

Using a train-the-trainer approach, the FPAHK conducted seminars and certificate training programs for teachers and social workers to help them conduct FLE and answer questions from their students and clients. FLE programs were also televised and broadcast, and regular newspaper columns were printed that answered readers' numerous questions.

Population education was a new concept at that time, which the FPAHK promoted. It sponsored the first "Seminar on Population Education" in 1973, stressing the messages of population awareness and responsible citizenship. The teacher participants unanimously agreed that population education should be introduced in secondary schools, but all felt handicapped by the lack of resource materials on the subject. The FPAHK again took the initiative by producing an information leaflet on the nature, scope, and rationale of population education for circulation among teachers and youth workers. It also prepared the *Teachers' Handbook on Population Education* for classroom teaching in conjunction with the Education Department's new social studies syllabus for secondary schools.

By 1975, the association had acquired an impressive collection of audiovisual materials on FLE and population education, including films, slides, charts, transparencies, tapes, periodicals, and books. Its own publications included pamphlets, booklets, and a newsletter with a wide distribution network. In 1972, the FPAHK set up a reference library to systematically file these resource materials for ready access by staff members, students, academics, members of the media, and the public.

Research and Monitoring

In addition to maintaining an extensive system of records on clients and services, the FPAHK conducted a series of surveys over the years. The earliest survey, in 1967, showed that 44 percent of couples where the wife was younger than age 45 were already using contraception. This figure rose to 54 percent in 1972 and to progressively higher levels in the next decade, with female sterilization and the pill dominating the method mix. The regular system of record keeping included the age and parity of women adopting contraception at the clinics and yielded trends that showed the movement toward adoption of contraception by younger couples with fewer children. The two-child family was becoming the norm.

A series of studies undertaken by the FPAHK with the University of Michigan showed that most (80 percent) of the fall in the birth rate from 1961 to 1965 was attributable to changes in the age and marital distribution of the population and 20 percent was attributable to declines in fertility rates within specific age groups of married women (marital age-specific rates) (Freedman and Lee 1989). However, during 1965 to 1968, when the birth rate declined more rapidly, increasing contraceptive use played a major role, reflecting the association's introduction of the recently invented intrauterine device (IUD), as well as considerable activity by pharmacies and private physicians.

The decline of the fertility rate in Hong Kong generated considerable international interest, as its experience had interesting parallels to other Asian populations that were experiencing fertility declines during the same period and for some of the same reasons (Coale and Freedman 1993). Hong Kong reached the replacement fertility level of approximately 2.1 children per woman in 1979 (Freedman and Lee 1989), and contraceptive use finally rose to 80 percent of couples.

Diversification to Meet Changing Needs, 1970s

Although this volume is concerned primarily with the early, formative years of large-scale family planning programs up to the mid-1970s, important changes occurred in Hong Kong thereafter. The 1970s heralded a change in the focus of the FPAHK's work. The government, recognizing the importance of family planning, began to absorb the family planning clinics into its maternal and child health centers. By 1975, the association had handed 32 clinics over to the government, but continued to operate 26 others. In the meantime, the FPAHK had also established a few special clinics for vasectomy, for marriage guidance and counseling, and for subfertility. A telephone answerline was set up, and in 1973, its number was changed to 722222, which was easy to remember, plus the string of twos signified that two children per family was the ideal. A postpartum family planning program was introduced, and women were encouraged to use contraception soon after delivery to space their pregnancies. Female sterilization was added, providing both minilaparotomy and culdoscopy. In 1979, a service for pregnancy termination was added that included counseling both before and after the procedure. With its tradition of pioneering services to meet the changing needs of the community, the association was no longer restricting its scope to birth control, but was actively branching out into other areas related to sexual and reproductive health care.

Subsequent years saw the development of other specialized services to address the needs of various sectors of the community. Youth services were added for counseling and clinic services for unmarried young people. A premarital checkup service was created that provided laboratory tests and educational seminars and was used by more than 150,000 people during 1979 to 1990. A service to help rape victims was established for trauma counseling, pregnancy prevention, and testing for disease. Special services were created for the disabled, the mentally handicapped, and the deaf. Migrant workers and Vietnamese boat people were also served, as well as new residents who arrived from the mainland after 1997 when China regained sovereignty.

The FPAHK celebrated its silver jubilee in 1975. Over the previous 25 years, the association had served more than 400,000 new clients, with total attendance exceeding 3 million visits. In the early 1970s, it successfully turned over responsibility for the bulk of routine services to the government, a transition that had also occurred elsewhere as the early innovative period led to a large volume of contraceptive users and extensive administrative burdens. The organization's role had evolved with the times: in the early postwar years, the focus was on providing accessible and affordable birth control services, which helped lead to a relatively stable rate of population growth. In the ensuing years, the association added programs on sex education, youth sexuality, and women's health. Finally, it engaged in a range of activities encompassing clinical services, information dissemination, and education to reach a wide segment of the community from youth through premarital couples to women of reproductive age. The "Two Is Enough" slogan, first introduced in 1975, became deeply-rooted in people's minds. The knowledge, attitude, and practice surveys continued to be carried out every five years, showing that the mean ideal family size and actual family size had declined from 3.2 and 3.3, respectively, in 1972 to 2.1 for both in 1981. With its large clinical client base, the association was in a unique position to carry out trials on new methods of fertility regulation, including a low-dose pill, a hormonal IUD, and, notably, emergency contraception in collaboration with the Department of Obstetrics and Gynaecology of the University of Hong Kong.

The jubilee paid tribute to some of the association's distinguished pioneer volunteers, including Li, who was president of the association at that time, and Laura Li, who had joined the association in 1952 and had taken up various positions, including chair and president, before retiring in 1980 while remaining as the association's patron. As 1975 was also International Women's Year, it was fitting for the FPAHK to celebrate its 25 years of work at that time.

References

Coale, Ansley J., and Ronald Freedman. 1993. "Similarities in the Fertility Transition in China and Three Other East Asian Populations." In *The Revolution in Asian Fertility: Dimensions, Causes, and Implications*, ed. Richard Leete and Iqbal Alam, 208–38. Oxford, U.K.: Clarendon Press.

FPAHK (Family Planning Association of Hong Kong). 1969. *Hong Kong*. Country Profiles Series. New York: Population Council.

———. 1975. *The Family Planning Association of Hong Kong Silver Jubilee*. Hong Kong: FPAHK.

Fan, Susan. 2002. "The Family Planning Association of Hong Kong: Half a Century of Voluntarism Dedicated to Sexual and Reproductive Health." *Hong Kong Journal of Gynaecology Obstetrics and Midwifery* 3 (1): 2–16.

Freedman, Ronald, and Joseph Lee. 1989. "The Fertility Transition in Hong Kong: 1961–1987." Research Report 89-159, University of Michigan, Population Studies Center, Ann Arbor, MI.

13 Singapore: Population Policies and Programs

YAP MUI TENG

Singapore's demographic transition from a young and rapidly growing population with a high rate of unemployment to one that is rapidly aging and is a net labor importer has been remarkable. The total fertility rate plunged from more than six children per woman at the height of the post–World War II baby boom in 1957 to below replacement level from 1977 onward. Projections indicate that Singapore's elderly population (aged 65 and over) will double, growing from 7 percent to 14 percent of the total population, during 1997–2018, that is, in less time than the 26 years taken by Japan, the most rapidly aging country to date (Kinsella and Gist 1995). Given the simultaneity of events, directly measuring the contribution of the government's population policies and programs, begun in the early stages of the country's independence to control the rate of population growth, is not possible, but those policies and programs have generally been considered successful. In particular, Singapore has been noted for the stringency of its National Family Planning Program, which included measures such as incentives and disincentives to reduce fertility. Today, however, Singapore is one of a handful of countries that have adopted pro-natalist policies.

The urgency with which the government has always regarded the population issue may best be understood in the context of the country's small size. As Paul Cheung, the former head of Singapore's Population Planning Unit, observed, "Population planning in Singapore is essentially one of managing population growth to meet economic needs, given the extreme land constraint" (Cheung 1995, p. 100). As an island city-state with no hinterland, Singapore lacks natural resources except for its people. Hence, its emphasis on maximizing its human resources is not surprising.

When the current government, led by the People's Action Party, came into power in 1959—the year Singapore became a self-governing state within the British Commonwealth—the annual population growth rate was about 4 to 5 percent. This high growth rate was attributable mainly to a high rate of natural increase, but it was augmented by net in-migration. The newly formed government faced problems of high unemployment, which persisted despite economic growth, and growing demand for social

This article is adapted from Mason (2001). The author wishes to acknowledge the kind permission given by Andrew Mason.

services, which it rightly attributed to the rapid population growth (S. Lee 1979). Singapore became a fully independent nation in August 1965, following the sudden end of a two-year merger with Malaysia, and with it a much-hoped-for common market. The British military withdrawal in 1968 heightened feelings of insecurity as jobs were lost.

Concerns since the mid-1980s have included issues of the growth of the labor force, the vibrancy of the workforce, and the country's ability to sustain economic growth in the face of persistent below-replacement-level fertility and population aging. A larger population is now considered desirable to provide the critical mass for future economic growth (Government of Singapore 1991; K. Lee 2005; Lian 2004). Planners consider the constraint of geographic size to be less critical than in the past, because they believe that the country can comfortably accommodate a much larger population of more than 5 million people,[1] compared with the 3 million thought desirable earlier (Wan, Loh, and Chen 1976). Cheung (1995), however, cautions against too rapid population growth to reach the larger population size, citing the momentum generated by pro-natalist population policies and the difficulty of reversing them (see also Yap 1995). Population planning has become a much more complex balancing act between the economy's needs for more and better qualified workers and such social and political considerations as the size of the dependent population and ethnic balance. Box 13.1 presents a timeline of the major events.

BOX 13.1 Timeline of Major Events

1949:   The Family Planning Association of Singapore is founded.

1959:   The People's Action Party comes to power, and Singapore becomes a self-governing state and a member of the British Commonwealth.

1965:   Singapore becomes fully independent from Malaysia.

1966:   The first official policy on family planning and fertility is promulgated.
         The National Family Planning Program is launched.
         The Singapore Family Planning and Population Board is established under the Ministry of Health.

1969:   Disincentives to large families are introduced.

1970:   Sterilization and abortion are legalized.

1972:   The two-child family norm is adopted.

1975–76: The total fertility rate reaches replacement level.
         Sterilization and abortion are liberalized.

1977:   The total fertility rate falls below replacement level.

1983:   Prime Minister Lee Kuan Yew raises issues of educational differentials in marriage and fertility, sparking what came to be known as the great marriage debate.

1984:   Incentives to encourage women with university degrees to have more children are introduced; however, a scheme offering priority in primary school registration to children of such women turns out to be controversial and has to be scrapped after a year.
         The Social Development Unit is set up to promote interaction among university graduates to help educated women find partners.

1987:   The anti-natalist policy is reversed with the adoption of a selectively pro-natalist policy using the slogan "have three, or more (children) if you can afford it."

Fertility Policies

The evolution of Singapore's fertility policies and programs can be divided into three phases: the phase of indirect government involvement in family planning activities (1949–65), the anti-natalist phase (1966–86), and the pro-natalist phase (1987–present).

Phase I: Indirect Government Involvement, 1949–65

Singapore had no official policy on family planning or fertility control until 1966. A group of volunteers motivated mainly by the high level of poverty in the aftermath of World War II and by concern about the deleterious effects of frequent childbearing on the health and welfare of mothers and their families introduced family planning in 1949 (Pakshong 1967; Saw 1980, 1991; Zhou 1996). They established the Family Planning Association of Singapore as a voluntary organization whose main goals were (a) to educate the public about family planning and provide contraceptive facilities to enable married couples to space and limit their families; (b) to promote the establishment of family planning centers at which, in addition to advice on contraception, women could obtain treatment for sterility and minor gynecological ailments and advice on marital problems; and (c) to encourage the birth of healthy children, who would be an asset to the nation if their parents were able to give them a reasonable chance in life (Family Planning Association of Singapore 1954).

From merely three clinics operated on premises owned by physician members of the association in 1949 and 1950, the number of clinics offering such services rose rapidly, reaching 34 in 1965. The number of new acceptors registered rose from 600 to nearly 10,000 during the same period. In 1965 alone, the clinics saw more than 94,000 repeat clients. Given this heavy demand, which the association's leaders felt was beyond the organization's ability to meet, they repeatedly requested the government to assume responsibility for its clinical services. This took place in 1966 with the establishment of the Singapore Family Planning and Population Board (SFPPB) and the launching of the National Family Planning and Population Program (henceforth called the National Family Planning Program), although the Family Planning Association continued to provide services at its own three premises until 1968. The association was renamed the Singapore Planned Parenthood Association in 1986 and henceforth focused on educational and advisory activities.

Even though the Family Planning Association was the main provider of family planning services from 1949 through 1965, the government (first the British colonial administrators and subsequently the government headed by Singaporeans) played an increasingly important role. It provided ever larger grants to the association that rose steadily from S$5,000 in 1949–50 to S$100,000 or more in 1957–65. Government clinics provided the association with increasing amounts of space to provide family planning services, including a piece of land at a prime location for the association's headquarters, charging a nominal S$1 annual rent. Funding for construction, equipment, and staff training came from the Ford Foundation. In November 1960, the government and the association launched a three-month nationwide family planning campaign as part of the government's Mass Health Education Program. The intent of the People's Action Party to spread the family planning message was part of the party's platform for the 1959 general elections. Its document, *The Task Ahead: PAP's Five-year Plan, 1959–1965*, also became the party's program of action after it won the elections and assumed governance of the island.

Phase II: Anti-Natalist Policy, 1966–86

The anti-natalist phase was characterized by the government's strong and direct assumption of family planning responsibilities. The catalyst for this change, aside from requests by the Family Planning Association for the government to take over, was the sudden attainment of independence in August 1965. The leaders of the People's Action Party did not believe that Singapore, a tiny island with no natural resources, could survive on its own, but the attempt at a merger with Malaysia had failed after only two years. Even though the annual rate of population growth had already slowed from the excessively high 4 to 5 percent per year in the late 1950s, it had remained quite high, around 2.5 percent, in the years immediately preceding independence. Control of immigration was easily achieved, as both Malaysia and Singapore introduced border controls soon after their separation, although low levels of selective immigration continued.

As concerns fertility control, Singapore was noted for its innovative, and in some views stringent, programs and policies.

The government launched the National Family Planning and Population Program in January 1966. Responsibility for the day-to-day running of the program was placed under the SFPPB, a statutory body under the Ministry of Health established by an act of parliament in December 1965. The board's objectives were (a) to act as the sole agency for promoting and disseminating information pertaining to family planning, (b) to initiate and undertake the population control program, (c) to stimulate interest in demography, and (d) to advise the government on all matters relating to family planning and population control (Saw 1991). The board's establishment followed a government review of the status of family planning activities in Singapore after yet another request by the Family Planning Association for the government to take over its family planning clinical services. The government accepted the recommendations of the review committee that it assume full responsibility for clinical work, research, and publicity, but deferred the takeover to January 1, 1966, instead of October 1 as the committee had recommended (Government of Singapore 1965). As in the past, the government provided space for family planning services at its island-wide network of maternal and child health clinics. Government personnel, from senior administrators (including several departmental heads) to physicians, nurses, midwives, and nonprofessional staff members, were shared with the board in a virtually seamless network of service provision.

The act establishing the board also provided that any person, association, or body "interested in promoting and disseminating information on family planning" or in "selling or distributing any medicine, preparation or article for such purpose" must register with the board. Accordingly, the Family Planning Association (except for a short break in 1968 and 1971) and the Catholic Medical Guild became registered bodies under the board beginning in 1966. Private medical practitioners, who were already registered with the Singapore Medical Council and allowed to prescribe and sell contraceptives, were not required to re-register with the Ministry of Health.

Initially, the National Family Planning Program promoted the message of the desirability of a small family without specifying the size. A two-child family norm was adopted in 1972, and with it, the goal to reduce fertility to replacement level and then maintain it at that level so as to achieve zero population growth. In 1977, as the prospect of the echo of the baby boom loomed, the program added the message to delay marriage and the first birth and to space the two children. Demographic and programmatic targets were defined in terms of reductions in births or fertility rates and the number of acceptors to be reached by the end of each five-year plan period (table 13.1). Most of these targets were achieved, and even exceeded, the most significant of which was the attainment of a replacement level total fertility rate in 1975, five years ahead of the original target date. The practice of developing five-year plans ended after 1980, as the total fertility rate continued to decline below replacement level. Activities in the early 1980s focused mainly on program maintenance.

TABLE 13.1 SFPPB Five-Year Plan Targets and Achievements

Plan	Targets	Achievements
First Five-Year Plan (1966–70)	To reduce the crude birth rate from 32 births per 1,000 population in 1964 to around 20 by 1970	Crude birth rate reduced to 22.1 births per 1,000 population by 1970
	To provide family planning services to 60 percent of all married women aged 15–44	A total of 156,556 women, or 62 percent of married women of reproductive age, accepted family planning from the board's clinics
Second Five-Year Plan (1971–75)	To reduce the crude birth rate from 22.1 births per 1,000 population in 1970 to 18.0 by 1975	Crude birth rate reached 17.8 births per 1,000 population in 1975
	To recruit 16,000 new acceptors per year from 1971 to 1975 for a total of 80,000 over the period	A total of 89,501 new acceptors were recruited, exceeding the target by 11.9 percent
	To retain the 156,556 acceptors already registered with the program	
	To promote male and female sterilization for those who have completed their family size	
	To create awareness of family planning and its benefits among young people, those of marriageable age, and newlyweds, particularly those in lower income and education groups	
Third Five-Year Plan (1976–80)	To maintain fertility at replacement level (2.0 births per woman) so as to achieve zero population growth by 2030	Total fertility rate reached 1.8 births per woman in 1980

Source: SFPPB various years.

TABLE 13.2 Sources of Contraceptive Supplies, Selected Years
percent

Source	1977	1982	1987	1992
Government clinics and hospitals	74.1	70.1	61.6	50.9
General practitioners	14.8	18.4		
Pharmacies and drug stores	4.9	5.0	38.4[a]	49.1[a]
Other	6.2	6.5		

Source: Ministry of Health, Population Planning Section data.

a. Includes all private sector sources.

While it lasted, the National Family Planning Program provided a wide range of contraceptive services through an island-wide network of family planning and maternal and child health clinics run by the government. Other services included home visits, a mobile clinic to reach rural areas, and a family planning clinic for men. In addition to offering reversible contraceptive methods, the government legalized sterilization in 1970. In 1975, it further liberalized the grounds for its use so that the procedure became available on demand and at an affordable cost of S$5 per procedure at government hospitals and the vasectomy clinic.

The results of knowledge, attitudes, and practices surveys carried out since 1973 showed that government hospitals and clinics were the main sources of contraceptive supplies for most women (table 13.2). Reliance on private sector sources has, however, grown over time.

Abortion was also legalized in 1970 and liberalized in 1975. According to Saw (1991, p. 233), the decision to liberalize abortion followed a review that found the 1970 law to have "worked satisfactorily," and moreover, "the Government had decided upon a comprehensive population control program to work towards replacement fertility." Following the liberalization of sterilization and abortion, private medical practitioners were allowed to perform these procedures as long as they and their premises were licensed by the Ministry of Health in accordance with the Abortion Act.

In addition to clinical services, the program also featured a strong, multifaceted communication program that reached out to practically every segment of the population, including students. When births began to increase and the fertility rate leveled off in the early 1970s, the Information, Education, and Communication Unit of the SFPPB was created in 1972 to reinforce the family planning message and acceptance of the two-child family norm. Virtually every mass communication medium was used, including radio, television, newspapers and magazines, movie theaters, billboards, and bus panels. Publicity materials of many kinds—posters, pamphlets, bumper stickers, coasters, key chains, calendars, and pens—were distributed free of charge. Lectures and seminars were organized for newlyweds, community leaders, union leaders, teachers, and school principals. Face-to-face motivation included a postpartum and postabortion contact service. A telephone information service was also established. The small size of the country and its highly urbanized population probably facilitated the outreach effort.

Perhaps the most distinguishing feature of Singapore's program, however, was the comprehensive package of social policies, or incentives and disincentives, used to promote the acceptance of sterilization and the small family and to discourage large families. First introduced in 1969, the incentives and disincentives were intensified over the years. According to Wan and Loh (1979, pp. 102–3), "The basic purpose of many of the social policies . . . was to reduce or eliminate heavy government subsidizing of certain services . . . The rationale is that individuals who use services paid for by other taxpayers should adopt a more responsible reproductive behavior."

Specific measures included restricting maternity leave initially to the first three children born, then to the first two; levying progressively higher delivery charges for higher-order births; restricting income tax relief to the first three children born; giving priority for the allocation of public apartments to families with fewer children; and giving priority for registering children in the first grade to children from families with three or fewer children. The incentives aimed at promoting voluntary sterilization included providing paid maternity leave for female civil servants who underwent sterilization after the third or higher-order birth, providing civil servants with seven days of fully paid leave in addition to normal leave allocations after sterilization, waiving delivery charges for patients whose hospital care was partly subsidized by the government if they accepted sterilization, and giving priority for registering for the first grade for children whose parents were sterilized before age 40 after no more than two children. No child was denied a place in school under the enrolment schemes, although parents of three or more children might not be able to register their younger children at the school of their choice. Similarly, given the expanding public housing program at that time, no family was likely to have been denied public housing if it met the housing authority's requirements.

In 1984, the government began to relax its strong anti-natalist stance and introduced selective measures to promote larger family sizes among better-educated women. This development followed public discussion by Prime Minister Lee Kuan Yew of the "lop-sided pattern of procreation." Better-educated women were, on average, having fewer than two children, whereas those with no educational qualifications were bearing an average of three children. In addition, the better-educated women were more likely than others to remain single (K. Lee 1983). The prime minister recommended amending existing policies "so that our better-educated women will have more children to be adequately represented in the next generation" (Saw 1990, p. 44). Although he acknowledged that nature determined an individual's performance more than nurture in the proportion of 80 percent to 20 percent, he believed that better-educated mothers were more likely to provide an improved nurturing environment.

The government amended its policies relating to first grade registration to give priority to children of women who were university graduates and who had at least three children (the graduate mother scheme). The level of income tax relief for mothers with certain academic qualifications was also increased (Saw 1990). At the same time, the government increased the charges for third and subsequent deliveries in government hospitals, making it relatively more expensive for lower-income groups to have more children, and also introduced a S$10,000 housing grant to encourage low-income parents with little education to become sterilized after having two children. A government agency was set up to promote interaction among men and women with university degrees with a view to increasing the marriage rate among them. The government abandoned the graduate mother scheme because of the controversy it had generated and the small number of children who were likely to benefit from the measure.

The SFPPB was dissolved in June 1986 after parliament repealed the act that had created it following a management rationalization exercise by the government's Management Services Department. The board's staff and functions were transferred to the Ministry of Health. For all intents and purposes, the anti-natalist phase of Singapore's population policy ended with the dissolution of the board, which had sole responsibility for the National Family Planning Program. The government, however, continued to provide family planning services at its maternal and child health clinics.

Phase III: 1987–Present

The third phase of Singapore's population policy began officially in March 1987, when Goh Chok Tong, then first deputy prime minister (later prime minister and currently senior minister) announced the new population policy, exhorting Singaporeans who could afford it to have larger families of three or more children. The promotion of marriage was also an integral part of the new policy. As before, the government backed up its exhortation for larger families with a package of financial and other incentives as follows: (a) incentives to ease the financial burden of childrearing (tax rebates for the third and fourth children and income tax relief for up to four children); (b) incentives to ease the conflict between work and childrearing roles for women (child care subsidy, rebates on maid levies, leave to take care of a sick child, leave without pay and part-time work in the public sector), and (c) modification of earlier two-child incentives in line with the new policy (priority in the allocation of housing and primary school registration for families with three instead of two children) (Yap 1995). Women with two or fewer children requesting an abortion or sterilization are now required to undergo counseling and asked to reconsider their decision. Low-income couples with a low level of education are encouraged through housing grants and children's education bursaries to practice family planning (though sterilization is not required) and to limit their families to two children. The incentive package has been revised and enhanced over the years, with the latest revision taking place in 2004.

Integration of Population and Development Policies

Singapore adopted an industrialization policy in the early 1960s, following reviews and recommendations by experts from institutions such as the United Nations and the World Bank. As Cheng (1991, p. 182) observes, "from an underdeveloped country heavily dependent on entrepot trade, Singapore joined the ranks of the newly industrialized countries and built up a diversified economy in which trade was supplemented by manufacturing, transport and communications, banking and finance, and tourism." Cheng (1991, p. 215) argues that the economy's dynamic performance during the postwar period, especially after independence, "was due to a great degree to the determined efforts of the Government," and that "to ensure that the fruits of development led to yet higher standards of living, the Government was very active and successful in promoting family planning." Fawcett and Chen (1979, p. 252) make the following observation in their appraisal of the Singapore experience: "Population growth, distribution, and composition are matters of strong concern and high salience throughout the government. . . . The political leadership has consistently stressed the importance of population control, based largely on arguments related to Singapore's small size and lack of natural resources. . . . In short, the physical and social characteristics of Singapore have facilitated, indeed demanded, that demographic considerations be given high priority in development planning, and the political leadership has not hesitated to articulate this as a key element of national policy."

The place of demographic changes, particularly fertility decline, in development planning in Singapore is perhaps best demonstrated by a speech given by pioneer Cabinet Minister Goh Keng Swee to members of the International Monetary Fund and the World Bank in 1969. According to Goh, who has been hailed as the architect of the Singapore economy, the declining birth rates in the late 1950s and early 1960s permitted increased expenditures on education "without dreading that the inevitable outcome would be to flood the labor market with unemployable educated school-leavers, as had happened in so many other developing nations. Further, there was hope of a leveling off of expenditure on education. . . . The problem had assumed a finite dimension, and it was possible to proceed with development planning with the hope that the resulting increment in GNP [gross national product] will not be eaten up by uncontrolled population increase" (K. Goh 1969, p. 131).

With characteristic candor, however, Goh admitted that the initial fertility decline was not the result of the government's development planning, but rather a useful discovery after the fact: "If regard had been taken to the demographic trends of the previous two decades, the [People's Action] Party might have hesitated to make [its electoral promise to provide free universal primary education]. But demographers are seldom consulted in the drafting of election manifestos" (K. Goh 1969, p. 130).

Be that as it may, the relationship between population growth and development and the effects of population growth on people's quality of life had not been lost on the government. The Singapore Development Plan for 1961–64 identified control of population growth, including both fertility control and control of immigration, as the solution to the problems of high unemployment and economic pressures that confronted Singapore. According to Soo Ann Lee (1979), however, the plan instead emphasized industrial development because of political constraints the government faced, particularly with regard to the control of immigration from Peninsular Malaysia. The White Paper on family planning (Government of Singapore 1965, para. 8.1), while proclaiming that the "chief purpose" of the proposed family planning program was to "liberate our women from the burden of bearing and raising an unnecessarily large number of children and as a consequence to increase human happiness for all," added the following statement (para 8.4, emphasis in the original):

We are already spending hundreds of millions of public funds each year to provide better social services for our people in Education, Housing, Health, etc. It will be almost impossible to maintain this standard in the future if our present rate of population growth continues unchecked. . . . By restricting the number of babies born each year, there will not only be increased happiness for mothers but also for their families and we can at the same time, improve the general welfare of our people by raising living standards, through channeling millions more of public funds into *productive economic development* of Singapore and thus to increase more job opportunities and prosperity, all round.

Former senior official of the SFPPB Margaret Loh explained the relationship between population control and economic development thus: "The National Family Planning and Population Programme in Singapore can be said to have been instituted firstly to improve the health and welfare of mother, child and the total family unit at the micro level and at the macro level to accelerate fertility decline to aid the socio-economic development process. Both objectives . . . meet the ultimate goal of improving the quality of life for the people" (Loh 1976, p. 26).

The participation of various sectors of the government in population planning and policy development occurred in two ways. First, members of the SFPPB included senior officials from government ministries and departments, such as the Ministry of Education, the Ministry of Social Affairs, and the Singapore Broadcasting Corporation, as well as academics and members of the medical community. Similarly, the permanent secretary for health headed the Inter-Ministerial Population Committee, appointed in the mid-1980s to advise the government on the new population policy, but committee members included counterparts from other government ministries and academics. In this way, the relevant sectors of government were made aware of the population issue, and various government ministries instituted their own incentives or disincentives to encourage couples to have small families. For example, the Ministry of Education instituted the incentives and disincentives relating to enrolment in the first grade, whereas the Housing and Development Board initiated those relating to public housing (Loh 1976).

Another way in which planners became involved in population planning was a colloquium organized by the SFPPB in April 1976 after the National Family Planning Program had completed its first decade. Administrators from various government ministries and academics were invited to examine the implications of various demographic scenarios for the country's economic development, physical development, environment, and so on. On the basis of their recommended demographic scenario, the board set specific programmatic targets (Ministry of Health 1977; Wan, Loh, and Chen 1976). Similarly, in the early 1990s, a population and housing subcommittee was included among the subcommittees that reviewed the Singapore Concept Plan, the blueprint for Singapore's physical development (Cheong-Chua 1995, annex 4.2).

In contrast with its previous strongly anti-natalist position, the government has more recently rationalized its new, pro-natalist population policy as necessary for the country's long-term development. Expressing his concern about Singapore's continued low fertility, Goh Chok Tong stated, "We have to pay close attention to the trend and pattern of births because of their consequences on our prosperity and security, in fact, on our survival as a nation" (C. Goh 1986).

From the beginning, the government's concern was not just about the size of the population or the rate of population growth, but also about its quality. Both its procreation and immigration policies have been important parts of its development strategy. In launching the National Family Planning Program, the health minister at that time, Yong Nyuk Lin, declared, "Family planning is . . . a matter of national importance and indeed, one of urgency for us. Our best chance for survival in an independent Singapore is [to lay] stress on quality and not quantity" (Saw 1980, p. 52). Former Prime Minister Lee Kuan Yew explained the government's strong anti-natalist stance in an interview in 1974 as follows: "The day we are able to break through this hard core, we shall have solved our population problem. We can achieve zero growth, possibly even negative population growth. Then we can make up for it by selective immigration of the kind of people we require to run a modern higher technology economy" (Fawcett and Chen 1979, p. 251). Hence, the new population policy of 1987, by being selectively pro-natalist, represents a continuation of the government's emphasis on population quality. Indeed, despite its desire to control the rate of population growth, Singapore has always permitted an inflow of those deemed to be net contributors to the economy (Yap 1993).

Singapore is stepping up immigration, referred to as the search for talent, as fertility has fallen to levels that place the country among the ranks of countries with the "lowest-low" fertility despite the pro-natalist incentives of recent years. Singapore now adopts a three-pronged strategy of encouraging marriage and procreation, increasing immigration, and engaging the Singaporean diaspora because, in the words of deputy prime minister Wong Kan Seng, who is also in charge of population issues, in an interview in August 2006: "We hope that we will be able to replace ourselves and eventually grow our population as we move towards becoming a vibrant, open and successful modern city."[2]

Demographic Impact

Singapore's fertility decline began before the advent of the National Family Planning Program. As former Cabinet Minister Goh Keng Swee noted, this might be attributed in large part to the work of the Family Planning Association in meeting the demand for services. Acceptance of family planning was such that the number of new contraceptive acceptors at the association's clinics jumped from 600 in 1949 to nearly 10,000 in 1965. Pakshong (1967) estimated that of all women at risk of an unwanted pregnancy, the proportion of new acceptors rose from 2 percent in 1957 to 4 percent by 1963–64. Pakshong also estimated that the clinics served about 9 to 10 percent of eligible women, with an unknown additional proportion obtaining contraceptives from other sources or practicing traditional methods such as coitus interruptus or periodic abstinence.

Table 13.3 shows the number of acceptors of reversible methods, sterilization, and abortion between 1966 and 1995. The data for reversible contraceptive methods refer to acceptors registered with the SFPPB, whereas those for sterilization and abortion include procedures performed in government and approved private facilities. Data on users of reversible contraceptive methods who obtained services from the private sector are not available. As mentioned earlier, the number of contraceptive acceptors exceeded even the board's ambitious target.

TABLE 13.3 Number of SFPPB New and Existing Acceptors, Sterilizations, and Abortions, 1966–95

Year	Family planning acceptors		Sterilization		Abortion[a]
	New	Existing	Female	Male	
1966	30,410	—	—	—	—
1967	30,935	—	—	—	—
1968	35,338	—	—	—	—
1969	35,643	—	—	—	—
1970	24,230	—	2,321	51	1,913
1971	17,749	—	3,871	99	3,407
1972	17,666	—	5,842	347	3,806
1973	19,102	—	8,964	374	5,252
1974	18,292	—	9,241	326	7,175
1975	16,692	—	9,495	453	12,873
1976	17,674	—	10,310	408	15,496
1977	15,158	—	8,236	351	16,443
1978	15,192	—	7,447	340	17,246
1979	15,266	—	6,768	495	16,999
1980	15,009	—	6,487	458	18,219
1981	14,534	—	6,312	486	18,890
1982	14,651	—	6,011	494	19,110
1983	13,741	—	5,571	456	19,100
1984	12,481	—	5,417	369	22,190
1985	12,686	69,772	5,233	257	23,512
1986	11,460	67,410	4,504	264	23,035
1987	8,573	59,416	3,524	128	21,226
1988	7,412	52,414	4,398	171	20,135
1989	7,436	44,976	4,367	172	20,619
1990	6,535	41,653	4,394	134	18,470
1991	6,575	42,019	4,697	163	17,798
1992	5,581	35,986	5,225	154	17,073
1993	5,061	33,621	5,549	128	16,476
1994	4,716	31,649	5,309	125	15,690
1995	3,892	29,024	5,410	152	14,504

Source: Ministry of Health data.

Note: — = not available.

a. Figures for 1970–75 exclude menstrual regulation.

Estimates of the prevalence of specific methods currently in use were obtained from periodic knowledge, attitudes, and practices surveys conducted between 1973 and 1992 (table 13.4). The total current practice rate rose from 60 percent of married women of reproductive age in 1973 to 74 percent in 1982. The latter figure is likely to be the saturation level of contraceptive prevalence, given that at any time some people will not require contraceptives because they are either planning to have a child, are pregnant, or are sterile. Contraceptive prevalence declined to 67 percent in 1987, coinciding with the introduction of the new, pro-natalist population policy

TABLE 13.4 Current Contraceptive Use by Method, Selected Years
percentage of currently married women aged 15–44

Method	1973	1977	1982	1987	1992
Total practice rate	60.1	71.3	74.2	67.4	64.8
Pill	21.7	17.0	11.6	7.3	6.9
Condom	17.0	20.8	24.3	17.3	21.7
Sterilization (male and female)	10.8	21.9	22.9	21.8	15.3
Intrauterine device	3.3	3.1	—	4.6	6.5
Traditional methods[a]	—	—	1.2	14.4	13.3
Other	7.3	8.5	14.2	2.0	1.1

Source: Ministry of Health, Population Planning Section data.

Note: — = not available.

a. Includes rhythm and withdrawal methods.

in March of that year. The contraceptive method mix also changed over the years. The proportion of couples sterilized rose sharply between 1973 and 1977, doubling from about 11 percent to 22 percent, and then remained at this level until 1987. A switch to the use of condoms and less reliable traditional methods accompanied the decline in contraceptive use after 1987.

Another reason for the decline in contraceptive use in 1987 might have been that many couples were planning to have babies the following year, which was deemed doubly auspicious because it was the Year of the Dragon in the Chinese lunar calendar and because the number 88 signifies double prosperity in Mandarin and Cantonese. The number of births was sharply higher in 1988, nearly 53,000, compared with about 44,000 in 1987 and 40,000 to 42,000 per year in the early 1980s.

The surveys also showed that the number of children born to married women of reproductive age fell from an average of 3.4 per woman in 1973 to 2.0 by 1987 (table 13.5). Remarkably, convergence was apparent among all three major ethnic groups. Actual and preferred family sizes had traditionally differed, with Malays wanting and having the most children and Chinese the least. Differentials by level of education also narrowed.

The number of children that survey respondents reported having was consistently lower than the number of children they desired, indicating an absence of unwanted fertility. Desired family size, which has remained fairly constant at about three children since 1977, has consistently been higher than the total fertility rate. Several possible explanations could account for this. It could be an indication of the effectiveness of government policies to promote the acceptance of the two-child family. For example, among survey respondents in 1982, the incentives and disincentives had variously affected the family size decisions of about 6 to 24 percent of those who had completed their families, and among respondents who had yet to complete their families, the policies were likely to affect the family size decisions of 11 to 35 percent of those with no children or only one child (Emmanuel and others 1984). As Cheng (1991) and Fawcett and Chen (1979), among others, have noted, increased female education and labor force participation, better health, and improved social security are likely to have affected families' calculations in relation to childbearing and the costs and value of children.

TABLE 13.5 Mean Number of Children Born and Desired by Ethnicity and Education, Selected Years

Category	1973	1977	1982	1987	1992
Mean number of children born by survey respondents' ethnicity					
All ethnic groups	3.4	2.8	2.2	2.0	2.0
Chinese	3.2	2.7	2.2	2.0	1.9
Malays	3.9	3.4	2.5	2.1	2.4
Indians	3.7	3.1	2.3	2.0	2.0
Mean number of children desired by respondents' ethnicity					
All ethnic groups	3.7	3.1	2.7	2.9	2.9
Chinese	3.6	2.9	2.6	2.8	2.7
Malays	4.5	3.7	3.2	3.6	3.6
Indians	3.8	3.2	2.7	3.0	2.9
Mean number of children born by respondents' education					
No formal education	4.5	4.0	3.4	2.7	2.4
Primary-level education	3.1	2.9	2.5	2.1	2.2
Secondary-level education	1.9	1.9	1.7	1.8	1.8
Tertiary-level education	1.7	1.7	1.4	1.2	1.4

Source: Ministry of Health, Population Planning Section data.

Another way to measure the effect of the National Family Planning Program is to estimate the number of births averted. Assuming a one-year lag between contraceptive use and an averted birth, Chen and Pang (1977) estimated that more than 250,000 births were averted during 1967 to 1976 and that the program accounted for nearly three-quarters of that figure. They estimated the proportionate contribution of the program to have risen from 27 percent (3,937 births) in 1967 to nearly 88 percent (35,725 births) in 1976. Among the methods used to avert births through the program, the pill made the greatest contribution (nearly 54 percent of averted births), followed by sterilization (19 percent), and condoms (15 percent).

Costs of Family Planning Activities

From the beginning, the program provided contraceptive services and supplies to users at low cost. The White Paper on family planning (Government of Singapore 1965) established the following subsidized fee structure for citizens: S$10 for the first insertion of a copper-T intrauterine device (IUD) and S$5 for each subsequent insertion, S$1.50 per monthly cycle of oral contraceptives, and S$25 for surgical ligation. Moreover, those on welfare received contraceptive services free of charge, but noncitizens were charged at unsubsidized rates (S$50 for the first IUD insertion and S$25 for subsequent insertions, S$4.50 per cycle of oral contraceptives, and S$100 for surgical ligation). Beginning in 1967, the fee for an IUD insertion was reduced to S$5 and it has remained at that level since, although users of the newer multiload IUD, introduced in 1983, pay S$30. The fees for condoms (S$0.50 for six) and diaphragms (S$2 each) have remained unchanged since 1966, and the fee for pills has remained at S$1 per cycle since 1968. Charges for sterilization (male and female) and abortions performed at government clinics and hospitals were initially pegged at S$5 per procedure, but these have been allowed to vary, as government hospitals were privatized in the mid-1980s.

As mentioned earlier, the government began providing financial support for family planning activities even before it established the national program. The value of its grants rose from S$5,000 in 1949–50 to S$120,000 by 1958, and then declined to S$100,000 per year during 1959 to 1965. Even after it assumed full responsibility for the National Family Planning Program in 1966, the government continued to provide an annual grant of S$10,000 to the Family Planning Association until 1968. With the establishment of the SFPPB, the government doubled its grants from S$100,000 to S$200,000 per year during the First Five-Year Plan period (1966–70). Its financial support for the board's family planning activities rose significantly in the 1970s, reaching S$1.5 million, and ultimately more than S$3.0 million in the 1980s (figure 13.1).

Figure 13.1 does not include the costs of the program to the Ministry of Health, which shared staff and premises with the SFPPB. As table 13.6 shows, the family planning budget represented less than 1 percent of the total government budget and less than 2 percent of the total health budget. As of March 1997, the Ministry of Health estimated that its current expenditure on family planning services amounted to about S$1.1 million annually.

Another measure of the costs of its population policy to the government is the revenue forgone because of various incentive schemes. According to the Ministry of Health, it does not monitor this information, because a variety of government agencies administer the incentives, making their total costs difficult to estimate.

FIGURE 13.1 SFPPB Income and Expenditure, 1966–84

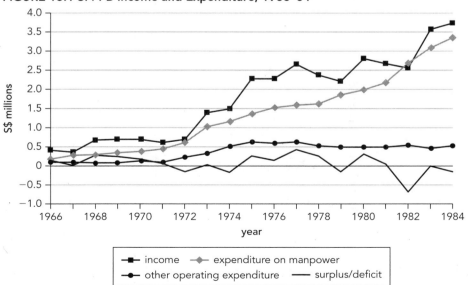

Source: SFPPB 1984.

TABLE 13.6 Family Planning, Health, and Total Government Budgets, 1978–83

Year	National Family Planning Program (S$ millions)	Ministry of Health (S$ millions)	Total government budget (S$ millions)	Family planning budget		Expenditure on health as a percentage of the total budget
				As a percentage of the total budget	As a percentage of the health budget[a]	
1978	2.8	177.6	3,668	0.08	1.6	4.8
1979	2.9	187.8	3,885	0.07	1.5	4.8
1980	3.3	217.0	4,113	0.08	1.5	5.3
1981	3.6	272.3	6,335	0.06	1.3	4.3
1982	3.7	318.7	7,638	0.05	1.2	4.2
1983	3.9	363.5	8,871	0.04	1.1	4.1

Source: Nortman 1985.

a. As the family planning budget is not included in the budget of the Ministry of Health, the figures shown are the ratio of the family planning budget to the health budget.

Various international agencies and overseas foundations have made cash and in-kind contributions to the program. Notably, the Ford Foundation provided funding for the construction of the National Family Planning Program's headquarters, which later became the headquarters of the SFPPB, and for training and equipment. The International Planned Parenthood Federation provided funding to the Singapore Planned Parenthood Association ranging from about S$235,000 (US$77,000) to nearly S$105,000 per year during 1985 to 1996. Funds raised locally complement this contribution. Compared with other countries, the amount of aid received by the program in Singapore is small.

Conclusion

Demographic management by the state has been more determined and more successful in Singapore than in most other countries. Once the government recognized that the population growth rate was unacceptably high, it took strong measures, including contraception, sterilization, abortion, public education, and incentives, as well as marriage and immigration measures. Later, when these, together with rapid social change, brought fertility to an unacceptably low level, the government modified its policies and introduced reverse incentives. Starting with concerns about human welfare, the policy rationale was closely intertwined with development objectives.

Population policies, both those relating to procreation and those directed at controlling immigration, continue to be an integral part of Singapore's development strategy. The prevailing view is that the fertility declines contributed to, or at least provided breathing space for, development in the early days of Singapore's independence, permitting resources that would otherwise have been spent on sustaining a rapidly growing population to be channeled into productive development. If, for example, the development of human capital has generally been instrumental in promoting economic development, as the World Bank (1993) suggests, then the stringent procreation control policies adopted by Singapore no doubt contributed to its economic growth, just as they are generally acknowledged to have contributed to its fertility decline. Singapore has adjusted its population policies to meet what planners consider to be the requirements for the next stage of its economic development, including more rapid labor force growth. The success of the new procreation policy remains to be seen, however, as the total fertility rate appears to be falling again after some initial rises. Because rapid augmentation of the population through immigration has social and political consequences, that aspect of population growth will have to be handled with care.

Notes

1. Urban Redevelopment Authority. "Concept Plan: Towards a Thriving World Class City in the 21st Century." Urban Redevelopment Authority, Government of Singapore. http://www.ura.gov.sg/conceptplan2001.
2. Channel NewsAsia. "Interview with DPM Wong Kan Seng on Population Issues." MediaCorp News. http://www.channelnewsasia.com/stories/singaporelocalnews/view/226426/1/.html.

References

Chen, Ai Ju, and Pang Swee Lan. 1977. "Births Averted by Ten Years (1966–1975) of the National Family Planning and Population Programme." Paper 48, Singapore Family Planning and Population Board, Singapore.

Cheng, Siok Hwa. 1991. "Economic Change and Industrialization." In *A History of Singapore*, ed. Ernest C. T. Chew and Edwin Lee, 182–216. Singapore: Oxford University Press.

Cheong-Chua, Koon Hean. 1995. "Urban Land-Use Planning in Singapore: Towards A Tropical City of Excellence." In *Environment and the City: Sharing Singapore's Experience and Future Challenges,* ed. Giok Ling Ooi, 108–29. Singapore: Times Academic Press.

Cheung, Paul, P. L. 1995. "Planning Within Limits: Population Policy and Sustainable Population Growth." In *Environment and the City: Sharing Singapore's Experience and Future Challenges*, ed. Giok Ling Ooi, 100–08. Singapore: Times Academic Press.

Emmanuel, S. C., S. B. Li, T. P. Ng, and A. J. Chen. 1984. *Third National Family Planning and Population Survey, 1982.* Studies on Health and Family Planning in Association of Southeast Asian Nations Countries, Phase II, Association of Southeast Asian Nations-Australian Population Programme. Singapore: Singapore Family Planning and Population Board.

Family Planning Association of Singapore. 1954. *Fifth Annual Report.* Singapore: Family Planning Association of Singapore.

Fawcett, James T., and Peter S. J. Chen. 1979. "Public Policy and Population Change: An Appraisal of the Singapore Experience." In *Public Policy and Population Change in Singapore*, ed. Peter S. J. Chen and James T. Fawcett, 243–58. New York: Population Council.

Goh, Chok Tong. 1986. "The Second Long March." Speech delivered at the Nanyang Technological Institute, August 4. Reproduced as Appendix D in Saw 1990.

Goh, Keng Swee. 1969. "Population Control." Speech delivered on October 1 at the International Monetary Fund and International Bank for Reconstruction and Development Annual Meetings, Washington, DC. Reproduced in Goh, Keng Swee. 1995. *The Economics of Modernization*, 2nd ed. Singapore: Federal Publications.

Government of Singapore. 1965. *Family Planning in Singapore.* White Paper. Singapore: Government Printers.

———. 1991. *Singapore: The Next Lap.* Singapore: Times Editions.

Kinsella, Kevin, and Yvonne J Gist. 1995. *Older Workers, Retirement and Pensions: A Comparative International Chartbook.* Washington, DC: U.S. Bureau of the Census.

Lee, Kuan Yew. 1983. "Talent for the Future." Speech delivered at the National Day Rally on August 14. Reproduced as appendix A in Saw 1990.

———. 2005. Speech in Parliament on the Proposal to Develop Integrated Resorts, April 19, Singapore.

Lee, Soo Ann. 1979. "Population, Industrial Development, and Economic Growth." In *Public Policy and Population Change in Singapore*, ed. Peter S. J. Chen and James T. Fawcett, 229–40. New York: Population Council.

Lian, Daniel. 2004. *A Bigger Singapore?* Singapore: Morgan Stanley Equity Research Asia/Pacific.

Loh, Margaret. 1976. "Beyond Family Planning Measures in Singapore." Paper 40, Singapore Family Planning and Population Board, Singapore.

Mason, Andrew, ed. 2001. *Population Policies and Programs in East Asia.* Occasional Papers, Population and Health Series 123. Honolulu, East-West Center.

Ministry of Health. 1977. *Population and Trends.* Singapore: Ministry of Health.

Nortman, D. 1985. *Population and Family Planning: A Compendium of Data through 1983.* New York: Population Council.

Pakshong, Dolly I. 1967. "Family Planning in Singapore 1949–1964." Diploma in Public Health dissertation, University of Singapore.

Saw, Swee Hock. 1980. *Population Control for Zero Growth in Singapore.* Singapore: Oxford University Press.

———. 1990. *Changes in the Fertility Policy of Singapore.* Institute of Policy Studies Occasional Paper 2. Singapore: Times Academic Press.

———. 1991. "Population Growth and Control." In *A History of Singapore*, ed. Ernest C. T. Chew and Edwin Lee, 219–41. Singapore: Oxford University Press.

SFPPB (Singapore Family Planning and Population Board). 1984, 1995, various years. *Annual Report.* Singapore: SFPPB.

Wan, Fook Kee, and Margaret Loh. 1979. "Fertility Policies and the National Family Planning and Population Program." In *Public Policy and Population Change in Singapore*, ed. Peter S. J. Chen and James T. Fawcett, 97–108. New York: Population Council.

Wan, Fook Kee, Margaret Loh, and Chen Ai Ju. 1976. "Population and Family Planning in Singapore." Paper 46, Singapore Family Planning and Population Board, Singapore.

World Bank. 1993. *The East Asian Miracle: Economic Growth and Public Policy.* New York: Oxford University Press.

Yap, Mui Teng. 1993. "Policy Options for Low Fertility Countries: The Singapore Experience." In *International Population Conference Montreal 1993*, vol. 4, 73–89. Liege, Belgium: International Union for the Scientific Study of Population.

———. 1995. "Singapore's 'Three or More' Policy." *Business Times*, Trends supplement, June 24.

Zhou, Mei. 1996. *The Life of Family Planning Pioneer, Constance Goh: A Point of Light.* Singapore: Graham Brash.

14 The Emergence of Thailand's National Family Planning Program

ALLAN G. ROSENFIELD AND CAROLINE J. MIN

Until the mid-1960s, the government of Thailand did not provide any family planning services beyond a special program funded by the Population Council that provided postpartum family planning services, including intrauterine devices (IUDs), oral contraceptives, and postpartum female sterilization, in four Bangkok hospitals. One of the hospitals, Chulalongkorn, developed one of the largest IUD clinics in the world, and by the late 1960s, women were coming to the clinic from almost every province, having heard about it by word of mouth (Rosenfield, Asavasena, and Mikhanorn 1973). In general, contraceptives could only be prescribed by physicians, most of whom practiced in Bangkok and other urban areas, leaving rural women with extremely limited access to services.

The government, reluctant to recognize the population problem, did not promulgate an official population policy promoting family planning until 1970. However, in late 1967, a new undersecretary of state for public health quietly initiated a nationwide family planning project that ultimately was the forerunner to a national family planning program. This enterprise began to significantly expand access to family planning services in previously underserved areas and established a framework for a national program that integrated family planning services within the exiting health care infrastructure.

The accomplishments achieved during this formative period are especially noteworthy given that the activities were conducted without an official mandate, public information campaigns, full-time family planning workers, targets, or incentives. The readiness of Ministry of Public Health officials to experiment with, and authorize, an expanded role for auxiliary midwives was a critical factor in scaling up family planning services so rapidly. At the same time, elements of Thai culture facilitated the adoption of family planning among couples (Rosenfield and others 1982).

Thailand in the 1960s

Like many other developing countries in the early 1960s, Thailand was a predominantly rural society with the majority of the population occupied in agricultural activities. While social and economic development was occurring in the larger cities, particularly Bangkok, change in rural areas was slow. Table 14.1 provides the socioeconomic context at the beginning and end of the decade. That two-thirds of women aged 20–44 were literate in 1960 demonstrates the relatively advanced social status of Thai women, although the percentage of women with more than a primary education, 4.2 percent, was low. Despite some regional and class differences with respect to language and lifestyle, Thais were culturally homogeneous in terms of their religious practices. More than 90 percent of the population observed Theravada Buddhism, which emphasizes individual autonomy and personal responsibility for behavior.

Government facilities provided most modern health care services, with the Ministry of Public Health being responsible for the majority of services provided outside the capital city. The nation's 71 provinces had 84 provincial hospitals ranging in capacity from 50 to 450 beds, and Bangkok had 3 large hospitals. In rural areas, the Ministry of Public Health offered curative and preventive health care services through a network of nearly 4,000 health centers; however, only about 175 of these centers had a physician on site. The remaining centers were staffed by an auxiliary midwife and a male health worker or by an auxiliary midwife alone. Midwifery centers, the smallest class of health centers, covered populations of 2,000 to 3,000 people each. Government nurses, like physicians, worked primarily in hospitals or urban health centers (Hemachudha and Rosenfield 1975).

According to the 1960 census, the total population at the start of the decade was approximately 27 million, with 45 percent of the population younger than age 15. The rate of population growth was more than 3 percent per year (Gille and Balfour 1964). Total fertility during this time was more than six children per woman (Institute of Population Studies and Population Survey Division 1977). Despite the rapid

TABLE 14.1 Socioeconomic Indicators, 1960 and 1970

Indicator	1960	1970
Literacy		
Percentage of total population aged 10 or older	70.8	81.8
Percentage of women aged 20–44	66.2	82.0
Secondary or higher education		
Percentage of total population aged 9–29	—	6.4
Percentage of women aged 20–44	4.2	5.8
Percentage of economically active population working in agriculture	82.3	79.3
Percentage of population living in municipal areas	12.5	13.2
Life expectancy (years)	53.0	57.6

Source: Knodel and Debavalya 1978.

Note: — = not available.

and unprecedented level of population growth, the government maintained an essentially pro-natalist position. Aside from the postpartum program in Bangkok, the government did not offer family planning services. In 1964, however, the Potharam Project demonstrated the interest of Thai women in a rural community in family planning services. Nonetheless, for much of the decade, most women in rural areas were, in effect, excluded from access to contraception.

Early Family Planning Activities: 1963–67

In 1959, a World Bank economic mission described the adverse consequences that Thailand's markedly high rate of population growth would have on economic development. Even though the government paid little attention to the population problem, the interest of key health officials and academics eventually prompted a series of seminars on the issue beginning in 1963. The First National Population Seminar, sponsored by the National Research Council of Thailand and funded by the Population Council, allowed for discussion about the high rate of population growth and recommended that the matter be studied more closely (Gille and Balfour 1964). National population seminars were held again in 1965 and in 1968.

Potharam Research Project

As an outgrowth of the first seminar, in 1964 the Ministry of Public Health and the National Research Council began a small demonstration project in Potharam, a rural district outside Bangkok (Hawley and Prachuabmoh 1966; Prachuabmoh and Thomlinson 1971). Family planning services were provided at a small number of health centers over an 18-month action period. Government health staff members, with assistance from some traditional midwives and a few field workers especially recruited for the project, were responsible for client education and motivation. A baseline knowledge, attitudes, and practices survey found that fewer than 5 percent of married women knew of any modern contraceptive method; fewer than 3 percent of couples were using contraceptives, including sterilization; and yet 70 percent of the women did not want additional children. During the action phase of the project, more than 30 percent of married women accepted contraception, the majority electing to use an IUD, with sterilization in second place. A follow-up survey found that more than 80 percent of women in the district knew about one or more modern methods of contraception. This project was instrumental in demonstrating to government officials that rural couples were interested in limiting their childbearing and would make use of family planning services if they were available.

Hospital-Based Family Planning Programs

In 1965, a few hospitals in Bangkok decided to open family planning clinics, including Chulalongkorn Hospital, whose clinic offered only the IUD. In 1966, four Bangkok hospitals joined the International Postpartum Program sponsored by the Population Council (Zatuchni 1970): Chulalongkorn Hospital and another medical school teaching institution, a large women's hospital of the Ministry of Public

Health, and a general hospital of the Bangkok municipality. This was part of a new international trend whereby hospitals in numerous participating countries provided family planning education to maternity patients in the prenatal and postpartum wards and offered contraception, primarily the IUD and sterilization, to women prior to discharge or in the months thereafter.

By mid-1970, the Thai postpartum program had expanded outside Bangkok to eight provincial hospitals and three maternal and child health centers of the Ministry of Public Health. From 1966 through November 1971, nearly 100,000 women accepted family planning services within three months of delivery or abortion, the majority accepting an IUD or sterilization prior to discharge from the hospital. The family planning clinic at Chulalongkorn Hospital became one of the world's largest IUD clinics at the time. Between 1965 and 1971, the clinic received 66,000 new IUD clients (Rosenfield and Varakamin 1972). During the clinic's first few years of oper-ation, women from 66 provinces came to obtain IUDs. This is especially notable given that the hospital did not conduct public information activities beyond its facil-ities. Rather, women learned about the services through informal word-of-mouth communication (Fawcett, Somboonsuk, and Khaisang 1967; Rosenfield, Asavasena, and Mikhanorn 1973).

The Family Health Project, 1968–70: Precursor of a National Program

In 1967, the undersecretary of state for public health, Dr. Sombun Phong-Aksara, quietly directed key Ministry of Public Health officials to develop a nationwide research project on family planning. The stated objective was to train Ministry of Public Health personnel to provide family planning information and services in preparation for a change in the government's population stance. Phong-Aksara and several senior ministry officials were also seriously concerned about Thailand's high rate of population growth and wanted to begin providing family planning services to poor women, especially in rural areas, who had limited access to services.

The ministry's Division of Family Health, led by Dr. Winich Asavasena, developed a three-year plan (1968–70)—the Family Health Project—that called for training at least one physician and one nurse from each of the 84 provincial hospitals and all physicians, nurses, and auxiliary midwives working in rural health centers. The train-ing courses were one week long and specific to each category of personnel. In gen-eral, the courses focused on population dynamics, including the impact of Thailand's rapid population growth on socioeconomic development, and methods of contra-ception to be used, mainly IUDs and oral contraceptives. The courses for auxiliary midwives emphasized information about methods of contraception to enable them to counter any fears or rumors that might develop. Between 1968 and 1970, approxi-mately 330 physicians, 700 nurses, and 3,090 auxiliary midwives were trained (Rosenfield and others 1971). In 1970, two-day courses were given to male health workers to allow them to assist with motivational aspects of the project.

Following personnel training, family planning clinics were to be opened in all hospitals and health centers staffed with a physician. Auxiliary midwives at health centers without a physician were charged solely with providing information to women, motivating them, and referring potential clients to family planning clinics. By mid-1970, some 350 family planning clinics had been established in hospitals and health centers (Hemachudha and Rosenfield 1975). Public information activities were prohibited during this time, and the project relied on communication between potential clients and satisfied clients as the main means of promoting family planning. No targets or quotas were set for the project as a whole or for individual staff members. In addition, no incentives of any kind were given to the staff or to potential clients. The Ministry of Public Health requested a small fee from women if they could afford to pay (up to US$0.25 for a cycle of pills and US$1 for an IUD).

Training Auxiliary Midwives to Distribute Oral Contraceptives

The stipulation that only physicians were allowed to prescribe oral contraceptives or insert IUDs severely limited rural women's access to family planning services. In 1968, more than 60 percent of Thailand's 6,000 physicians worked in Bangkok and most of the rest practiced in other urban areas (Bryant 1969). The physician-to-patient ratio in more rural areas at this time was estimated to be one physician for approximately 110,000 people (Hemachudha and Rosenfield 1975). Working as an adviser to the Ministry of Public Health, one of the authors (Rosenfield) helped the ministry experiment with alternative methods of delivering contraceptive services. After a thorough review of the medical issues involved, a pilot study was initiated in 1969 to test the ability of auxiliary midwives to safely prescribe the pill (Rosenfield and Limcharoen 1972). In four provinces used as experiments, auxiliary midwives were trained to use a specially developed checklist, which included a simple medical history and examination, to screen for women for whom use of the pill was contraindicated. A pelvic examination was not required. Women who answered yes to any of the medical history questions were referred to a physician.

The number of women accepting the pill in the experiment provinces quadrupled during the first six months of the study compared with the six months prior to the study, and the percentage of women accepting the pill in the experiment provinces was significantly higher than in the control provinces. In addition, 12-month continuation rates were found to be higher among women who received the pill from an auxiliary midwife compared with the rates among women who received the pill from a physician. The incidence of side effects did not increase for women who received the pill from an auxiliary midwife (Rosenfield and Limcharoen 1972).

In mid-1970, the Ministry of Public Health reviewed the evidence and ruled that all auxiliary midwives could prescribe the pill, a pivotal decision that coincided with the cabinet's announcement of an official population policy. The basic training that auxiliary midwives had already received in population dynamics and family planning was deemed sufficient to prepare them for this new responsibility. Thus, the ruling immediately increased the potential number of family planning outlets from fewer than 350 clinics to almost 3,500, predominantly in rural areas, allowing the national program to accelerate at a much faster rate than expected.

Undertaking Monitoring and Evaluation Activities

In addition to special research projects such as the foregoing study, a central research and evaluation unit was created to routinely monitor project performance. All clinics were expected to submit specially developed patient record forms and a monthly activity report to the unit. Family planning clinics not run by the Ministry of Public Health, including clinics run by the Bangkok Municipal Health Bureau and private agencies, were also expected to submit the same information. The unit carried out sample analyses of patient characteristics for three different time periods during 1969 to 1970 and did not observe any significant differences over time. Approximately 80 percent of all new clients lived in rural areas, more than two-thirds were from agricultural households, more than 90 percent had four years or less of formal schooling, and roughly 80 percent had never used any contraceptive method before. For the total sample, more than 50 percent of new clients were under 30 years of age. The vast majority of women, more than 90 percent, obtained information about family planning services mainly from friends and relatives and, to a lesser degree, from health personnel (Rosenfield and others 1971).

The number of new clients in rural areas relative to urban areas increased during this time. During 1965 to 1968, 56 percent of all new family planning clients lived in Bangkok, compared with only 17 percent in 1970. That is, only 14 percent of new clients received services from rural health centers compared with 61 percent in 1970.

Table 14.2 breaks down family planning clients by method during the course of the Family Health Project. An impressive increase is apparent in the number of clients between 1968 and 1970. The increase in the number of women accepting the pill by 1970 reflects the Ministry of Public Health's ruling on auxiliary midwives in the middle of that year.

Organizing and Financing the Project

Given the lack of an official mandate for family planning activities, creating a separate family planning infrastructure was not feasible. In addition, ministry officials believed that integrating family planning activities within the national health care infrastructure made sense, both to make use of existing resources and personnel and

TABLE 14.2 Family Planning Clients by Method, 1968–70

Method	1968[a] Number	1968[a] Percent	1969 Number	1969 Percent	1970 Number	1970 Percent	Total Number	Total Percent
IUD	35,300	62	54,496	42	74,404	33	164,200	40
Pill	10,000	17	60,459	46	132,387	59	202,846	49
Female sterilization	12,000	21	15,265	12	18,648	8	45,913	11
Total	57,300	100	130,220	100	225,439	100	412,959	100

Source: Rosenfield and others 1971.

a. The reporting system was not in place until midyear, and thus, the numbers are approximate.

to help improve the maternal and child health care system more generally. Project operations and the central evaluation unit were placed under the jurisdiction of the Family Health Division of the ministry's Department of Health, while medical research and hospital operations were placed under the Provincial Hospital Division of the ministry's Department of Medical Services.

No funds were specifically allocated for family planning activities in the national budget. Rather, project costs were indirectly incorporated in the budgets of the various ministry divisions through expenditures for existing staff members and facilities. In addition, the Population Council provided a small amount of local currency needed at the beginning of the project for training (supplemented in 1969 by the United Nations Children's Fund), hiring of local staff members, and other expenses. The U.S. Agency for International Development provided a significant amount of commodity support, including oral contraceptives, clinic and research equipment, and vehicles (Rosenfield and others 1971). By the early 1970s, the U.S. Agency for International Development had become the largest donor. Other organizations, including the International Planned Parenthood Federation and the Ford and Rockefeller foundations, also provided support for family planning activities to institutions other than the Ministry of Public Health during this time. The technical and financial assistance provided by these agencies was important for the successful launch of family planning efforts in Thailand.

Overcoming Political Constraints

During this period, the military leader at the time and other military and government officials did not believe that Thailand had a serious population problem and were opposed to encouraging family planning. While this did not prevent the Ministry of Public Health from moving forward with its provisional efforts, such opposition did constrain programmatic options. A key limitation was the restriction on public communications promoting family planning. Even though the success of early activities demonstrated the effectiveness of person-to-person communication, the ministry believed that educational campaigns were necessary to reach a greater number of women (Rosenfield Asavasena, and Mikhanorn 1973). The women who accepted family planning services when they first became available were likely the most self-motivated, and changing the reproductive behavior of the broader population would require additional efforts. In general, however, the Ministry of Public Health was able to experiment with and implement innovative approaches to delivering family planning services without formal support.

In 1968, the National Economic and Social Development Board established a Population Unit within its Manpower Planning Division, with financial and technical assistance from the Population Council. At the request of the cabinet, the Population Unit's first task was to review the population issue and submit recommendations. The unit presented its conclusions in 1970, which, along with the endeavors of the Ministry of Public Health, quickly led to the cabinet's declaration of an official population policy, and the first national campaign to promote family planning was initiated in 1972.

The National Family Planning Program: 1970–80

The new population policy called for lowering the population growth rate by providing family planning information and services. The government developed a five-year plan (1972–76) with the goal of reducing the rate of population growth from more than 3.0 percent per year to 2.5 percent per year by the end of 1976. The Family Health Project became the National Family Planning Program (NFPP), and family planning activities continued to be integrated within the existing health care infrastructure. Box 14.1 provides a timeline of key milestones.

In the 1970s, the NFPP expanded the range of available contraceptive methods. In 1972, Thai surgeons developed the minilaparotomy, a modified sterilization technique that required only a small abdominal incision to access the fallopian tubes and could be carried out in rural or provincial areas where many physicians had neither the equipment nor the training to perform laparoscopic sterilizations. This became an important sterilization method in Thailand and throughout the world. In 1977, the Ministry of Public Health officially approved the injectable contraceptive depot medroxyprogesterone acetate (known commercially as Depo-Provera). Over time, its use grew substantially.

Building upon past results, the NFPP continued to expand the role of auxiliary midwives to meet demand. The Ministry of Public Health reviewed the practicality of using nurses and midwives to insert IUDs and found the approach to be safe (Wright and others 1977). However, as most nurses and midwives worked in hospitals or urban health centers, training them did not have a major impact on IUD use. The ministry then studied the effectiveness of using auxiliary midwives to insert IUDs and found that they performed the task as well as physicians and midwives (Sujpluem, Bennett, and Kolsartsanee 1978). The ministry also undertook studies to determine whether auxiliary midwives could provide depot medroxyprogesterone acetate injections and perform sterilization procedures, which were generally supportive.

The demonstrated safety of using auxiliary midwives to distribute the pill also led the Ministry of Public Health to agree to the concept of community-based

---

BOX 14.1 Key Milestones in the Emergence of the NFPP

1963:   The First National Population Seminar is convened to discuss population issues.

1964:   A family planning demonstration project is initiated in Potharam.

1966:   Four Bangkok hospitals join the International Postpartum Program.

1967:   The undersecretary of state for public health creates the Family Health Project

1970:   The Ministry of Public Health authorizes auxiliary midwives to distribute oral contraceptives.
        The cabinet declares a population policy promoting voluntary family planning.
        The Family Health Project becomes the NFPP.

1972:   Thai surgeons develop the minilaparotomy.

1974:   The first community-based distribution program is initiated by a nongovernmental organization.

1977:   The Ministry of Public Health approves the use of an injectable contraceptive.

distribution programs. A privately operated organization, Community-Based Family Planning Services, later renamed the Population and Community Development Association, one of the developing world's most successful nongovernmental organizations for community development and family planning, introduced the first such program in 1974. One of Thailand's most charismatic individuals, Mechai Viravaidya, created the organization in the early 1970s. One of his first efforts was to desensitize people's attitudes toward condoms through condom balloon blowing contests and other activities, and he was so successful that in many parts of the country the condom became known as the Mechai. As the ministry's national program moved forward, the Population and Community Development Association assisted with the provision of community-based family planning education and services.

The NFPP was extraordinarily successful in providing services to Thai women. According to NFPP service statistics, the number of new family planning clients climbed from 225,000 in 1970 to 1.12 million in 1980 (Rosenfield and others 1982). Contraceptive use increased steadily during this period as well. The proportion of married women aged 15–44 who used contraception increased from 14 percent in 1969–70 to 53 percent in 1978–79 and to more than 70 percent by 1993 (figure 14.1).

The percentage of married women using different methods of contraception varied over time (figure 14.2). In 1996, 23 percent were using the pill, with female sterilization a close second (22 percent) and the injectable in third place (18 percent), while use of the IUD had declined to 3 percent. By 1978–79, the rural-urban differential in contraceptive use had almost disappeared. More than 80 percent of rural women and 66 percent of urban women reported that they obtained their contraceptives from a government facility (Kamnuansilpa, Chamratrithirong, and Knodel 1982).

The population growth rate peaked at more than 3 percent per year during the 1950s and early 1960s, but declined to less than 2 percent per year by the first half of the 1980s (Chayovan, Kamnuansilpa, and Knodel 1988). This change reflected a rapid and substantial decline in fertility that began at the end of the 1960s and was

FIGURE 14.1 Prevalence of Contraceptive Use, 1969–96

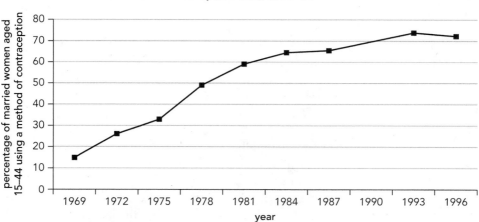

Source: Ross, Stover, and Adelaja 2005, table A.1.

FIGURE 14.2 Use of Different Methods of Contraception, 1969–96

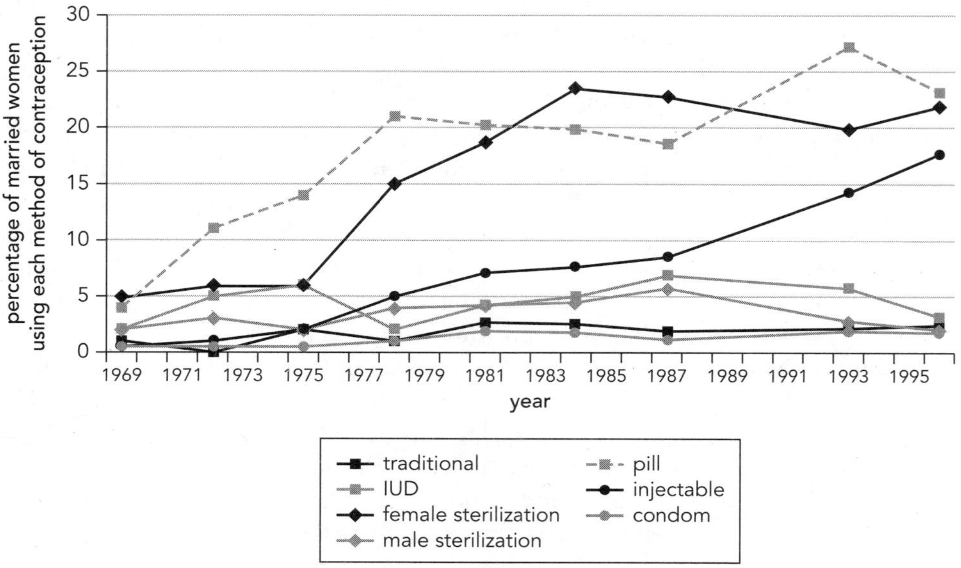

Source: Ross, Stover, and Adelaja, 2005, table A.1.

largely attributable to reductions in marital fertility rather than to changes in marital patterns (Knodel and Debavalya 1978). Between 1969 and 1979, marital fertility decreased by almost 40 percent (Kamnuansilpa, Chamratrithirong, and Knodel 1982). Observers credit the NFPP with having played a significant role in Thailand's "reproductive revolution" (Knodel and Debavalya 1978).

The Influence of Thai Culture

The early success of family planning efforts in Thailand in the absence of government support or widespread socioeconomic development can be attributed in part to aspects of Thai culture. The higher status of women in Thailand relative to that in other developing countries may have contributed to the rapid rise in contraceptive use. As noted earlier, a large proportion of women were literate in the 1960s. They were also free to engage in social and economic activities, thereby exposing them to new ideas and lifestyles. The liberalism of Buddhist culture in Thailand also enabled women and men to more readily adopt modern attitudes and behaviors concerning reproduction (Knodel and Debavalya 1978). Buddhist doctrine is not particularly pro-natalist and has no bans on the use of contraception. In addition, because Theravada Buddhism, the form of Buddhism practiced by the vast majority of the population, emphasized that each individual is responsible for her or his own salvation, Thais tended to be nonjudgmental of each other's actions. A sense of individual autonomy and privacy fostered by Thai Buddhism also dispelled any type of social pressure for or against family planning. In villages, neither the extended family nor the broader community exerted control over individual behavior. For example,

Thailand has no tradition of arranged marriages that enables the kinship group to exert control over the next generation. Furthermore, while Buddhism links its adherents to the past, it also promotes a sense of pragmatism that allows followers to be responsive to social change (Rosenfield and others 1982). This pragmatism was apparent not only in couples' behavior with respect to family planning, but also in the Ministry of Public Health's decision to experiment with the professional responsibilities of auxiliary midwives. Recognizing the shortage of physicians in rural areas, ministry officials did not hesitate to make evidence-based rulings that promoted access to family planning services nationwide.

Use of Nonphysicians in Service Delivery Programs

The Thai experience demonstrated that alternative approaches to delivering services are both safe and imperative, a lesson that still holds true today. Preventive and curative health care services do not necessarily require physicians or highly specialized personnel. The shortage of physicians, and even of nurses, in rural areas of developing countries has not improved since the 1960s, and the current burden on available health care workers is great, especially in light of the HIV/AIDS epidemic. If a principal goal of global health programs is universal access, then expanding and using all levels of the health care workforce is critical.

Thailand's family planning program was one of the earliest to break down the physician barrier. The concept of using auxiliary health care workers soon spread to family planning programs in many other countries. More recently, in some countries, programs to reduce maternal mortality and morbidity have used nurses and paraprofessionals to provide emergency obstetric care. Programs aimed at addressing the global HIV/AIDS epidemic are also reexamining the roles of various health workers in testing, treatment, and care. This approach does not imply a lower standard of care. Rather, health officials must consider whether a highly trained physician or nurse is uniquely qualified to perform certain tasks or whether others can do so. Countries must develop human resource policies based on risk-benefit assessments that ensure widespread access to care.

Conclusions

Activities during the late 1960s positively shaped the future of family planning efforts in Thailand. With no official mandate, the Ministry of Public Health initiated the training of its personnel to address the serious population problem that threatened Thailand's social and economic development. Rather than creating a separate infrastructure, the ministry successfully used existing resources and health care workers to carry out family planning activities. Responsiveness to the local context and to people's needs was a guiding principle from the start, and ministry officials were quick to expand the responsibilities of auxiliary midwives to provide family planning services nationwide. In its three years of operation, the Family Health Project provided contraceptives to an impressive number of clients without setting targets, providing incentives to staff members or potential clients, or being able to conduct public information campaigns. When a formal population policy was finally announced in 1970, the NFPP was well positioned to intensify its efforts. From the late 1960s through the 1970s, changes in contraceptive use and fertility in Thailand made it one of the biggest family planning success stories in Asia. A spirit of innovation and pragmatism within the Ministry of Public Health, coupled with the openness of Thai culture, fostered the dramatic achievements in family planning. Thailand's population growth rate in 2005 was just under 1 percent, compared with 3 percent in 1965.

References

Bryant, John. 1969. *Health and the Developing World*. Ithaca, NY: Cornell University Press.

Chayovan, Napaporn, Peerasit Kamnuansilpa, and John Knodel. 1988. *Thailand: Demographic and Health Survey, 1987*. Bangkok: Chulalongkorn University, Institute of Population Studies.

Fawcett, James T., Aree Somboonsuk, and Sumol Khaisang. 1967. "Thailand: An Analysis of Time and Distance Factors at an IUD Clinic in Bangkok." *Studies in Family Planning* 1 (19): 8–12.

Gille, Halvor, and Marshall C. Balfour. 1964. "National Seminar on Population Problems of Thailand: Conclusions of the Seminar." *Studies in Family Planning* 1 (4): 1–5.

Hawley, Amos H., and Visid Prachuabmoh. 1966. "Family Growth and Family Planning in a Rural District of Thailand." In *Family Planning and Population Programs,* ed. Bernard Berelson, Richmond K. Anderson, Oscar Harkavy, John Maier, W. Parker Mauldin, and Sheldon J. Segal, 523–44. Chicago: University of Chicago Press.

Hemachudha, Chitt, and Allan Rosenfield. 1975. "National Health Services and Family Planning: Thailand, a Case Study." *American Journal of Public Health* 65 (8): 864–71.

Institute of Population Studies and Population Survey Division. 1977. *The Survey of Fertility in Thailand: Country Report (1975)*, vols. I and II. Bangkok: Chulalongkorn University and National Statistical Office.

Kamnuansilpa, Peerasit, Aphichat Chamratrithirong, and John Knodel. 1982. "Thailand's Reproductive Revolution: An Update." *International Family Planning Perspectives* 8 (2): 51–56.

Knodel, John, and Nibhon Debavalya. 1978. "Thailand's Reproductive Revolution." *International Family Planning Perspectives and Digest* 4 (2): 34–49.

Prachuabmoh, Visid, and Ralph Thomlinson, eds. 1971. *The Potharam Study*. Research Report 4. Bangkok: Chulalongkorn University, Institute of Population Studies.

Rosenfield, Allan, Winich Asavasena, and Jumroon Mikhanorn. 1973. "Person-to-Person Communication in Thailand." *Studies in Family Planning* 4 (6): 145–49.

Rosenfield, Allan, Anthony Bennett, Somsak Varakamin, and Donald Lauro. 1982. "Thailand's Family Planning Program: An Asian Success Story." *International Family Planning Perspectives* 8 (2): 43–51.

Rosenfield, Allan, Chitt Hemachudha, Winich Asavasena, and Somsak Varakamin. 1971. "Thailand: Family Planning Activities 1968 to 1970." *Studies in Family Planning* 2 (9): 181–92.

Rosenfield, Allan, and Charoon Limcharoen. 1972. "Auxiliary Midwife Prescription of Oral Contraceptives: An Experimental Project in Thailand." *American Journal of Obstetrics and Gynecology* 114 (7): 942–49.

Rosenfield, Allan, and Somsak Varakamin. 1972. "The Postpartum Approach to Family Planning: Experiences in Thailand, from 1966 to 1971." *American Journal of Obstetrics and Gynecology* 113 (1): 1–13.

Ross, John A., John Stover, and Demi Adelaja. 2005. *Profiles for Family Planning and Reproductive Health Programs: 116 Countries,* 2nd ed. Glastonbury CT: Futures Group.

Sujpluem, Chusie, T. Bennett, and W. Kolsartsanee. 1978. *Auxiliary Midwife IUD Insertion: Results of a Comparative Study.* Bangkok: Ministry of Public Health, Family Health Division.

Wright, Nicholas H., Chusie Sujpluem, Allan Rosenfield, and Somsak Varakamin. 1977. "Nurse-Midwife Insertion of the Copper T in Thailand: Performance, Acceptance, and Programmatic Effects." *Studies in Family Planning* 8 (9): 237–43.

Zatuchni, Gerald I., ed. 1970. *Post-Partum Family Planning: A Report on the International Program.* New York: McGraw-Hill.

15 Formative Years of Family Planning in Indonesia

TERENCE H. HULL

While the histories of national family planning programs around the world differ, they also have common threads that provide complementary lessons. Whether one considers the debates about incentives in Bangladesh, the one-child policy in China, or the attempt by an authoritarian ruler to push population control in India, explanations for behavioral change must be looked at in a cultural or historical framework, yet the themes that emerge can often be generalized to quite different settings.

A family planning program is an outcome of deliberate actions by key individuals and this results in the formation of institutions, in logistics systems, and in various health and social resources. At the same time, the population must experience a radical transformation of beliefs that leads them from a preference for large families to a preference for small families. This is the experience of Indonesia, where actions by some remarkable individuals, combined with dramatic social changes, shifted a high-fertility nation to replacement-level fertility over the course of four decades.

The Indonesian state was born in 1945–49 (box 15.1). Relations with Western countries were normalized over the ensuing years, leading to some international involvement in family planning in Indonesia and the establishment of a private family planning association following President Sukarno's announced opposition to government assistance. Then in 1965 the government changed, opening the door to what would become one of the most prominent family planning programs in the world.

Political Commitment to Family Planning, 1965–94

The period of government transition following an attempted coup and countercoup in 1965–66 marked the crucial nexus in the politics of family planning. Contemporary histories sometimes reduce the events to a simple series: President Sukarno had forbidden family planning throughout his presidency (1950–65). Under the so-called New Order (new regime) that came to power in 1966, President Suharto signed the World Leaders' Declaration on Population in 1967, set up the Family Planning

BOX 15.1 Timeline of Major Events

1945:	Sukarno and Hatta declare Indonesian independence from the Netherlands, thereby starting a revolutionary struggle that lasted until 1949, when formal independence was agreed upon at the United Nations.
1956:	The U.S. Agency for International Development funds Indonesian doctors to train in family planning techniques in New York.
	President Sukarno refuses to consider government support for family planning.
1957:	The voluntary Indonesian Planned Parenthood Association is established as a private, nonprofit, nongovernmental organization to offer contraception to women through a network of largely urban clinics.
1965:	An attempted coup triggers the fall of the Sukarno regime and the emergence of the New Order government of General Suharto, who becomes acting president in March 1967.
1967:	The Jakarta Pilot Project is the first government-supported activity related to the mass promotion of birth control.
	The National Family Planning Institute, which in 1970 becomes the National Family Planning Coordinating Board, is established.
Early 1970s:	The National Family Planning Coordinating Board embarks on a strategy of village-based contraceptive delivery using local fieldworkers and a hierarchical logistics and management structure. This system is supported by international donors and starts in Java and Bali, then spreads to a select number of outer island provinces, and is finally adopted throughout the nation.
Early 1980s:	Family planning is increasingly criticized by a minority of Islamic leaders in conflict with the Suharto regime.
	The first indications of substantial fertility decline become apparent across the nation.
1997:	The rupiah collapses, bringing the Asian economic crisis to Indonesia.
1998:	The New Order government falls, and the reform era starts.
1999–2001:	Attempts are made to reform the National Family Planning Coordinating Board under the Ministry of Women's Empowerment.
2001–07:	The board is placed under the direction of the minister of health, although the board's chair still has some direct access to the coordinating minister for people's welfare.

Institute in 1968, and raised the status of the Family Planning Institute to that of a coordinating board with a chair directly responsible to the president in 1970. Family planning was viewed formalistically and in terms of institutional change.

President Suharto's central role in the formation of the family planning program and his unswerving support for its implementation was internationally recognized in 1989, when the United Nations gave him its Population Award. While Suharto clearly made an outstanding contribution to the program over two decades, the details of the events surrounding the initiation of the government program are important because of the insight they provide into the difficulties of overcoming government inertia and hostility toward family planning. They also clarify some of the dynamics encountered in Indonesian politics at a time when the structures of governance were undergoing substantial renovation.

The two key political actors involved in the initiation of the government's family planning program were General Suharto (later president) and General Ali Sadikin, governor of Jakarta. In 1966–68, Suharto was engaged in an enormously delicate attempt to gradually assume de jure recognition of the de facto power he had attained in the aftermath of the 1965–66 coup (Liddle 1985). High on his list of priorities was resuming formal relations with the United Nations, which had been broken off during Indonesia's earlier confrontation with Malaysia and its previous attempts to expel the Dutch from West Papua. Such diplomatic recognition was needed to increase the flow of foreign assistance. The advice from technocrats staffing Suharto's Planning Board and from various donors returning to Jakarta was the same: to gain development funding, he had to control the growth of Indonesia's population. Suharto, like Sukarno, thought this would be impossible given religious opposition to what was widely regarded as a morally objectionable practice, but it was advice he could not simply ignore.

In April 1966, during his fading days, a politically besieged Sukarno appointed Sadikin to the sensitive position of governor of Jakarta. This was obviously not a move he could make without the tacit agreement of Suharto, who held the real reins of power. Sadikin was a marine whose previous responsibilities had been in the area of logistics and the formulation of battle strategy. The sprawling, poverty-filled city offered a substantial challenge, and he approached it with the zeal of a military campaigner, assembling his "troops," setting his goals, and making frequent tours of the "battlefield" (Ali Sadikin, interview by T. Hull and N. Widyantoro, July 25, 1989). Suharto's problems involved political jockeying and grand strategy, but Sadikin was daily confronted with the practical problems of administering a city's needs. The demands of the residents of the rapidly growing national capital were growing even more rapidly than the city and included housing, sanitation, water, education, and infrastructure.

Population issues, though relevant to both Sukarno and Sadikin, had a different meaning in the two settings, national and city (Sadli 1963). The New Order was concerned with economic growth and political stability, with the stress on economic restructuring and social control. The street demonstrators who in 1966 had been instrumental in pushing Sukarno aside and crushing communism were reined in and told to resume their normal activities under the guidance of the military-dominated government. Political competition was regarded as the enemy of economic growth, and all political parties were told to toe the government line. Most were eventually merged into two large parties substantially controlled by the government.

Numerous people in the new government's councils were pressing for birth control, including U.S.-trained planning officials (technocrats), Ford Foundation advisers, Indonesian Planned Parenthood Association leaders, doctors, and members of World Bank missions. Suharto was cautious in his consideration of these urgings. At the same time, the hard-driving governor of Jakarta was quickly learning demographic lessons in his attempts to renovate a city with poor housing, schooling, transport, and basic services. The rapidly growing population meant that no matter how fast the new administration worked, the problems always seemed to grow at a faster rate. By mid-1966, Sadikin was regularly making speeches linking urban problems to rapid population growth.

Toward the end of 1966, Sadikin challenged the Indonesian Planned Parenthood Association to devise a project that would help ease the rate of natural population increase in the capital. The association had developed a network of private clinics and training centers for family planning in the previous decade, but these did not have sufficient resources to meet the population's huge needs. At most, they stood as symbols of what could be achieved if the government could supplement the association's resources. Sadikin was the first political leader to commit those resources. The Jakarta Pilot Project, the country's first government-funded family planning program, was up and running by April 1967. The governor frequently assisted its activities by making strong speeches of support at the opening of clinics and seminars and by encouraging the integration of family planning activities with activities undertaken by the city's Health Department. Between 1966 and 1968, most official family planning initiatives were taken under the aegis of the city government, and later, as programs began in other areas, the example of Jakarta was cited as proof that strong, responsive leadership could overcome the problems of religious opposition and community intransigence (Hull 1987).

Concentrating on actions by individuals such as Suharto and Sadikin prevents an understanding of the environment in which the debate took place and changing attitudes in the broader community. One example illustrates how fragile the situation was and how important the political factor was in the development of family planning in Indonesia. One of the key activities leading to the establishment of an official family planning program in 1968 was the compilation and publication of a pamphlet on "Views of Religions on Family Planning" (Panitya Adhoc Keluarga Berentjana [Ad Hoc Committee for Family Planning] 1968). Based on a panel discussion that included government representatives and religious leaders in February 1967, the purpose of the pamphlet was to document the general acceptance of principles of family planning by four of the five officially recognized religions: Islam, Protestant Christianity, Catholic Christianity, and Balinese Hinduism. The consultations did not include Buddhists, as at that time many Indonesians did not recognize Buddhism as a religion. The discussion and the pamphlet captured an important moment in social change, a tipping point when national consensus around the morality of birth control was turning from strongly negative to strongly positive.

Those who contributed to these discussions made many points that remain controversial decades later. The pamphlet repeatedly condemned abortion, yet the implied definition of abortion was often vague and contradictory. The acceptable motivations for family planning were couched in terms of the welfare of the family, and the pamphlet assumed that having "too many" children was a threat to both mothers and offspring. Yet at the same time, it stated that the "use of birth control for selfish reasons, just to have a luxurious lifestyle and the like, obviously cannot be accepted by religion" (Panitya Adhoc Keluarga Berentjana 1968, p. 8). In summary, while religions could be accepting of birth control, it was only acceptable in the context of a philosophy of family planning that was responsible, unselfish, and moral. The definitions adopted by this national consensus left a wide range of key reproductive health issues unresolved—along with human rights issues that persist to this day—ranging from abortion and assisted reproductive technologies to services for teenagers and unmarried people, to the whole panoply of issues surrounding sexuality and sexual identity. Nonetheless, the social breakthrough of 1967–68 provided the foundation for a change of approach by the government that led directly to a major fertility decline.

Following the successful example of Sadikin's Jakarta program, in 1967 and 1968, the Suharto regime made political decisions to initiate a national family planning program. As a result, a completely new set of issues came to the fore as the program established its place in the bureaucracy. A number of administrative complexities were involved. The most obvious were budgets and staffing issues, but other important issues related to the exercise of authority, including who was to control clinics and outreach services, how research priorities were to be set, who would set the terms of evaluation, and who would have the right to administer foreign assistance. In a general sense, the answers to these questions were contained in the subsequent mandate of the National Family Planning Coordinating Board (NFPCB) as the agency charged with coordinating activities implemented by line departments and nongovernmental organizations. However, from the outset, the NFPCB was much more than a coordinating agency. In 1968, the Indonesian Planned Parenthood Association transferred its clinics, equipment, and supplies in Java and Bali to the NFPCB through the Department of Health. Foreign donors invested heavily in the NFPCB to build a strong bureaucracy capable of handling the logistics, training, and promotion tasks they believed were beyond the capability of the established departments of Health and Information. As the NFPCB took on more responsibilities for implementation, the coordination became more directive and took on the characteristics of control, with a growing staff increasingly involved in setting up and running projects, often with generous foreign funding.

Family planning fieldworkers were hired and outfitted by the NFPCB rather than the Department of Health, and as time passed, with their numbers growing to more than 6,000, the fieldworkers pressed for and received permanent status within the government structure. All of this justified an expansion of the NFPCB's presence in provincial and regency governments, and after a decade of growth, the NFPCB had become a quasi-departmental institution with a large staff; a huge fleet of vehicles; and impressive buildings in Jakarta, the provincial capitals, and many regency and subdistrict towns.

Understandably, the rapid growth of the NFPCB and the organization's ready access to foreign assistance resulted in jealousy among the more established government departments, in particular, the Department of Health and the Central Bureau of Statistics. From ministerial suites to district offices and clinics, complaints were voiced about the NFPCB's tendency to become involved in activities that were well beyond the scope of coordination (Warwick 1986). Meanwhile, the NFPCB saw its mission as addressing a problem of great urgency—a population explosion—and justified its activism as a necessary way to circumvent complex and moribund bureaucracies.

Foreign review teams regularly reinforced the NFPCB's argument, although over time the review teams realized that long-term development would require the family planning program to be well integrated into the work of line departments and strongly rooted in the community (see, for example, Snodgrass 1978). By the end of the 1970s, the NFPCB was making greater efforts to involve departments and community groups in implementing foreign-financed projects and was using U.S. Agency for International Development and United Nations Population Fund assistance to train the staff of departments and nongovernmental organizations at both the central and the provincial levels (Haryono and Shutt 1989; Moebramsjah 1983; Moebramsjah, D'Agnes, and Tjiptorahardjo 1982; Sumbung 1989).

Nevertheless, the conflict was not completely diffused. Rivalry was apparent between the NFPCB and the Central Bureau of Statistics concerning the methods and purposes of measuring fertility levels and rates of contraceptive use. The gap between NFPCB and Central Bureau of Statistics estimates of current use was often huge, with the NFPCB claiming at one stage that contraceptive use was around 60 percent, compared with a 40 percent Central Bureau of Statistics estimate, and with little attempt by either organization to adjust its estimation techniques to make valid comparisons. Because of the demands of international funding agencies, the NFPCB staked its reputation on its estimates of the proportion of women actually using contraceptives, so those differences were of more than academic interest. Indeed, Indonesian and foreign academics involved in evaluating data sometimes found their efforts thwarted, ignored, or inhibited (see, for example, Streatfield 1985) if they questioned the validity of the data produced by the NFPCB or promoted interpretations that failed to credit the official program as primarily responsible for fertility decline.

The official interpretation of events depicted Indonesia as a case where rapid fertility decline preceded major economic improvement, which could therefore be attributed largely to the efforts of the government's family planning program (Freedman, Khoo, and Supraptilah 1981; Sinquefield and Sungkono 1979). While many demographers interpreted the role of the NFPCB as that of a catalyst rather than the prime causative mechanism of fertility change, the political and popular interpretation of the situation was simplified down to the notion that the government had engineered a remarkable change through force of policy, planning, and logistics management. The financers of the program—the World Bank and the U.S. Agency for International Development—welcomed and often promoted this somewhat naïve idea, and many development agencies embraced Indonesia as the model for other developing countries, including awarding numerous prizes and awards to the NFPCB and to Suharto.

In the early 1980s, the NFPCB, seeing itself as the central authority on all forms of population policy, was actively pursuing an agenda formulated by its deputy for population. This included forays into such issues as labor force development, urbanization, and resettlement.

In 1984, the establishment of the State Ministry of Population and Environment under the leadership of Professor Emil Salim, a feisty and experienced minister, soon cut back the NFPCB to a narrower mandate whereby it coordinated specific fertility control efforts. This was a masterful management of bureaucratic politics by the president, as by means of one decision he both reinforced the NFPCB's responsibility for family planning and reduced policy wrangles between the NFPCB and the departments of Labor, Transmigration, and Public Works; the Central Bureau of Statistics; and the National Planning Board.

Ten years later the tables were turned. The chief architect of the family planning program, Dr. Haryono Suyono, was appointed as minister for population, while environment was split off into a separate ministry. The new Population Office was established in the NFPCB's buildings, and a full complement of assistant ministers was given responsibility for monitoring population movement and evaluating family planning efforts. Even though they were officially separate entities, the Ministry of Population was popularly seen as having validated the position and the reputation of the NFPCB.

The NFPCB achieved legitimation through the development of a large establishment and the vertical and horizontal integration of its activities in the government structure, often involving connections with sectors not normally associated with family planning service delivery. During 1970 to 1990, it became a ubiquitous feature of Indonesian society, with the blue NFPCB symbol adorning posters, houses, and vehicles across the archipelago and family planning slogans cited daily on television and radio; in traditional forms of theater; and among scouts, women's groups, and school classes and referred to regularly in presidential speeches. A wide range of social organizations, such as religious groups, manufacturing establishments, cultural troupes, and youth groups, were active in promoting the messages of family planning, and assisting with the organization of services.

The Indonesian family planning program thus represented one of the most effective collaborations between government and society in Southeast Asia, a true collaboration because the program emphasized institutions not normally associated with family planning, but did so in a way that was both socially acceptable and socially invigorating.

Even though program messages frequently originated from the departments of Information, Education, Health, or Women's Affairs, it was a sign of the entrenchment of the NFPCB that whatever the source, people identified them as KAH-BAY (KB, the acronym for family planning) and saw them as a seamless fabric. In reality, the program has been far from seamless, often torn and stretched in the tussle of bureaucratic politics, but the leadership was brilliant in repairing the outward signs of conflict and maintaining the illusion of perfect balance between governmental and social interests.

Emergence of Religious Objections, the 1980s

Denied other means of criticizing the secular Suharto government, Islamic groups sometimes turned to family planning as an issue that could be attacked on religious and moral grounds. They forced the government to at least appear to be taking action in response to religious sensitivities (Aidid 1987). This was apparent in a variety of contexts. For example, the so-called Priok affair of 1984 consisted of large street demonstrations, violent military intervention, and numerous arrests and killings in the port area of Jakarta. These were precipitated by sermons by religious leaders who, among other things, criticized the implementation of the family planning program. A few years later, police in East Java banned a number of Islamic books that condemned certain birth control practices. As a prominent government program fraught with moral sensitivities, family planning was a natural target for any group opposed to the regime, but the situation became particularly important as the New Order government pushed Islamic political parties into a single, powerless, conglomerate political grouping (the United Development Party), and major Islamic religious groups withdrew from overt political activity. In this setting, family planning was one of the few issues that could be criticized in a relatively nonpolitical context.

In the early days of the program, various religious leaders expressed dissatisfaction with specific family planning methods, especially the intrauterine device, condoms, and abortion, and some conservative leaders questioned the presumptuousness of the notion that parents, rather than God, would decide family size (Akbar 1959). As the program became more widely accepted in society, and as the NFPCB became larger and more powerful, religious objections shifted to specific actions or policies. For example, in 1983, articles in the widely distributed Islamic magazine *Panji Masyarakat* alleged that the NFPCB was using coercion and inappropriate birth control methods.

The magazine's reports of decisions of the 1983 Congress of Islamic Scholars included condemnation of sterilization and pregnancy termination except in the case of an emergency. This was a direct criticism of government support for the former and tacit acceptance of the menstrual regulation techniques of abortion used by members of the medical profession. The Congress of Islamic Scholars only accepted the intrauterine device on the condition that it be inserted by a woman doctor, or, in emergencies, by a male doctor in the presence of the woman's husband or another woman. Such complaints not only served to shape public attitudes about the family planning program; they also established notional boundaries to the NFPCB's policies and activities, preventing official acceptance of sterilization and inhibiting program strategies for community mobilization and campaigns involving incentives and disincentives.

The Islamic challenges to family planning also highlighted the potential danger to the program of major changes in the domestic political constellation through the reemergence of conservative Islamic political parties. Even though the Suharto government was active in building up the strength of Islam by financing mosques, promoting religious education in government schools, and injecting Islamic rituals into secular ceremonies and government meetings and through mass communications, Muslim leaders remained critical of many aspects of the New Order (Suryadinata 1989). Muslim opposition was not particularly strong in the 1980s and early 1990s, but conservative Islam emerged as a major force to be reckoned with after the fall of Suharto in 1998, and the family planning program came under increasingly critical scrutiny.

During the 1990s, the family planning program was transformed in response to changing political ideologies and structures.

Family Planning in a Changing Political Order, 1980–2000

Even as the international community was feting Indonesia as a model, it was obvious that much more was changing than simply the spread of contraception and the fall of fertility. By 1980, the rapid pace of broad economic progress had become clear and the social changes that were accompanying this progress were dramatic. Nevertheless, many evaluations continued to treat the family planning program in isolation. This was exemplified by the Lapham and Mauldin (1985) framework of analysis as critiqued by Entwisle (1989) and Hernandez (1984, 1989) (see also Mauldin and Ross 1991). If observers adopted a broader perspective, the family planning program was seen as an instrumental means of achieving a wide range of economic and social changes through stressing income-generating projects, family welfare goals, or so-called acceptor groups (Giridhar, Sattar, and Kang 1989; Haryono and Shutt 1989; Warwick 1986). Only rarely was the program analyzed in the context of the more extensive ideological and political changes occurring in Indonesia (see, for example, Hull 1987; Hull and Hull 1997; Hugo and others 1987; McNicoll 1997).

This pattern of analysis is strange, as the political setting, especially the ideological underpinnings of political changes, was crucial in determining the establishment, development, and results of government programs, including family planning, health, education, and social development. Even those elements of the program credited with carrying contraception and population education to villages, such as the establishment of community-based distribution systems, were ultimately products of changes to village structure rooted in the colonial period and developed in an accelerated form under the New Order (MacAndrews 1986; Warren 1986). The central government succeeded in developing tight lines of control that reached through the various levels of political administration to a cadre of village officials who owed their livelihoods and their loyalties to the Department of Internal Affairs. The family planning program represented development at the margin (albeit an important margin) of new forms of governance and socialization in a society that was grappling with different options for building a monolithic national identity on a heterogeneous foundation.

The social change witnessed between 1965 and 1990, the time when the fertility rate was essentially halved, was incremental, and was a process of transformation through a series of mutually reinforcing marginal movements. The engine of that change was less the formal institution of the family planning program than it was the oil boom that began in the 1970s and nourished economic development, along with the political controls that established stability. Those, in turn, underlay the bureaucratic reforms and communications innovations that made regions responsive to central direction. Without these more basic changes, the NFPCB would not have had a firm foundation on which to implement actions to achieve the logistics and informational goals for promoting contraceptive use.

These key political and administrative changes were attributable to the nature of the New Order. The change from the old to the New Order involved a rearrangement of political power such that the major inhibitions to family planning, namely, political Islam and nationalistic economic planning, were replaced by forces supporting birth control, that is, secular authoritarianism and modernizing technocratic planning. The new agenda included high-profile institution building with large investments in improving central government departments, strengthening control of regional and local governments, and directing all social organizations to a goal of development under the common ideological banner of the Panca Sila (Five Principles of National Ideology). The Panca Sila were created in 1945 at the dawn of Indonesian independence to lay the foundation of a secular state. The five pillars can be summarized as belief in God, national unity, humanitarianism, social justice, and rule by consensus (van Ufford 1987). At the time of the formulation of the ideology, and frequently and increasingly since that time, many leaders from the conservative Muslim stream of politics have pushed for modifying or abandoning the Panca Sila in favor of a religious-based ideology supportive of an Islamic state. The family planning program has grown as a product of a secular state, even as it has included policies formulated to be sensitive to Islamic values and teachings (Fathuddin 1993).

The call for an Islamic state is based on the argument that the vast majority of the population is Muslim, and advocates often quote figures indicating that adherence is as much as 95 percent, rather than the census figure of 87 percent or the more pragmatic realization that a substantial proportion of those listed as adherents to Islam are "statistical Muslims" who cite Islam as their religion merely as a convenient option for their official identity cards. Resistance to such religious politics prevailed under the leadership of Sukarno in 1945 and was maintained by Suharto through 1998. While the leaders who replaced Suharto—B. J. Habibie (1998–99) and Abdurrahman Wahid (1999–2001)—were more religiously oriented than Suharto, conservative religious forces increased their pressure between 2000 and 2006. Habibie and Wahid refused to support moves to an Islamic state because they had visions of the nation as a technocratic powerhouse or a humanistic democracy, respectively. Their successor, Megawati Sukarnoputri (2001–04), the daughter of Sukarno, maintained a commitment to secular government against growing pressure from many national legislators and local leaders, who wanted a charter to institute a religious state with a range of laws and legal procedures for Muslims while respecting the political rights of other religions. President Susilo Bambang Yudhoyono, elected in 2004, maintained this commitment to secularism in the face of more outspoken calls from religious groups. The fear of many secularists was that challenges to the ideology of the secular state would fracture society and, specifically, would place the family planning program on the firing line because of issues related to morality, women's roles, the family, and particularly the issue of the reproductive health of adolescents.

During the period from the early 1980s through the fall of Suharto and into the current so-called reform period, social changes related to marriage and family relations rode on a wave of globalization that was the hallmark of developmentalism and consumerism. As Indonesia entered the 1990s, the family planning program had been transformed in response to changing political ideologies and structures. Moves to deregulate and privatize state enterprises and the financial sector were mirrored in the Family Planning Self-Sufficiency Program for privatizing contraceptive services and a variety of initiatives to reduce government spending on health care in favor of private sector development. The rise of private and secular forces challenged the exclusionary type of authoritarianism of the early New Order period and, after 1989, accompanied calls for more openness in government, a greater role for parliament, and increased pluralization of power. The demand for greater participation in government and enhanced responsiveness from the bureaucracy spawned an investigative approach in the press and among professionals and led to the public airing of complaints of undue pressure to ensure public compliance with family planning targets (Hull 1991). Having the NFPCB take a quality-of-care line in defining a more comprehensive reproductive health approach in the year leading up to and following the 1994 International Conference on Population and Development in Cairo was therefore not surprising. Hearing complaints from donors and nongovernmental organizations that the quality-of-care initiatives seemed to be more window dressing than sincere commitments was also not surprising.

Slogans could not overcome authoritarian habits, and the political forces to challenge and ultimately defeat the New Order and usher in a reform agenda could not be mobilized until 1997–99. While these transformations were widely regarded as signs of strengthened democratic processes, they also demonstrated the persistence of debilitating conflicts within the national elite. In such a context, it was difficult for the nation to focus on issues such as the reproductive health needs of women.

Achievements in Contraceptive Use and Fertility Decline

However unsteady the ship of state may have appeared in 1999, the year President Wahid came to power, the demographic situation provoked none of the fear and concern that had bothered technocrats three decades earlier. Instead, the news about family planning and fertility seemed quite good, at least in terms of the direction of trends. The new leadership inherited prior family planning achievements (table 15.1). By the early 1990s, the majority of married couples were using birth control, largely reflecting the easy availability of a wide range of methods of contraception throughout the country. The lack of gender equity is highlighted by the persistent low levels of reported use of condoms, vasectomy, and withdrawal, which ranged from 3.1 percent of couples in 1987 to 2.8 percent in 2003.

Had the program placed more emphasis on male methods of contraception during this period, Indonesia may have achieved even higher rates of contraceptive prevalence. Instead, the bureaucracy faltered. Leaders in the community and the family planning program were remarkably conservative about the idea of promoting male methods. Increasingly, they questioned the efficacy of condoms and the acceptability of vasectomy, opting to ignore the fact that the public was quite interested in trying male methods. It seemed to be a matter of frightening the horses: once a few conservative leaders had expressed concerns about the morality or efficacy of male methods, the herd began running with unfounded ideas based on primordial male fears of castration and pinhole leaks in vulcanized rubber. As a result, Indonesia saw a steady decline in reported condom use for family planning (and for HIV prevention) and the failure of relatively inexpensive male sterilization to reach even one-ninth of the

TABLE 15.1 Reported Use of Methods of Birth Control, Selected Years
percentage of currently married women aged 15–49

Method	1976	1987	1991	1994	1997	2003
Official program methods	17.2	40.7	43.7	48.4	51.3	52.4
Intrauterine device	4.1	13.2	13.3	10.3	8.1	6.2
Pill	11.6	16.1	14.8	17.1	15.4	13.2
Injectable	—	9.4	11.7	15.2	21.1	27.8
Implant	—	0.4	3.1	4.9	6.0	4.3
Condom	1.5	1.6	0.8	0.9	0.7	0.9
Promoted by the program but not official methods	0.1	3.3	3.3	3.8	3.4	4.1
Female sterilization	0.1	3.1	2.7	3.1	3.0	3.7
Male sterilization	0.0	0.2	0.6	0.7	0.4	0.4
Traditional methods	1.0	6.0	2.7	2.7	2.7	3.7
Rhythm	0.8	1.2	1.1	1.1	1.1	1.6
Withdrawal	0.1	1.3	0.7	0.8	0.8	1.5
Other, including herbs and massage	0.1	3.5	0.9	0.8	0.8	0.6
Current use of any method	18.3	49.8	49.7	54.7	57.4	60.2
No method being used	81.7	52.3	50.3	45.3	42.6	39.7

Source: Intercensal population survey 1976; contraceptive prevalence survey 1987; demographic and health surveys 1991, 1994, 1997, 2003.

Note: — = not available.

number of female sterilizations. Indonesian women were less prone to panic than men, or at least they were more accepting of the side effects and discomfort they suffered in their attempts to control their fertility. In a relatively unsupportive environment, they persevered with birth control by changing methods on a fairly regular basis.

Over time, the patterns of contraceptive use tended to show a broad mix of methods, with most users choosing one or another formulation of hormonal methods, but a substantial minority persisting with the intrauterine device. A few women reported the use of traditional methods such as the rhythm method or herbal preparations. Where in 1970 women were rounded up for mass lectures on the need for birth control, by 1997, virtually all Indonesian women knew how to obtain and use a number of contraceptive methods and were acting on that knowledge. Young women in particular saw the methods as key to delaying and spacing pregnancies so they could participate in the formal labor force. Moreover, in the rapidly developing economy, people were increasingly shifting from the government's contraceptive supplies to the private sector, with the result that many were paying for injectables and implants provided by midwives operating small but lucrative clinics. A deep change in attitudes about childbearing had taken place. Couples approached by survey researchers no longer quoted the Javanese proverb "each child brings its own fortune" (Hull 1975), but instead detailed the fortune required to raise a child well in a rapidly changing world filled with consumer temptations and expensive schooling requirements.

While the rising trend of contraceptive use appeared to signal a change in the reproductive desires of Indonesian women, many policy makers continued to fear that any faltering in the pressure exerted by the official family planning program could see a reversal of that trend. Essentially, the elite believed that Indonesian women needed continual guidance to control their fertility. At the same time, other observers feared that the logistics system delivering contraceptives across the nation was fragile, and that any blow to the government budget could result in the collapse of services. The 1997 economic crisis produced just the conditions these observers had feared: economic decline struck the budget for family planning and political change carried with it calls for an end to authoritarianism. New leaders in the family planning program set about constructing new strategies to meet the needs of a mission statement revised to promote voluntarism and quality of care. Table 15.1 shows that in the years following the crisis, contraceptive use rose rather than fell, even though this was accompanied by a substantial shift in the methods women used, and despite the regular publication by several key national daily newspapers of stories speculating that the economic crisis would produce a baby boom.

Perhaps the key point is that by the time of the economic crisis, family planning had become a universally accepted practice among virtually all political, religious, and social groups. In addition, the NFPCB was widely regarded as one of the strongest government departments in terms of planning, administration, and evidence-based policy making. When the crisis hit, the staff of the NFPCB was ready to identify areas of need and could justify immediate support for intervention. Donors moved quickly to meet requests for help in providing supplies. The result was that from 1998 through 2003, no national crisis in relation to contraception occurred, though some isolated regions did experience logistics problems and attendant shortfalls in the supply of some methods (Hull 1998).

The steady growth of contraceptive use over three decades was related to major changes in the lives of Indonesian women. Focusing on the crucial decision-making years of adolescence and young adulthood, censuses show that women's participation in schooling had increased markedly as had their participation in the formal workforce. In 1970, about 50 percent of girls aged 10 to 14 were able to go to school, but by 1990, 80 percent were attending school, and in 2000, 92 percent were doing so. At the same time, this age group's involvement in the formal labor force declined, a trend that matches the observations in community studies showing that young adolescents were much less likely to participate in any form of household or informal work than previous generations, in part because they were enrolled in school. Another major factor changing the roles of girls aged 10 to 14 was their mothers' lower fertility in the 1970s and 1980s, which meant that pubescent girls had fewer young siblings to care for. With high-parity births becoming rarer, children reaped benefits in terms of free time, increased shares of family resources, and encouragement to study.

The situation of maturing adolescents was somewhat different. While they were more likely to continue in school, the proportion of girls aged 15 to 19 who were currently enrolled had only reached 33 percent of the age group in 1990, up from less than 20 percent in 1971, while another 33 percent was active in the formal labor force. About 20 percent of the age group was married in 1990. At that time, this group seemed suspended in a series of incomplete changes. While they might have wished to continue school, they faced barriers in relation to either availability of places or the cost of enrolment. Employment might have been attractive, but good jobs in the formal workforce required training. Increasingly, late adolescence was defined as not yet an adult (a status bestowed with marriage), and no longer a child, but this meant a life of informal labor and confusion about options for the future. Certainly marriage figured prominently in the picture, but the search for a partner became more problematic, with young people increasingly searching for love matches, while their parents continued to have an important role in arranging what they saw as appropriate matches for their children. By 2000, the 15- to 19-year-old group had changed considerably. Fifty percent of the girls were attending school, only 25 percent were in the formal workforce, and just 12 percent had ever been married.

Young adults found that the social changes opened new options, depending on their social class (Hull 2002). For the elite and growing middle class, the rapid expansion of the tertiary education sector meant that they could prolong their studies in various professional and academic pursuits. The private sector ran many of the tertiary institutions that prepared young men and women for careers in services or administration, while others produced teachers and health sector workers. Few tertiary-level students could combine marriage with their studies, but some could work and study at the same time. The idea of a career made young women reconsider the timing and style of their marriages. Increasingly, marriage did not necessarily mean early childbearing, both because the marriage might be delayed until they had completed their tertiary education and because the initiation of a career competed with motherhood. Like women throughout the developed world, young Indonesian women struggled with their competing expectations of their families and their tentative ambitions for personal development. In the large cities, an increasing number of women resolved the tensions by simply deciding to remain single and devote themselves to their careers. For most women though, marriage was the firm expectation, and they attempted to achieve career goals and motherhood goals by using family, servants, and leave conditions to support them in the early difficult years of childrearing.

The age-specific fertility rates presented in figure 15.1 and in table 15.2 show the impact of these changes. Successive groups of 15- to 19-year-olds have been less likely to be married and have children, to the extent that the fertility of the group dropped by 67 percent between 1965 and 2000. Young adult women were less than half as likely to give birth in 2000 as were the same age group in the late 1960s. For these women, the pattern of delayed childbearing was followed by fewer children later on. In all age groups, each successive survey showed steady fertility declines, with an overall decline of 56 percent in the total fertility rate between the late 1960s and 2000. This demonstrates that policy makers' fears that the 1997 economic crisis would produce a baby boom were totally unfounded.

Figure 15.1 should be interpreted with some care, because the data sources and the methods of estimating the total fertility rate are less than ideal. Indonesia's birth registration system is incomplete, so fertility must be estimated through periodic censuses and surveys whose estimation techniques are not precise. Some rely on mothers' reports of dates of recent births, and these mothers are subject to memory

FIGURE 15.1 Reduction in Fertility Rates by Age Group, 1965–70 to 1999–2002

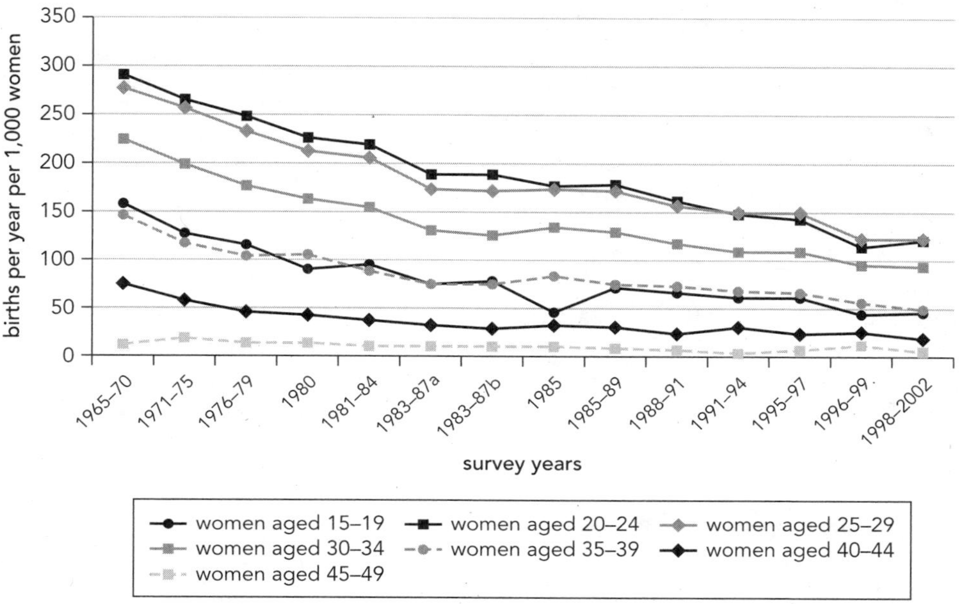

Source: Census 1971; intercensal population survey 1976; contraceptive prevalence survey 1987; demographic and health surveys 1991, 1994, 1997, 2002/3; national social and economic survey compilation for 2002, 2003, 2004 added together.

Note: X axis is not to scale.

lapses. Others calculate recent fertility by looking at the total number of children ever born to women of specific age groups, sometimes applying statistical techniques to convert one form of report into an estimate of annual fertility. Weaknesses of reporting and estimation techniques combine to skew results in different directions, making each data source and method potentially incomparable with others. Nevertheless, the fertility rates shown in figure 15.1 all show declines in a fairly consistent pattern, which raises confidence in the conclusion that fertility really has fallen substantially and is continuing to fall. The recent trend of the TFR in table 15.2 is irregular and not fully understood. After falling from 3.0 to 2.9 to 2.8 in successive surveys it suddenly dropped to 2.3 in the next two surveys, which is improbable. In the latest survey it is back on the long-term trend, at 2.6. National surveys have been done by somewhat different agencies, so methodological differences may be at work; programmatic or demographic shifts may also contribute to irregularities.

With all the political uncertainties in Indonesia today, saying that fertility will never rise again would be unwise, but at the same time, there are no indications to suggest that either the government or the public would welcome higher fertility. Fertility is likely to continue its long-term decline, even if the rate of decline slows because of the impact of economic mismanagement and political conflict on the provision of health and contraceptive services; however, this is a proposition that needs careful examination.

TABLE 15.2 Age-Specific and Total Fertility Rates, 1964–2002

Reference period	Age group in years							Total fertility rate (births per woman)
	15–19	20–24	25–29	30–34	35–39	40–44	45–49	
1965–70	158	290	277	224	146	75	12	5.9
1971–75	127	265	256	199	118	57	18	5.2
1976–79	116	248	232	177	104	46	13	4.7
1980	90	226	213	163	105	43	14	4.3
1981–84	95	220	206	154	89	37	10	4.1
1983–87a	75	189	174	130	75	32	10	3.4
1983–87b	78	188	172	126	75	29	10	3.4
1985	46	176	173	134	83	32	10	3.3
1985–89	71	179	171	129	75	31	9	3.3
1988–91	67	162	157	117	73	23	7	3.0
1991–94	61	148	150	109	68	31	4	2.9
1995–97	62	143	149	108	66	24	6	2.8
1996–99	44	114	122	95	56	26	12	2.3
2000 (average 1998–2002)	46	120	123	93	50	19	5	2.3
2000–03	51	131	143	99	66	19	4	2.6
Percentage decline	67	55	48	55	55	75	67	56

Source: Census 1971; intercensal population survey 1976; contraceptive prevalence survey 1987; demographic and health surveys 1991, 1994, 1997, 2002/3; national social and economic survey compilation for 2002, 2003, 2004 added together.

The Future of Reproductive Health in Unpredictable Times

Just as views of the past differ depending on the interpretations that can be applied to events, then the future also holds different possibilities in accord with the wide variety of reasonable assumptions that can be made about the likely course of events. This view seems all the more apt as Indonesia struggles with the challenges of building democracy on the foundations of authoritarianism. Predicting the political future of reproductive health requires going into more detail about the potential of the current political process than is possible here, but there are signs that some valuable legacies of the New Order may be preserved and that the more egregious errors of authoritarianism may be overcome. In this context, the nature of population trends and the challenges of population policies must be understood with reference to the history of the family planning program.

Hayes (2006) summarizes recent discussions about the future of family planning in Indonesia in work carried out as part of the Sustaining Technical Achievements in Reproductive Health/Family Planning project of assistance funded by the U.S. Agency for International Development. The starting point of this work is the question of whether levels of contraceptive prevalence make any difference at a time when fertility seems inevitably headed to replacement level. Drawing on projections prepared by John Ross in 2003, Hayes argues that the government still faces a major challenge in terms of overall population growth. If the contraceptive prevalence rate (CPR) were to falter by as much as 0.5 percentage points per year, the total population would grow by nearly 50 million by 2015. If during the same period the CPR were merely stagnant, the population would grow less, by 40.5 million. If the CPR actually grew by 0.5 percentage points per year, the population would increase by only 30.9 million. In fact, the NFPCB would like to see the CPR grow faster than this, and careful study of the unmet demand for contraceptive services and of the many provinces that have CPRs well below the national average indicates that higher growth of the CPR is feasible. If then the CPR were to grow by a full 1.0 percentage point per year, the increment added to the total population would be only 22.8 million. That is far below (by 27.2 million) the addition of 50 million under the worst projection based on a 0.5 percentage point per year decline in CPR. The lesson is clear. Even when considering the relatively small margins of change found in a nation with a relatively high CPR and low fertility, those changes have major impacts on overall population numbers and consequent demand for education and health spending.

From this starting point, Hayes has tried to unravel the question of how the CPR could best be increased. In other words, how the evident demand for fertility control by couples can best be satisfied. The scenarios sketched out in the paper cover the short term (2004–06), medium term (2005–10), and long term (2005–15). The priority of the short term is to develop strong institutions at the local level to promote family planning under the decentralized governance system established in 2001. This would have at its core a system of early warning and rapid response to any failures of logistics systems to distribute a wide range of contraceptives. The medium-term strategy is to identify areas of unmet need, poverty, and unserviced demand and promote better-quality services with the aim of achieving replacement-level fertility. Finally, in the longer term the NFPCB would need to be overhauled to carry out the quite different roles of broad population policy making and of stewardship of a system of regulation and monitoring of programs run by local governments.

To a large degree, these ideas have been overtaken by political maneuverings in the legislature and in political parties. The NFPCB has never had an appetite for reinvention that would strip it of a wide range of implementation roles and the attendant budgets. As a regulatory and policy body, it would essentially be converted into a technical institution, with requirements for a different human capital profile than it has accumulated over four decades. Similarly, the medium-term notion of targeting the poor and underserved was not conceived of in a way that distinguished clearly between the implementation responsibilities of local governments and innovation by a central agency. Instead, again looking to the potential flow of funds through the agency, the central NFPCB office saw itself as the key innovator and implementer. By 2007, many of the closest advisers to the NFPCB had begun to wonder if the agency had become irrelevant. This was not because the fertility transition had run its course as argued by Caldwell, Phillips, and Barkat-e-Khuda (2002), but rather because the democratic transition that had produced decentralization had left the organization floundering in an uncertain search for new roles and functions.

The health reform initiatives of the Ministry of Health in 1998–2000, and the more exuberant embrace of decentralization by that ministry (Hull and Iskandar 2000; Lieberman and Marzoeki 2000), offer the strongest hope that both women and men will continue to have access to contraceptive services, irrespective of the fate of the NFPCB. After all, during the course of development of the national family planning movement, medical personnel were assisted by paid or volunteer outreach workers to provide most basic services for the bulk of the population. The longstanding commitment to preventative health care offers a firm foundation for sustainable family planning services and could be used to improve services for the prevention of sexually transmitted diseases and of the morbidity and mortality associated with pregnancy. A network of factories and distribution channels that make a wide variety of contraceptives available to all Indonesians constitutes a major industrial resource worthy of preservation. Conservative politicians could in time question the maintenance of a specialized family planning promotional service in the NFPCB, but society generally welcomes the work of such an organization as a facilitator of community mobilization, even when some people may question certain specific activities.

Past errors arising from patrimonialism and authoritarianism may be resistant to correction to the extent that cultural factors underpin many unhealthy practices, as those are not easily changed. Complaints of coercion, insensitivity, lack of male participation or responsibility, lack of adequate information, and disrespectful treatment of clients can often be traced back to gender relations, class relations, and organizational cultures that may require years, if not generations, to redress (Hull and Hull 1997). Nonetheless, when President Wahid appointed Khofifah Indar Parawansa as minister for women's affairs in 1999, many observers were startled that two of her first actions were to rename her position as the minister for women's empowerment and to claim authority to oversee the NFPCB. She clearly had the desire to face issues of gender and morality in providing directions for the reproductive health program and to set out a feminist agenda to ensure that women took an active role in shaping the program and that men took on some of the burdens of contraceptive use. In the two years of her tenure in the post she steered the NFPCB to adopt a new "vision and mission statement." The vision was for "quality families in 2015" and the mission was to "empower and motivate the community to build small, quality families," where the word small was not given a numeric value, but was accompanied by a statement that families should be brought to an understanding that the best ages for childbearing are 20 to 30 and that a healthy pattern of birth spacing needs to be maintained. Effectively this implies a two- or three-child family, if one assumes a woman begins childbearing at age 20, but as noted earlier, women are increasingly delaying marriage and childbearing for education and work reasons. Indonesia is certainly maintaining goals consistent with further fertility decline, even as the government moves to empower women.

Beyond the correction of errors and the preservation of valuable legacies of family planning are the challenges of big arena politics facing Indonesia. Discussions of reproductive health go quiet when newspapers headline murders in city streets, religious battles in neighborhoods, and intractable corruption on an enormous scale.

Loss of self-confidence is a problem for an individual, but it can become a tragedy for a nation. It drains the mental resources needed to address issues, including citizens' reproductive health needs. Even worse, the loss of a sense of common purpose erases all realistic formulations of health goals from the national consciousness. In eastern Indonesia and Aceh, the new millennium was greeted with demands for separation from the state rather than plans for cooperation to overcome HIV/AIDS, maternal mortality, or unwanted pregnancies. While unemployable youths fought in the streets over ethnic and religious slights, spectators to the violence learned that national unity was fragile, humanitarianism was conditional, social justice was problematic, and rule by consensus was impossible. Since then, the resolution of the conflict in Aceh has given the government some hope that conflicts in Papua and Sulawesi and among religious groups might be overcome.

For many people, the only pillar of the Panca Sila left standing was belief in God, and with all the other pillars weakened, that belief is open to manipulation in unpredictable directions. Without social justice, humanitarianism, or rule by consensus, religion could justify intolerance. Without national unity, a reliance on religion could promote destruction. Hope lies in the fact that Indonesia's alternative futures remain open, the five pillars set out in the 1945 revolution can be defended, and the commitment to citizens' welfare could become a reality if both the leadership and the citizenry are committed to these values. If that were to happen, the reproductive health program could return to improving the implementation of activities rather than being caught in dealing with threats of disintegration.

For most Indonesians, the time horizon for thinking about the future has shrunk since 1997. Economic crisis, political turmoil, and concerns about the emergency support mechanisms available in society have come to dominate people's thinking. Politicians have a time horizon measured in terms of days or weeks, with a limit defined by the next general election. Economists focus on the release of key economic indicators and breathe hefty sighs of relief each time a positive growth estimate is released and deep sighs of depression when they think of the national debt, the banking crisis, and low foreign investment. While macroeconomic indicators are dismissed as the parochial interests of men in suits, clear links exist between these myopic visions and the factors shaping the plans and aspirations of young women entering the years of potential motherhood. Each woman who fails to progress to higher levels of education risks having parents urge marriage on her as an alternative future. Each female worker laid off from a factory risks finding the most feasible alternative to be staying at home to engage in the work of the household, including raising children. Women without education and without work find their negotiating position in the family potentially undermined. In such situations, elite Indonesians fear that poor women will simply retreat to childbearing to put meaning in their lives. The poor may, however, reject that option because they still desire education for their children and see economic problems as barriers to be overcome by investing more in each child rather than gambling that many children will produce some natural winners. However the national political and economic problems work out, the thinking of individual Indonesians has changed in ways that imply moderate to low fertility, depending on the changing context in which they live and make their decisions. The prediction of future fertility levels means that we have to predict future society. Students of Indonesia have struggled to do this over the past decade. By all accounts, the next decade will not pose a lesser challenge.

References

Aidid, Hasyim. 1987. "Islamic Leaders' Attitudes towards Family Planning in Indonesia (1950's–1980's)." Master of Arts thesis, Asian Studies, Australian National University, Canberra.

Akbar, Ali. 1959. "Birth Control di Indonesia." *Madjalah Kedoktoran Indonesia* 9 (4): 198–215.

Caldwell, John C., James F. Phillips, and Barkat-e-Khuda, eds. 2002. "Family Planning Programs in the Twenty-First Century." *Studies in Family Planning* 33 (1) (special issue).

Entwisle, Barbara. 1989. "Measuring the Components of Family Planning Program Effort." *Demography* 26 (1): 53–76.

Fathuddin, H. Usep. 1993. *The Muslim Ummah and Family Planning Movement in Indonesia.* Jakarta: National Family Planning Coordinating Board in cooperation with the Department of Religious Affairs. (Translation of a 1990 version entitled *Umat Islam dan Gerakan Keluarga Berencana di Indonesia.*)

Freedman, Ronald, Siew-Ean Khoo, and Bondan Supraptilah. 1981. *Modern Contraceptive Use in Indonesia: A Challenge to Conventional Wisdom.* Scientific Reports 20. London: World Fertility Survey.

Giridhar, G., E. M. Sattar, and J. S. Kang. 1989. *Readings in Population Programme Management.* Singapore: International Committee on the Management of Population Programmes.

Haryono, Suyono, and Merrill M. Shutt. 1989. "Strategic Planning and Management: An Indonesian Case Study." In *Strategic Management of Population Programmes*, ed. Gayl Ness and Ellen Sattar, 257–84. Kuala Lumpur: International Council on the Management of Population Programmes.

Hayes, Adrian C. 2006. "Towards a Policy Agenda for Population and Family Planning in Indonesia 2004–2015." *Jurnal Kependudukan Indonesia* I (1): 1–11.

Hernandez, Donald. 1984. *Success or Failure? Family Planning Programs in the Third World.* Westport, CT: Greenwood Press.

———. 1989. "Comment." *Demography* 26 (1): 77–80.

Hugo, Graeme, Terence H. Hull, Valerie Hull, and Gavin Jones. 1987. *Demographic Dimensions of Indonesian Development.* Kuala Lumpur: Oxford University Press.

Hull, Terence H. 1975. "Each Child Brings Its Own Fortune." Ph.D. thesis in demography, Australian National University, Research School of Social Science, Canberra.

———. 1987. "Fertility Decline in Indonesia: An Institutionalist Interpretation." *International Family Planning Perspectives* 13 (3): 90–95.

———. 1991. *Reports of Coercion in the Indonesian Vasectomy Program: A Report to AIDAB.* Development Paper 1. Canberra: Australian International Development Assistance Bureau.

———. 1998. "Indonesia's Family Planning Program: Swept Aside in the Deluge?" *Development Bulletin* 46 (winter): 30–32.

———. 2002. "Caught in Transit: Questions about the Future of Indonesian Fertility." Paper delivered at the Expert Group Meeting on Completing the Fertility Transition, March 11–14, United Nations Secretariat, Department of Economic and Social Affairs, Population Division, New York. http://www.un.org/esa/population/publications/completingfertility/RevisedHULLpaper.PDF.

Hull, Terence H., and Valerie J. Hull. 1997. "Culture, Politics and Family Planning in Indonesia." In *The Continuing Demographic Transition*, ed. Gavin W. Jones, Robert Douglas, John C. Caldwell, and Rennie D'Souza, 383–421. Oxford, U.K.: Oxford University Press.

Hull, Terence H., and Meiwita B. Iskandar. 2000. "Indonesia." In *Promoting Reproductive Health: Investing in Health for Development*, ed. Shepard Forman and Romita Ghosh, 79–109. London: Lynne Rienner.

Lapham, Robert J., and W. Parker Mauldin. 1985. "Contraceptive Prevalence: The Influence of Organized Family Planning Programs. *Studies in Family Planning* 16 (3): 117–37.

Liddle, R. W. 1985. "Soeharto's Indonesia: Personal Rule and Political Institutions." *Pacific Affairs* 58 (1): 68–90.

Lieberman, Samuel S., and Puti Marzoeki. 2000. *Indonesia Health Strategy in a Post-Crisis, Decentralizing Indonesia*. Report 21318-IND. Washington, DC: World Bank.

MacAndrews, Colin, ed. 1986. *Central Government and Local Development in Indonesia*. Singapore: Oxford University Press.

Mauldin, W. P., and J. A. Ross. 1991. "Family Planning Programs: Efforts and Results, 1982–89." *Studies in Family Planning* 22 (6): 350–67.

McNicoll, Geoffrey. 1997. "The Governance of Fertility Transition: Reflections on the Asian Experience." In *The Continuing Demographic Transition*, ed. Gavin W. Jones, Robert Douglas, John C. Caldwell, and Rennie D'Souza, 365–82. Oxford, U.K.: Oxford University Press.

Moebramsjah, J. 1983. "Management of the Family Planning Programme in Indonesia." In *Views from Three Continents*, ed. Ellen Sattar, 6–21. Kuala Lumpur: International Council on the Management of Population Programmes. (Edited reprint of Moebramsjah, D'Agnes, and Tjiptorahardjo 1982).

Moebramsjah, H., Thomas R. D'Agnes, and Slamet Tjiptorahardjo. 1982. *The National Family Planning Program in Indonesia: A Management Approach to a Complex Social Issue*. Jakarta: National Family Planning Coordinating Board.

Panitya Adhoc Keluarga Berentjana (Ad Hoc Committee for Family Planning). 1968. *Pandangan Agama terhadap Keluarga Berentjana* (Views of Religions on Family Planning). Jakarta: Pertjetakan Hidajah.

Sadli, Mohammad. 1963. "Indonesia's Hundred Millions." *Far Eastern Economic Review* 42 (4): 21–23.

Sinquefield, J. C., and Bambang Sungkono. 1979. "Fertility and Family Planning Trends in Java and Bali." *International Family Planning Perspectives* 5 (2): 43–58.

Snodgrass, D. R. 1978. *The Integration of Population Policy into Development Planning: A Progress Report*. Development Discussion Paper. Cambridge, MA: Harvard Institute for International Development.

Streatfield, Peter Kim. 1985. "A Comparison of Census and Family Planning Program Data on Contraceptive Prevalence, Indonesia." *Studies in Family Planning* 16 (6): 342–50..

Sumbung, Peter. 1989. "Management Information System: The Indonesian Experience." In *Readings in Population Programme Management*, ed. G. Giridhar, E. M. Sattar, and

J. S. Kang, 13–28. Singapore: International Council on the Management of Population Programmes.

Suryadinata, Leo. 1989. *Military Ascendancy and Political Culture: A Study of Indonesia's Golkar.* Southeast Asia Series 85. Athens, OH: Ohio University, Center for International Studies.

van Ufford, Philip Quarles. 1987. *Local Leadership and Programme Implementation in Indonesia.* Amsterdam: Free University Press.

Warren, Carol. 1986. "Indonesian Development Policy and Community Organization in Bali." *Contemporary Southeast Asia* 8 (3): 213–30.

Warwick, Donald. 1986. "The Indonesian Family Planning Program: Government Influence and Client Choice." *Population and Development Review* 12 (3): 453–90.

16 The Family Planning Program in Peninsular Malaysia

NAI PENG TEY

This chapter focuses on Peninsular Malaysia, because the National Family Planning Program only began to operate in Sabah and Sarawak in 2003, although a family planning association (FPA) was set up in 1963 in Sarawak and in 1967 in Sabah. The discussion is centered on the early stages of the program, as family planning has been de-emphasized since 1984.

Sociopolitical and Economic Background

Malaysia covers an area of 332,762 square kilometers, with 131,675 in Peninsular Malaysia and 201,087 in Sabah and Sarawak (formerly North Borneo). The Federation of Malaya, consisting of 11 states in what is now Peninsular Malaysia, became independent from British rule in 1957. Sabah, Sarawak, and Singapore joined the federation to form Malaysia in 1963. Singapore left the federation to become an independent nation two years later. In 2000, the total population was 23.3 million, 79.6 percent living in Peninsular Malaysia, 11.2 percent in Sabah, 8.9 percent in Sarawak, and 0.3 percent in Labuan.

The country has been ruled by a coalition government comprising ethnic-based component parties since independence. The United Malay National Organization, which represents the Malays, has been the dominant party in the coalition government.

The Malaysian population is characterized by a great diversity of ethnicity and culture. In Peninsular Malaysia, the Malays and a small number of other indigenous populations comprise 60.1 percent of the population, up from 50 percent in 1957, with the share of Chinese and Indians declining correspondingly from 37.0 and 11.0 percent, respectively, to 26.4 percent and 9.1 percent, respectively. With the large inflows of foreign workers since the 1990s, noncitizens now constitute about 4 percent of the population in Peninsular Malaysia.

Each community maintains its own sociocultural way of life in terms of religion, language, dress, and cuisine. The Malays profess Islam, the official state religion; the Chinese are mainly Buddhist or Taoist; the Indians are mainly Hindus; and a significant number of both Chinese and Indians are Christians. The family system and marriage and divorce laws and practices differ for the various ethnic groups, but most adhere to the traditional Asian way of life that stresses strong family ties. Two systems of laws govern marriage and the family: Islamic laws, which are only applicable to Muslims, and another set of laws that applies to non-Muslims.

The diverse ethnic groups also differ in terms of occupation, place of residence, level of education, and economic status. Traditionally, Malays lived predominantly in rural areas, working as paddy farmers, fishermen, and rubber tappers. The Chinese have been dominant in trade and commerce and other urban activities. The Indians have been the mainstay of the labor force on rubber plantations, although some are involved in trade and commerce and in professional occupations in urban centers (Leete 1996). Since the launch of the new economic policy in 1970, the rate of urbanization among Malays has been increasing rapidly. Between 1970 and 2000, the rate of urbanization of the Malays increased from 14.9 percent to 54.2 percent, while that of the Chinese and Indians increased from 47.4 and 34.7 percent, respectively, to 85.9 and 79.7 percent, respectively.

Until the 1960s, the main economic activities were the production of rubber and tin for export and of a variety of food crops. In 1970, slightly more than half the labor force was employed in agriculture, but this had declined to 15 percent by 2000. With industrialization and rapid economic growth, gross domestic product per capita (in constant 1995 U.S. dollars) increased from US$950 in 1960 to US$4,708 in 2001 (World Bank 2003). Malaysia has been one of the success stories among developing countries. Since 1970, Malaysia's development plans have been guided by the new economic policy (1970–90), the national development policy (1990–2000), and the national vision policy (2000–10). These policies were aimed at restructuring society, eradicating poverty, and ensuring equitable distribution of income.

Malaysia has also achieved remarkable progress in human development. Life expectancy increased from 54.3 years in 1960 to 72.7 years in 2001. Enrolment in primary school stands at about 95 percent and in secondary school at about 58 percent (Department of Statistics 1999). Gender differentials in educational attainment are narrower than in the past, and the female labor force participation rate has hovered at around 47 percent (Department of Statistics 2001). Concomitant with socioeconomic development, the age of marriage has been rising rapidly. The singulate mean age at marriage among females (an indirect measure based on the proportion never married at each age group) increased from 18.5 years in 1947 to 25.1 in 2000. Chinese women are marrying later, at about age 27.0, compared with Malays (24.8) and Indians (25.4). The proportion ever married among males and females in their 20s and 30s has decreased substantially over the years. All these social changes, along with policy shifts, have significantly affected the implementation of the National Family Planning Program.

Demographic Trends and Patterns

For the bulk of the 20th century, the population of Peninsular Malaysia increased at more than 2.4 percent per year, rising from about 3.8 million in 1931 to 18.5 million in 2000. Prior to World War II, population growth was characterized by large-scale immigration of Chinese and Indians. While the Chinese were attracted by employment opportunities in the tin mines and in commerce, the Indians were recruited to work in the rapidly expanding rubber industry.

With the cessation of immigration, natural increase began to play a dominant role in population growth. From the late 1950s, Peninsular Malaysia was poised for rapid population growth resulting from high fertility as the large cohort of postwar baby boomers began to marry and have children. The crude birthrate declined from about 46 live births per 1,000 population in the late 1950s to about 39 in the mid-1960s and less than 25 by 1998 (Department of Statistics various years).

The fertility transition has not been uniform across the various ethnic groups. The total fertility rate among the Chinese and Indians had already declined relatively sharply before the launching of the National Family Planning Program in 1967. Between 1957 and 1967, the total fertility rate for the Chinese fell from 7.2 children per woman to 5.0 and that for the Indians fell from 7.7 to 6.1. In contrast, Malay fertility had declined much more gradually from 6.0 to 5.7 during the same period. By 2000, the total fertility rate of the Malays had declined to 3.5, while that of the Chinese and Indians was 2.4, just above replacement level (Department of Statistics various years). Preliminary estimates for 2005 show that the total fertility rate of the Chinese and Indians had dipped below replacement level (1.7 and 1.8, respectively), while that of the Malays had declined to 2.8.

Socioeconomic development and comprehensive health care programs have contributed to the remarkable decline in mortality rates. The crude death rate fell from 19.4 deaths per 1,000 population in 1947 to less than 5.0 by 1990. The infant mortality rate also declined rapidly, from 39.4 deaths per 1,000 live births in 1970 to 7.7 in 1998. In addition, ethnic differentials in mortality rates have been narrowing.

The Voluntary Family Planning Movement

A voluntary family planning movement began in 1938, when Dr. A. E. Doraisamy, a government obstetrician in Kuala Lumpur, formed a 10-member family planning committee to provide family planning advice and services (see box 16.1 for a timeline of the main events in relation to family planning in Malaysia). The first FPA was set up in Kuala Lumpur in 1953, followed by the setting up of associations in various other locations. By 1962, FPAs had been set up in each of the 11 states in Peninsular Malaysia. The Federation of Family Planning Associations (FFPA) was formed in 1958 to liaise with the government and the International Planned Parenthood Federation. The FFPA became a full member of the latter in 1961. The founder members and supporters of the FPAs and the FFPA included many prominent expatriates;

BOX 16.1 Development of the National Family Planning Program

1938:   Voluntary family planning activities begin.

1953:   FPAs are set up in Kuala Lumpur and Selangor.

1958:   The Federation of Family Planning Associations (FFPA) is created.

1961:   The FFPA becomes a member of the International Planned Parenthood Federation.

1962:   FPAs are set up in all states of Peninsular Malaysia.

1962–63:   Economic problems resulting from falling rubber prices and rising unemployment spur a change in official attitudes toward family planning.

1964:   A cabinet subcommittee headed by Khir Johari is set up to review population trends and their impact, which leads to the adoption of a family planning policy.

1965:   The recommendations of the cabinet subcommittee to implement the National Family Planning Program are accepted.

1966:   Family Planning Act No. 42 is enacted and the National Family Planning Board is set up under the Prime Minister's Department.

            The west Malaysia family survey is conducted to provide baseline information for program planning and evaluation.

1967:   The National Family Planning Board opens its first clinic to deliver contraceptive services.

1970:   The Central Coordinating Committee is established to integrate family planning with rural health services.

1971:   Family planning services are integrated with the maternal and child health services of the Ministry of Health, the Federal Land Development Authority, and the estates.

1973:   The Population and Health Project (1973–78) is launched.

1974:   The main clinics introduce Pap smears.

1976:   The Urban Improvement Program is launched.

            The Association of Southeast Asian Nations Population Program is launched with financial assistance from the United Nations Population Fund.

1977:   Pilot projects to integrate family planning with parasite control are implemented.

1978:   The Specialist and Reproductive Research Centre is set up.

1979:   The Population and Family Health Project (1979–82) is launched.

            Fertility clinics are set up.

1989:   The National Population and Family Development Board is moved from the Prime Minister's Department to the Ministry of National Unity and Social Development.

1996:   The cabinet decides that the roles and functions of the National Population and Family Development Board should be reviewed and that the organization should be restructured to reflect three main thrusts: population, family development, and reproductive health.

2001:   The Advisory and Coordinating Committee for the Reproductive Health Program replaces the Central Coordinating Committee.

            The National Population and Family Development Board comes under jurisdiction of the Ministry of Women, Family, and Community Development.

medical professionals; and wives of influential businessmen and politicians, such as Sharifah Rodziah, the prime minister's wife, who was the first patron of the FFPA (Lee, Ong, and Smith 1973).

With an annual grant of RM 200,000 from the government since 1962, the FFPA was in a position to enlist human resources to expand and accelerate family planning activities. The total number of new and repeat patients served increased from 19,463 in 1962 to 182,590 in 1966 (Lee, Ong, and Smith 1973). The FFPA and its affiliates remain one of the main family planning agencies in the country, along with the National Population and Family Development Board (NPFDB) and the Ministry of Health. The FFPA has now broadened its scope to provide a wider range of services, such as Pap smears, breast examinations, minor gynecological treatments, and annual checkups by doctors. Services relating to menopause, subfertility, and other reproductive health services are now available in most of the state FPAs.

Changes in Official Attitudes toward Family Planning, 1960s

Until the early 1960s, family planning was not incorporated into development plans. Malaysia was perceived to be relatively underpopulated and the government did not see population growth as an obstacle to development. However, emerging economic problems and growing awareness of the long-run social, economic, and health implications of the high rate of population growth spurred the government to change its stand on family planning.

After World War II, growth in the use of synthetic rubber had a serious negative effect on the price of natural rubber. With a rate of population increase of 3.2 percent per year resulting from high fertility, per capita incomes declined between 1960 and 1962. The government also realized that the large income disparities among the various ethnic groups were growing. The 1962 survey on employment, unemployment, and underemployment showed that the unemployment rate in urban areas had reached 10 percent and that the problem was more serious among the young. In reviewing the Five-Year Development Plan in 1963, the Economic Planning Unit in the Prime Minister's Department expressed grave concerns about the adverse effects of rapid population growth. A report submitted by Dr. Lyle Saunders, a Ford Foundation consultant, showed that all available land would be used up within 15 years. This report expedited the adoption of a family planning policy, which would also address the adverse effects of frequent births on both maternal and child health (Lee, Ong, and Smith 1973). M. Khir Johari, the minister for agriculture and cooperatives from 1962 to 1965 and later the minister of education, was the first cabinet minister to express concern about the population problem, and he called for the government to take vigorous and positive efforts to incorporate the National Family Planning Program into the national development plan (Lee, Ong, and Smith 1973).

The prime minister and his cabinet colleagues advocated family planning as a way of life by making it part of a health package to improve the health of mothers and children and the welfare of families. Contrary to earlier beliefs of the possibility of widespread religious opposition to family planning, religious objections to family planning were minimal and came primarily from the Catholic Church. No objections were raised to the government's support of the voluntary work of the FPAs. In addition, the medical profession had assured the government that it would actively support and participate in the national program. The availability of good medical and health facilities across the country also facilitated the provision of family planning services (Khir Johari 1969).

Malay opposition to family planning was concerned primarily with the question of whether family planning was against the teachings of Islam. Responding to these concerns in parliament on March 28, 1966, Khir Johari stated that other Islamic countries had also adopted family planning policies and reassured his listeners that the government had no intention of compelling anyone, Muslims or non-Muslims, to accept the government's family planning facilities (Lee, Ong, and Smith 1973).

Launch of the National Family Planning Program, 1965–67

In November 1964, a cabinet subcommittee was formed to review population trends and their impact on the country's social and economic development. The subcommittee suggested ways to obtain popular support for fertility reduction and recommended an integrated approach for effective implementation of the National Family Planning Program.

The cabinet accepted the subcommittee's report in mid-1965. In March 1966, the Family Planning Bill was presented to parliament and enacted as Family Planning Act No. 42 of 1966 and received Royal assent. Following passage of the act, the National Family Planning Board (NFPB or the board) was established in June 1966 under the Prime Minister's Department as an interministerial statutory body with a certain degree of autonomy. The three main objectives of the National Family Planning Program were as follows:

- Improving families' health and welfare through voluntary acceptance of family planning

- Increasing the average annual per capita income from RM 950 in 1966 to RM 1,500 by 1985

- Reducing the population growth rate from about 3 percent in 1966 to 2 percent by 1985.

Khir Johari was appointed as the first chair of the NFPB, and Dr. Ariffin Marzuki, a government obstetrician who had been a strong supporter of the various FPAs, was appointed as the first director general. The NFPB had 21 members, with 10 members representing government ministries and departments and 11 prominent members from the nongovernmental sector. The establishment of the NFPB permitted detailed objectives, strategies, and plans concerning population and family planning to be developed and implemented.

The west Malaysia family survey was conducted in 1966 to provide benchmark information for program planning and implementation. The survey showed that

70 percent of married women of reproductive age approved of family planning and that 36 percent did not want any more children. Among those who wanted to stop childbearing, only 14 percent had used a birth control method. Survey findings indicated both the absence of strong opposition to family planning and a substantial unmet need for family planning. The FPAs were the only source for family planning services and were limited to urban areas.

The NFPB opened it first clinics in May 1967. Program expansion involved the use of existing health facilities in cooperation with government and private hospitals, health clinics, private practitioners, and FPAs.

Foreign assistance played an important role in the early stages of the Malaysian family planning program. International agencies and foreign foundations, such as the Ford Foundation, the Population Council, the Swedish International Development Cooperation Agency, and the United Nations Children's Fund, provided various types of assistance. With the implementation of the Population Project (1973–78) and the Population and Family Health Project (1979–82), the United Nations Population Fund and the World Bank also provided significant financial and technical assistance for the implementation of population, family planning, and family health programs (Noor Laily and others 1982).

Functions and Organizational Structure of the NFPB

The functions of the NFPB, as stipulated in the National Family Planning Act No. 42 of 1966, were as follows:

- Formulating policies

- Devising methods for promoting family planning knowledge and practice on the grounds of the health of mothers and children and the welfare of the family

- Programming, directing, administering, and coordinating family planning activities

- Training those involved in family planning extension work

- Conducting research on medical and biological methods of family planning

- Promoting studies and research into the interrelationship between social, cultural, economic, and population changes and into fertility and maternity patterns

- Setting up a system of evaluation to assess the program's effectiveness and the progress made toward attaining national objectives.

The NFPB began operation in 1966, with six staff members. The number of staff increased to 73 in 1967 and 216 in 1968. Thereafter, the number increased less rapidly to 544 in 1975 and even more gradually in the following years, reaching 750 in 2004 (NFPB various years).

At the start of the program, the NFPB was headed by a director general, who was assisted by division heads. A deputy director general was appointed in 1974. Initially, the board had four divisions: General Administration and Finance; Research,

Evaluation and Planning; Service, Supply, and Training; and Information. The organizational structure has undergone changes, with the expansion of the program and the changing roles of the board over the years. By 1982, the board had six divisions at headquarters: Administrative, Finance, and Supply; Training and Manpower Development; Information, Education, and Communication; Research, Evaluation, and Management Information; Service, Specialist, and Biomedical Research; and Planning and Development. More changes were made to the organizational structure of the NFPB following the shift in program thrust in 1984, when the board was renamed the National Population and Family Development Board (NPFDB). Currently, the three main thematic divisions of the board relate to population, family development (such as marriage and parenting counseling), and reproductive health.

As the program's overall coordinator, the board is responsible for organizing, directing, administering, and coordinating family planning and population-related activities. Since its inception, the board has set up the following committees to coordinate implementation of the National Family Planning Program:

- The Executive Committee, which makes decisions about policy, implementation, financial, and administrative matters

- The National Family Planning Committee and its various subcommittees on service, training, information, education, communication, and evaluation, at the central and state levels

- The Central Coordinating Committee, which works on integrating family planning services with rural health services at the central and state levels

- The Medical Advisory and Medical Research Committee

- The National Joint Research Committee

- The National Advisory Committee on Religious Issues

- The Project Steering Committee, which coordinates and monitors activities of the Population and Family Health Project funded by the World Bank and the United Nations Population Fund.

The organizational structure of the board has facilitated smooth implementation of the National Family Planning Program. The board also benefited greatly from the support of and cooperation by other government agencies, international organizations, and nongovernmental organizations. Private practitioners have also been involved in providing family planning services.

Contraceptive services are currently provided through an extensive network of 2,924 clinics (50 NPFDB clinics, 2,822 Ministry of Health clinics, 47 FPA clinics, and 5 army clinics) and 312 mobile clinics (24 NPFDB mobile clinics, 40 Ministry of Health mobile clinics, and 248 FPA mobile clinics). In urban areas, family planning services are available at general and district hospitals, urban health centers, factory clinics, and the offices of private practitioners. Services in rural areas are provided mainly by the integrated family planning and maternal and child health centers of the Ministry of Health.

Evolution of the National Family Planning Program, 1967–84

At its inception, the National Family Planning Program adopted a clinical approach, using medical and paramedical personnel as well as specially trained family planning workers to provide services and information. Since 1973, the clinical approach has gradually been transformed into a multisectoral and multidisciplinary approach with greater emphasis on family development and family welfare (Noor Laily and others 1982; Tey 1991; United Nations 1987).

The NFPB drew up a 10-year plan (1967–76) to implement the National Family Planning Program in phases, beginning in metropolitan areas, where health facilities were much better than elsewhere, to serve couples who were receptive to the concept of fertility regulation. Table 16.1 summarizes the different phases of the plan.

The expansion of the program into rural areas in the early 1970s encountered several problems related to shortages of trained personnel, facilities, and resources. As a means to overcome these problems, family planning services were functionally integrated with the Ministry of Health's maternal and child health services. The Central Coordinating Committee was established in 1970 to coordinate the efforts of the Ministry of Health, the NFPB, and the FFPA in relation to the provision of family planning services. A tripartite agreement between the Federal Land Development Authority, the Ministry of Health, and the NFPB resulted in the integration of family planning services with the social programs of the Federal Land Development Authority. Under this arrangement, the NFPB trained midwives to provide family planning services along with other social and health services offered under land development schemes. In addition, private practitioners, traditional birth attendants, rubber plantations, and the industrial sector were enlisted to participate in the program. In 1976, an urban improvement program was launched to provide services to those migrating to underserved urban areas, especially those in squatter settlements, where family planning and health facilities were lacking.

In 1972, a World Bank appraisal mission recommended further strengthening of the family planning program and the introduction of population, nutrition, and health education programs, particularly for the rural population. Consequently, the Population Project (1973–78) was launched, with total funding of US\$14.76 million:

TABLE 16.1 Phases for Implementing the National Family Planning Program, 1967–76

Phase	Activities
Phase I (1967–68)	Covering large municipalities that had maternity hospitals, selected rural health centers, and pilot study areas
Phase II (1969)	Covering small towns and adjoining rural health centers
Phase III (1970–72)	Covering the remaining health centers and integrating family planning services with the Ministry of Health's maternal and child health services
Phase IV (1973–75)	Providing additional coverage in relatively remote rural areas through the use of mobile units and involving traditional birth attendants as motivators and service providers

US$5.0 million from the World Bank, US$4.53 from the United Nations Population Fund, and US$5.23 from the government of Malaysia. This was followed by implementation of the Population and Family Health Project (1979–82), with funding of US$17.0 million from the World Bank, US$6.5 million from the United Nations Population Fund, and US$20.70 million from the government of Malaysia (Noor Laily and others 1982).

The Population Project initiated a multidisciplinary approach to the population problem with the aim of enlarging the scope of family planning from simple fertility reduction to improvement of the overall welfare of families and society. The project was designed to strengthen and intensify the family planning program and maternal and child health services and to incorporate family life education and population education into the education system. The Population Studies Unit was established at the University of Malaya to conduct research on the interrelationships between population and development. To achieve its objectives, the Population Project provided for infrastructure development for providing specialized family planning services, including marriage and genetic counseling, investigation and treatment of infertility, cancer screening, and an effective follow-up system for promoting biomedical research.

The multidisciplinary approach of the National Family Planning Program also supported related social programs and activities aimed at raising the quality of life, including improving the status of women. Attempts have been made to integrate family planning services with other social services. Pilot projects to integrate family planning with parasite control were implemented to cover underprivileged segments of the urban and rural populations. A three-pronged approach involving improvements in the environment, health, and social welfare services and the promotion of greater community participation to improve the condition of the urban poor have also been attempted (Noor Laily and others 1982).

Incorporation of the National Family Planning Program into Development Plans

Since the inception of the National Family Planning Program, family planning and population issues have been incorporated into successive development plans. Until the late 1970s, the demographic objective was to reduce the rate of population growth by reducing the crude birthrate through the recruitment of an increasing number of new acceptors.

The First Malaysia Plan (1966–70) stressed the importance of family planning for successful economic and social development. It recognized that a high rate of population increase would pose challenging problems of finding productive employment for each year's new entrants into the labor force. Furthermore, the plan document also noted that resources that might have been used to increase levels of welfare would instead be devoted to supporting the growing population at the existing standard of living. Thus, one of the plan's objectives was to lay the groundwork for less rapid population growth by instituting an effective family planning program. The demographic target was to reduce the crude birthrate of 37.3 live births per 1,000 population to 35.0 during the plan period. This called for recruiting 345,350 new acceptors. In addition, family planning was considered to be vitally important from the point of view of maternal and child heath and was to be implemented in conjunction with the extension of medical facilities and public health services (Government of Malaysia 1966).

As noted earlier, the program has evolved toward encompassing an integrated approach to population and development. While the First Malaysia Plan merely acknowledged the implications of a high rate of population growth in terms of job creation and social costs, subsequent plans included considerations of the impact of population growth.on education, health, housing, and the provision of basic needs. The crude birthrate was to be further reduced to 30 live births per 1,000 population by the end of the Second Malaysia Plan period (1971–75) with the recruitment of 535,000 new acceptors, and to 28.2 by the end of the Third Malaysia Plan period (1976–80) with the recruitment of at least 1 million new acceptors.

The Second Malaysia Plan placed greater emphasis on population factors by including an analysis of population trends and structure and detailed population projections, including of the school-age population and the working-age population, as a basis for planning. During the 1970s, problems associated with population increase, such as the need for increasing public expenditure on social services and pressures on employment creation, continued to occupy planners' attention (Government of Malaysia 1971).

The Third Malaysia Plan widened the scope of the family planning program from a purely health-oriented and clinic-based method to a welfare-oriented and community-based approach, and the introduction of population education further exemplified the growing importance of population factors within the socioeconomic development framework. The plan stated that the best approach to family planning, apart from the clinical approach, was to combine a strong program with efforts to create the social, economic, cultural, and political conditions conducive to the acceptance of a small family norm (Government of Malaysia 1976).

The Fourth Malaysia Plan period (1981–85) witnessed a major shift in family planning policy. While the plan continued to emphasize the importance of population factors, statements about the adverse effects of population growth on economic growth and the socioeconomic infrastructure were conspicuous by their absence. Instead, the emphasis was on labor planning and the need to upgrade the quality and productivity of the labor force to provide the critical inputs into the socioeconomic development effort. Given the optimistic economic outlook during that time and the expected deceleration in the growth of the population and the labor force, the plan also envisaged a fall in the unemployment rate and expressed concern about the possibility of emerging labor shortages (Government of Malaysia 1981).

The New Population Policy, 1984–the Present

Several developments in the late 1970s and early 1980s led to a drastic reversal of official policy from anti-natalist to pro-natalist. These developments included a revival of Islamic fundamentalism; the emergence of labor shortages following rapid industrialization; and the installation of Dr. Mahathir Mohamad as the nation's fourth prime minister.

Malaysia witnessed a resurgence of Muslim fundamentalism in the 1970s led by Malays returning from foreign universities and reacting to the cultural shock they had experienced abroad and to Westernization. In response, the government took several measures to raise the public profile of Islam (Leete 1996). The resurgence of Islamic fundamentalism probably contributed to a change in official policy on family planning, as Islamic teaching was interpreted to be pro-natalist.

With the economy expanding at more than 8 percent per year, various sectors were facing labor shortages, which had resulted in an influx of foreign workers since the early 1980s. The tightening of the labor market was another main reason for government's call for a review the country's demographic targets.

On becoming prime minister in 1981, Mahathir, a former radical and government critic, made drastic changes to the country's foreign and domestic policies and pursued rapid industrialization. In his address to the General Assembly of the United Malays National Organization in 1982, Mahathir suggested that Malaysia could support a population of up to 70 million. This change in official policy was stated in the midterm review of the Fourth Malaysia Plan, which suggested that a larger domestic market was necessary for industrial development (Government of Malaysia 1984).

Population projections based on past trends suggested that the population would stabilize at about 40 million by 2050. Therefore, achieving a population of 70 million would require a review of family planning policy and demographic targets. The NFPB set up an ad hoc committee to examine various scenarios for achieving the target of a population of 70 million and its social economic implications, and recommended a deceleration in the rate of fertility decline by allowing it to drop by 0.1 child every five years so as to reach replacement-level fertility in 2070. With the adoption of the new policy, the NFPB was renamed the NPFDB. Subsequently, family planning has been de-emphasized, and the emphasis has been shifted to family development and reproductive health. The information, education, and communication programs were withdrawn. These changes in program thrust resulted in a temporary decline in family planning acceptance; however, the impact of the new population policy on the fertility rate was evident only for Malays and only for about five years. The forces of social changes, including delayed marriage, have also resulted in a relatively rapid decline in Malay fertility, even in the state of Kelantan, where the Islamic influence has been the strongest.

The NPFDB was moved out of the Prime Minster's Department and placed under the Ministry of National Unity and Social Development. With the dissolution of the Ministry of National Unity and Social Development after the 2001 general elections, the board has since been placed under the Ministry of Women, Family, and Community Development.

Impact of the National Family Planning Program

The effectiveness and impact of the National Family Planning Program can be assessed from the contraceptive prevalence rate and the decline in fertility. In addition to providing contraceptive services, the NFPB played an important role in informing and educating the public about contraceptives and the benefits of family

TABLE 16.2 Family Planning Knowledge and Practice, Selected Years
percentage of currently married women aged 15–49

Year	Know how to use at least one method	Had ever used contraception	Currently using a method	
			Any	Modern
1966	22	14	8	8
1970	85	27	16	16
1974	92	53	38	30
1984	99	77	62	35
1994	—	73	55	39
2004	—	68	49	41

Source: Chander and others 1977; Hamid and others 1988; NFPB 1967; author's tabulations based on the 1994 and 2004 population and family surveys.

Note: — = not available.

planning, which would also have affected family planning practice. Table 16.2 shows trends in contraceptive knowledge and practices.

Knowledge of Family Planning

At the beginning of the program, 22 percent of married women of reproductive age knew how to use one or more methods of family planning (table 16.2). The proportion who knew how to use a method ranged from 13 percent among rural women to about 45 percent among urban women. Large differentials were found across ethnic groups (10 percent among Malay women, 12 percent among Indian women, and 47 percent among Chinese women).

The effectiveness of the information, education, and communication activities, including the use of mass media, resulted in a sharp increase in the level of family planning knowledge. In the 1970 postenumeration survey, 85 percent of married women of reproductive age reported that they knew how to use at least one contraceptive method. Rising levels of education would also have contributed to the improvement in family planning knowledge, which has become nearly universal since 1984.

Attitudes toward Family Planning

The 1966 west Malaysia family survey found that 70 percent of respondents approved of family planning, ranging from 68 percent among rural women, 73 percent among those from metropolitan areas, and 77 percent among those from small towns. Among women aged 35–44, the proportion who approved of family planning was lowest among Indian women (49 percent) and highest among Chinese women (73 percent), with the Malays falling in between (64 percent).

The same survey found that the proportion of women wanting no more children ranged from 12 percent among those aged 15–24, to 34 percent among those aged 25–34, to 61 percent among those aged 35–44. In terms of location, 81 percent of women aged 35–44 in metropolitan areas and small towns wanted to stop childbearing, compared with 52 percent of their rural counterparts. The high proportion of women wanting to terminate childbearing revealed that demand for family planning services was substantial.

Contraceptive Practice

In 1966, 14 percent of married women of reproductive age in Peninsular Malaysia had used one or more birth control methods. The pill was the most popular method. More than half of those who used a method of contraception did so before their fourth pregnancy. A large percentage of women had used family planning to space their children rather than to limit the number of births. Sixty-four percent of women who knew how to use a method had used one. The lack of knowledge about family planning was a major reason for the low rate of contraceptive use at the start of the National Family Planning Program.

Following the launching of the program, the proportion of married women of reproductive age who had ever used a method of contraception almost doubled from 14 percent in 1966 to 27 percent in 1970, peaking at 77 percent in 1984 (table 16.2). The proportion currently using a modern contraceptive method increased to 30 percent in 1974 and 41 percent in 2004, while the proportion using any method started declining after 1984, presumably because of the change in official policy to de-emphasize family planning since the early 1980s. Overall, contraceptive prevalence is lower in Peninsular Malaysia than in many other Asian countries.

The expansion of the National Program to rural areas resulted in a substantial increase in the contraceptive prevalence rate just after the launching of the program, but it began to show a downward trend as of 1984. The contraceptive prevalence rate in rural areas has always lagged behind that in the urban areas. In addition, table 16.3 shows that the contraceptive prevalence rate has always been higher among the Chinese and Indians than the Malays. Malays were also more likely to use traditional methods. The 1994 Malaysian population and family survey showed that 27.6 percent of married Malay women were using a modern method and 18.3 percent were using a traditional method, while the corresponding percentages were 66.5 and 6.3 percent, respectively, among Chinese women.

At the start of the program, the pill was the most popular method of contraception and was made readily available at the low price of RM $1 per cycle (US$0.33). Since the integration of family planning with other activities, the Ministry of Health has supplied rural women with pills free of charge. Nevertheless, household surveys show that the proportion of contraceptive users relying on the pill had declined from

TABLE 16.3 Percentage of Married Women Aged 15–49 Currently Using Any Contraceptive Method, Selected Years

Category	1974	1984	1994	2004
Place of residence				
Metropolitan	55	69	58	51
Small town	48	69	67	57
Rural area	32	56	49	40
Ethnicity				
Malay	26	51	46	40
Chinese	55	74	73	65
Indian	49	76	64	51

Source: Chander and others 1977; Hamid and others 1988; author's tabulations based on the 1994 and 2004 population and family surveys.

TABLE 16.4 Percentage Distribution of Contraceptive Users Among Currently Married Women, by Type of Method, Selected Years

Method	1974	1984	1994	2004
Pill	50.7	23.0	24.3	27.0
Intrauterine device	2.2	4.0	7.1	8.6
Condom	9.1	15.0	9.8	14.5
Other female methods	0.4	1.0	1.4	3.2
Sterilization (male and female)	10.6	15.0	12.6	12.7
Rhythm	10.8	14.0	16.1	17.9
Withdrawal	5.7	8.0	12.6	7.9
Abstinence	4.3	4.0	2.3	2.4
Other traditional methods	6.2	17.0	13.8	5.8
Total	100.0	101.0	100.0	100.0

Source: Chander and others 1977; Hamid and others 1988; author's tabulations based on the 1994 and 2004 population and family surveys.

TABLE 16.5 Number of New Acceptors in the National Family Planning Program, 1967–83

Year	Number of acceptors	Year	Number of acceptors
1967	20,726	1976	75,210
1968	74,075	1977	75,774
1969	69,416	1978	75,439
1970	54,957	1979	71,263
1971	54,033	1980	66,354
1972	55,843	1981	62,297
1973	56,902	1982	60,083
1974	61,644	1983	63,467
1975	69,344		

Source: NFPB various years.

about 50 percent in 1974 to around 25 percent in subsequent years as couples switched to other methods, particularly the rhythm method (table 16.4). In 2004 close to 13 percent of all users had opted for sterilization.

Family Planning Acceptors

As noted before, in the early stages of the National Family Planning Program, one of the main objectives was to reduce the birthrate by recruiting new acceptors. The program achieved 63 percent of the target number of acceptors under the First Malaysia Plan (1966–70) and 56 percent of the target under the Second Malaysia Plan (1971–75). The trend in the number of new acceptors shows an erratic pattern, exceeding 70,000 in 1968 and falling below 60,000 per year during 1970 through 1973 (table 16.5). The number of new acceptors then increased to more than 75,000 annually during 1976 to 1978 and declined to around 60,000 in 1982, the year the prime minister first called for a revision of the population policy.

In 1967, the highest proportion of acceptors was recruited by the FPAs (48.9 percent), followed by the NFPB (39.8 percent), the rubber plantations (8.7 percent), and others (2.6 percent). The NFPB took the lead in 1968 with 57.4 percent, while the FPAs' share dropped to 33.5 percent. From 1969 to 1972, the NFPB extended its lead, recruiting about two-thirds of new acceptors. NFPB clinics accounted for about 60 percent of new acceptors during 1967 to 1975, but with the shift in the program's thrust and the integration of family services with maternal and child health services, the board now accounts for fewer than 10 percent of new acceptors (table 16.6).

The program initially concentrated on postpartum women. Of new acceptors in the last quarter of 1969, 63.7 percent had had a child earlier that same year and 17.5 percent had had one in 1968. During 1967 to 1969, relatively more acceptors

TABLE 16.6 Number of New Acceptors by Agency, 2000–04

Year	Ministry of Health clinics	NPFDB clinics	FPA clinics	Army clinics	Total
2000	33,351	9,283	5,024	370	48,028
2001	30,850	7,658	4,345	190	43,043
2002	57,726	6,864	11,458	85	76,133
2003	58,088	6,199	11,019	165	75,471
2004	65,188	7,189	10,391	196	82,964

Source: NPFDB various years.

TABLE 16.7 Percentage Distribution of Acceptors by Fertility Intention, 1967–72

Year	Fertility intention			
	Wanted more children	Wanted no more children	Uncertain	Total
1967	38.3	53.5	8.2	100.0
1968	40.8	50.9	8.3	100.0
1969	44.4	45.1	10.5	100.0
1970	48.8	39.1	12.1	100.0
1971	53.5	34.6	11.9	100.0
1972	56.5	31.3	12.2	100.0

Source: NFPB various years.

TABLE 16.8 Percentage Distribution of Acceptors by Parity, 1967–72

Year	Number of births						Total
	0	1	2	3	4	5+	
1967	1.0	12.3	14.0	13.8	13.4	45.5	100.0
1968	1.1	11.4	14.7	13.9	13.8	45.1	100.0
1969	1.5	12.7	16.0	14.2	13.2	42.4	100.0
1970	1.6	15.5	17.0	14.3	12.8	38.8	100.0
1971	1.6	18.0	18.1	14.6	12.2	35.5	100.0
1972	1.6	19.9	19.2	14.6	12.1	32.6	100.0

Source: NFPB various years.

were practicing family planning to limit births rather than to space births, but in subsequent years more women were practicing family planning to space rather than to limit births (table 16.7) and were increasingly doing so at lower parity (table 16.8).

Among program acceptors, the pill was by far the most popular method, accounting for about 90 percent of acceptors during 1967 to 1972. This was followed by sterilization (5.4 percent), condoms (2.1 percent), intrauterine devices (1.8 percent), and other methods (1 percent).

Ethnic Differences in the Impact of the National Family Planning Program

The National Family Planning Program had different effects on family planning acceptance and fertility levels of the three main ethnic groups in Peninsular Malaysia. In the decade following the program's implementation (1966–75), fertility among the Malays declined by 1.0 child per woman to 4.6, that of the Chinese declined by about 1.3 children per woman to 3.5, and that of the Indians declined by 1.5 children per woman to 3.9. The late 1970s saw a retardation in the decline of fertility among the Malays, while that of the non-Malays continued to decline. The slowing of the fertility decline among the Malays was attributable to a slight increase in the fertility rate among women aged 25–34, probably because of the upsurge in Islamic fundamentalism.

The extension of paid maternity leave from the third to the fifth child under the 70 million population policy has been viewed as pro-natalist. The 1984 Malaysian population and family survey found that 25 percent of the Malay respondents reported that they would revise their desired family size upward in line with the policy, but fewer Chinese and Indians said that they would do so (Hamid and others 1988). Govindasamy and Da Vanzo (1992) argued that the benefits accruing to the politically dominant Malays from the 1971 new economic policy had encouraged them to raise their desired family size in response to the pro-natalist policy.

Following the adoption of the pro-natalist policy in the early 1980s, Malay fertility rose to 4,820 births per 1,000 women in 1985, and then dropped to 4,115 in 1990 and 3,524 in 2000 (table 16.9). Data from the 1994 and 2004 Malaysian population and family surveys show that the mean number of children born among Malay women aged 15–49 had declined from 3.7 in 1994 to 3.4 in 2004, while that of the Chinese and Indians had declined from 2.9 and 3.0, respectively, to 2.7 each during the same period. The fertility rate of the non-Malays continued to decline in the 1980s, notwithstanding the official policy and incentives for having children, but reversed slightly to remain at above replacement level in the 1990s. The latest estimates showed that total fertility rates among the Chinese and Indians had dipped below replacement level in 2005, while that of the Malays had declined to about 2,800 births per 1,000 women. An examination of the age-specific fertility rate shows that the decline in fertility has been most pronounced among younger women as a result of rising age at marriage and among older women as family planning has become more widespread.

TABLE 16.9: Total Fertility Rates and Age-Specific Fertility Rates, by Ethnicity, Peninsular Malaysia, 1957–2000
number of births per 1,000 women per year

Ethnic group and age group	1957	1966	1970	1975	1980	1985	1990	1995	2000
Malays									
TFR	6.04	5.66	5.06	4.64	4.45	4.82	4.11	3.97	3.52
15–19	163	97	71	60	40	32	23	19	11
20–24	342	266	243	212	187	185	152	144	107
25–29	279	266	257	242	248	269	231	234	222
30–34	208	251	222	200	207	235	201	197	185
35–39	146	158	148	149	143	169	147	136	125
40–44	55	75	57	57	59	67	66	57	49
45–49	16	20	15	9	7	7	3	3	5
Chinese									
TFR	7.33	4.78	4.61	3.52	3.11	2.67	2.25	2.51	2.45
15–19	38	20	25	24	22	12	9	10	10
20–24	280	193	190	141	148	107	75	80	72
25–29	412	261	280	231	217	198	164	193	173
30–34	355	241	222	170	151	145	135	149	156
35–39	239	152	136	97	63	60	58	59	68
40–44	117	71	59	37	19	11	10	10	12
45–49	26	18	11	5	2	1	0	0	1
Indians									
TFR	7.95	5.36	4.78	3.86	3.34	2.89	2.55	2.65	2.42
15–19	209	113	68	52	43	30	23	22	16
20–24	429	259	270	212	193	151	126	124	100
25–29	441	320	254	248	225	200	178	189	166
30–34	283	231	198	145	140	133	121	127	127
35–39	159	112	115	84	52	55	51	56	61
40–44	60	23	44	27	14	8	11	11	13
45–49	10	14	8	4	2	1	0	0	1

Source: Department of Statistics, Vital Statistics, various years.

Note: TFR denotes the total fertility rate. It is obtained by multiplying by five the sum of age-specific fertility rates divided by 1,000.

Conclusions

The emergence of economic problems related to the fall in rubber prices and to rising unemployment prompted the government of Malaysia to launch the National Family Planning Program in 1966. The program was designed to reduce the birth rate, in order to safeguard maternal and child health and to increase per capita income. The change in official policy represented the triumph of economics and health over politics in a multiethnic country, with Islam as the national religion.

Upon achieving Independence in 1957, Malaysia depended primarily on agriculture, and there was a concern that with rapid population growth all available land would be used up within 15 years. A number of factors had facilitated the implementation of the national program. The family planning associations had stressed the benefits of planned parenthood, as well as the considerable demand for family planning services. Several community and political leaders, notably Khir Johari, had advocated strongly for family planning, without much opposition. By the early 1970s, family planning services had been extended to all parts of the country, through integration with the maternal and child health programs of the Ministry of Health.

Even though the national family planning program did not fully achieve its rather ambitious target for the number of acceptors or its demographic targets, it had done reasonably well in the initial period despite constraints in finance, staff, and facilities. As a statutory body, the board had been able to harness the support and cooperation of relevant agencies and partners, in particular the Ministry of Health, the family planning associations, and the private practitioners in delivering contraceptive services.

In 1981, the government under the leadership of Prime Minister Mahathir Mohamad adopted different development strategies with great emphasis on the industrialization program, to be supported by a larger population and a larger domestic market. Subsequently, with rapid industrialization, labor shortages began to emerge. Malaysia is now a major destination for foreign labor, which constitutes about 10 percent of the labor force.

In a speech to a political gathering in 1982, the Prime Minister announced a new demographic target, to achieve a population of 70 million by 2100. That became an official policy in the Midterm Review of the Fourth Malaysia Plan (1981–85). The National Family Planning Program was renamed the National Population and Family Development Program. With the de-emphasis of family planning following the shift from an anti-natalist to a pro-natalist policy, greater emphasis has been placed on marriage and parenting counseling, reproductive health, and gender issues. Great emphasis has also been placed on human resource development and improved status of women. The de-emphasis of family planning has resulted in a substantial decline in family planning acceptance among the Malays, who have always been more likely to respond positively to government policies than the non-Malays.

The thrust of Malaysia's population program, to make family planning part of a broader approach in population and development, is consistent with the program of action adopted at the 1994 International Conference on Population and Development in Cairo. Some countries that have undergone very rapid fertility declines are now having difficulty reversing the trend. Malaysia can learn from the experience of these countries by implementing programs to achieve a more harmonious balance between population and development.

References

Chander, R., Venugo T. Palan, Aziz Noor Laily, and Boon Ann Tan. 1977. *Malaysian Fertility and Family Survey: First Country Report*. Kuala Lumpur: Department of Statistics and National Family Planning Board.

Department of Statistics. 1999. *Social Statistics Bulletin*. Kuala Lumpur: Department of Statistics.

————. 2001. *Labor Force Survey Report*. Kuala Lumpur: Department of Statistics.

————. Various years. *Vital Statistics*. Kuala Lumpur: Department of Statistics.

Government of Malaysia. 1966. *First Malaysia Plan (1966–70)*. Kuala Lumpur: National Printing Department.

————. 1971. *Second Malaysia Plan (1971–75)*. Kuala Lumpur: National Printing Department.

————. 1976. *Third Malaysia Plan (1976–80)*. Kuala Lumpur: National Printing Department.

————. 1981. *Fourth Malaysia Plan (1981–85)*. Kuala Lumpur: National Printing Department.

————. 1984. *Midterm Review of Fourth Malaysia Plan (1981–85)*. Kuala Lumpur: National Printing Department.

Govindasamy, Pavalavelli, and Julie Da Vanzo. 1992. "Ethnicity and Fertility Differentials in Peninsular Malaysia: Do Policies Matter?" *Population and Development Review* 18 (2): 243–68.

Hamid, A. 1988. "The New Population Policy." In *Proceedings of the Seminar on Findings of Population Surveys and Policy Implications*. Kuala Lumpur: National Population and Family Development Board.

Hamid, Arshat, Boon Ann Tan, Nai Peng Tey, and Murugappa Subbiah. 1988. *Marriage Family Formation in Peninsular Malaysia: Analytic Report on the 1984/85 Malaysian Population and Family Survey*. Kuala Lumpur: National Population and Family Development Board.

Khir Johari, M. 1969. "Malaysia: A Bold Attack." In *Population: Challenging World Crisis*, ed. Bernard Berelson. Voice of America Forum Lectures. Washington, DC: Government Printing Office.

Lee, Eddy, Michael Ong, and T. E. Smith. 1973. "Family Planning in West Malaysia: The Triumph of Economics and Health over Politics." In *The Politics of Family Planning in the Third World*, ed. T. E. Smith, 256–90. London: George Allen & Unwin.

Leete, Richard. 1996. *Malaysia's Demographic Transition: Rapid Development, Culture and Politics*. Oxford, U.K.: Oxford University Press

NFPB (National Family Planning Board). 1967. *Report on West Malaysia Family Survey, 1966–1967*. Kuala Lumpur: NFBP.

Noor Laily, A., B. A. Tan, O. Ramli, and L. C. Kuan. 1982. *Facts and Figures: Malaysia National Population and Family Development Programme*. Kuala Lumpur: National Family Planning Board.

NPFDB (National Population and Family Development Board). Various years. *Annual Report*. Kuala Lumpur: NPFDB.

Tey, Nai Peng. 1991. "Population Policy Formulation, Implementation and Evaluation: The Case of Malaysia." In *The Utilization of Demographic Knowledge in Policy Formulation and Planning*, ed. Rudolf Andorka and Raul Ursua, 389–432. Liege, Belgium: International Union for the Scientific Study of Population.

United Nations. 1987. *Case Studies in Population Policy: Malaysia*. New York: United Nations.

World Bank. 2003. *World Development Indicators*. Washington, DC: World Bank.

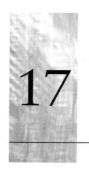

17 Development of the Philippines' Family Planning Program: The Early Years, 1967–80

ALEJANDRO N. HERRIN

In the late 1960s, the president and Congress of the Philippines were strongly committed to policy to reduce population growth through fertility reduction, with family planning as the principal instrument. Awareness of the implications of rapid population growth for development was high among top government officials, academics, influential people from the private sector, and local media. However, the sector of society represented by the Catholic Bishops Conference of the Philippines (CBCP) did not fully agree with the formers' assessment or with family planning that involved the use of artificial methods of contraception and sterilization.

A number of factors facilitated the implementation of a family planning program to operationalize the fertility reduction policy. The first was the existence of a fairly extensive health infrastructure consisting of hospitals, rural health units, puericulture centers (maternal and child health care centers established in rural areas by nongovernmental institutions and financed by the Philippine Charity Sweepstakes, few of which remain in existence today), and private hospitals and clinics. These facilities were complemented by highly trained physicians, nurses, and midwives. The delivery of family planning services could be added to the wide range of services already offered. Second, the concept of family planning and the provision of services had been already introduced as early as the prewar years by voluntary organizations, private institutions, and private physicians. These, together with technical personnel from the College of Medicine of the University of the Philippines and from the Department of Health, were a readily available group of trainers who could train various family planning service providers in clinical settings. Third, donors were available that were willing to provide financial support and technical assistance for the implementation of a nationwide family planning program.

Given the high-level government support and the various facilitating factors, expectations were high that the evolving family planning program was on its way toward achieving the goals of moderating population growth and stimulating socioeconomic development. However, while other countries in the region did achieve

The author gratefully acknowledges the helpful comments and suggestions provided by Carol Carpenter-Yaman and Warren Robinson during the preparation of this chapter.

such success, the Philippines is still grappling with the issue of population growth and development and debating the issue of family planning. The rate of population growth has remained high at 2.3 percent per year; total fertility, pegged at 3.5 births per woman, has not declined as rapidly as in other countries; and the use of modern methods of family planning has peaked at only 33 percent of married couples.

In looking back at what appeared initially to be a promising family planning program, one can see several discordant notes. Stresses and strains were present at the program level, and the program's favorable features—multisectoral approach, participation by multiple agencies and the private sector, and donor support—also contained inherent disadvantages. The rapid expansion of activities involving numerous participants and funded by different donors taxed the administrative capacity of the Commission on Population (POPCOM) in relation to management and coordination. The structure of the POPCOM board itself, whose board consisted of cabinet secretaries who had many other responsibilities, was not conducive to maintaining a steady focus and providing guidance to the program. The POPCOM secretariat, whose staff initially consisted of dedicated and committed members, was soon unable to develop the capacities needed for the more complex tasks of managing and coordinating a wide-ranging program. In addition, the leadership of the POPCOM secretariat changed often, compromising continuity. At the same time, while the funding for many activities was assured by a number of donors, their number and their different mandates and requirements made coordination difficult. As the family planning program began to decentralize and outreach activities became more extensive, local governments were expected to finance and implement the outreach activities in their respective jurisdictions, but whether local financing would actually be forthcoming in a sustained and adequate manner in view of the different financing capacities and commitments of individual local government units was not clear.

Perhaps the major factor in the entire story of the family planning program is the underlying opposition of the CBCP and of influential conservatives. This prevented the implementation of a stronger and sustained program that involved the use of modern contraceptives. Indeed, the government's commitment to fertility reduction reversed in 1986, when the political influence of the leaders of the Catholic Church hierarchy reached its peak. Thus, what appeared to be the beginnings of a strong program to reduce fertility in the late 1960s and early 1970s was actually a fragile program that could be stopped in its tracks by inaction emanating from the Office of the President.

Box 17.1 presents a timeline of major events in relation to family planning in the Philippines.

BOX 17.1 Timeline of Major Events

1939–48: Individual efforts by Presbyterian, Congregational, and other Protestant ministers to spread information about birth control increase.

1957: The National Council of Churches establishes the Family Relations Center, a counseling clinic.

The Children's Medical Center Foundation is established. One of its semi-autonomous units is the Institute of Maternal and Child Health, which is responsible for extending services to rural areas.

1964: The Population Institute is established at the University of the Philippines to undertake population studies and train graduates in demography.

1965: The Family Relations Center is reorganized into the Planned Parenthood Movement in the Philippines.

The Family Planning Association of the Philippines is established to provide education, information, and clinic services.

The University of the Philippines Population Institute organizes the first Conference on Population with support from the Population Council.

1967: President Ferdinand Marcos and 17 other heads of state sign the United Nations Declaration on Population.

The Institute of Maternal and Child Health sets up the National Training Center for Maternal Health Service in accordance with an agreement between the National Economic Council, the Institute of Maternal and Child Health, and the U.S. Agency for International Development.

1968: The government starts to participate in population and family planning efforts by creating the Project Office for Maternal and Child Health in the Department of Health to coordinate family planning activities.

1969: An executive order creates a study group known as the Commission on Population to undertake population studies and formulate policy and program recommendations on population as they relate to economic and social development.

The Family Planning Association of the Philippines and the Planned Parenthood Movement in the Philippines are merged to form the Family Planning Organization of the Philippines.

Congress approves a resolution to establish basic policies aimed at achieving economic development and social justice. Such policies include a policy on population and family planning.

The Catholic bishops issue a statement disagreeing with the government's intervention in couples' fertility decisions and objecting to the promotion of family limitation as a measure to reduce population growth.

The secretary of justice liberalizes the interpretation of an existing ruling to permit the importation of contraceptives.

1970: In his State of the Nation speech, President Ferdinand Marcos states that he will propose legislation making family planning an official policy of his administration.

1971: Republic Act 6365 establishes the national population policy and creates the national agency in charge of population, which is also called the Commission on Population (POPCOM).

President Ferdinand Marcos instructs the Department of Health to add family planning services in all of its 1,400 rural health units. By 1973, 1,070 rural health units are offering family planning services.

1972: President Ferdinand Marcos declares martial law.

The Population Center Foundation is set up to forge a stronger partnership between the government and the private sector.

Presidential Decree no. 79 revises Republic Act 6365. The decree authorizes nurses and midwives, in addition to physicians, to provide, dispense, and administer all acceptable methods of contraception to those who desire to avail themselves of such services as long as these health workers have been trained and properly authorized by the POPCOM board.

The Population Education Program is established within the Department of Education Culture to provide instruction in population education for elementary and high school children by training teachers to develop curriculum materials.

(Continued)

BOX 17.1 Timeline of Major Events (*Continued*)

	General Order no.18 enjoins all sectors to promote the concept of family planning and responsible parenthood.
	Letter of Instruction no. 74-A directs the secretary of the Department of Public Information and the postmaster general to help implement the POPCOM board programs by disseminating information on family planning.
1973:	Presidential Decree no. 69 amends the National Internal Revenue Code to reduce the number of children for which additional tax exemptions can be claimed from an unlimited number of children to four. Decentralization of the Population Program starts with the establishment of 11 POPCOM regional offices.
	Presidential Decree no. 166 appoints two members from the private sector to the POPCOM board for three-year terms.
	The Catholic hierarchy issues a pastoral letter on the population problem and family life. The letter objects to the use of artificial contraceptives to solve the population problem and notes that the government reneged on its earlier pledge not to encourage sterilization.
	A Department of Justice ruling permits sterilization.
1974:	Presidential Decree no. 34 exempts contraceptives and supplies necessary for the family planning program from payment of customs duties.
	Presidential Decree no. 1202 reduces the number of paid maternity leaves to four.
	Presidential Decree no. 442 requires private companies to provide their female employees with family planning services.
1975:	The orientation of the Population Program shifts because of the operationalization of the total integrated development approach that is piloted in provinces.
	The Department of Justice removes the requirement for prescriptions for oral contraceptives, thereby permitting widespread distribution of pills through nonclinical channels by trained field workers.
1976:	Presidential Decree no. 965 requires applicants for marriage licenses to receive instruction on family planning and responsible parenthood.
	The National Population and Family Planning Outreach Project is initiated.
	Letter of Instruction no. 433 authorizes provincial governors and city mayors to gradually assume the responsibility of funding the cost of all activities related to population and family planning and of projects agreed to by the POPCOM board and provincial officials for their respective jurisdictions.
1977:	The National Population and Family Planning Outreach Project begins implementation. Between 1977 and 1979, 30,000 volunteers are recruited to provide contraceptive supplies and referrals.
1978:	Letter of Instruction no. 661 creates the Special Committee to Review the Philippine Population Program in the context of the overall development goals of the country and to recommend policy and program directions for the future.

Population Policy Development, 1967–80

In December 1967, Philippine President Ferdinand Marcos and 17 other heads of state signed the United Nations Declaration on Population. The declaration proclaimed that "the population problem must be recognized as a principal element in long-range national planning if governments are to achieve their economic goals and fulfill the aspirations of their people" (SCRPPP 1978, p. 4). This event can be seen as the beginning of official recognition in the Philippines that rapid population growth was a problem that was affecting the nation's socioeconomic development.

Subsequently, a series of policy issuances culminated in Republic Act 6365 of 1971 and Presidential Decree no. 79 of 1972 that established the national population policy to address the challenge of rapid population growth by undertaking a national program of family planning involving both the public and the private sectors. The government's role in population was later enshrined in the 1973 Philippine Constitution, Article XV, section 10, which stated as follows: "It shall be the responsibility of the State to achieve and maintain population levels conducive to the national welfare."

Policy Articulation in Legislation

In February 1969, Ferdinand Marcos created by executive order a group to undertake population studies and to make recommendations on population policy and programs called the Commission on Population (referred to as the commission to distinguish it from another body created by law known as the Commission on Population and referred to as POPCOM, a body tasked to implement the national population policy and family planning program). A major feature of the commission was its multi-agency, multisectoral composition. The commission's board had 22 members from both the public and the private sectors and included representatives from religious organizations, such as the CBCP, the National Council of Churches, and the Muslim Association of the Philippines (SCRPPP 1978). The commission completed its task in less than a year. The task of studying all aspects of population was facilitated by prior work on population that became widely available at that time as a result of work carried out at Philippine universities and as an outcome of various conferences. The commission's recommendations addressed a broad range of population concerns that included not only population growth and family planning, but also concerns regarding morbidity, mortality, internal migration, and spatial distribution of the population. In December 1969, Ferdinand Marcos approved the commission's statement on population policy and a family planning program (Concepcion 1970).

Meanwhile, in June 1969, Congress approved a joint House resolution on basic policies to achieve economic development and attain social justice. This resolution contained the following statement on population policy: "A high rate of population growth poses grave social and economic challenges. The state shall meet these challenges both by positive social and economic measures that will increase the productivity of human work, so as to promote economic growth, and by programs of family planning which respect the religious beliefs of the individuals involved, so as to increase the share of each Filipino in the fruits of economic development" (Concepcion 1970, p. 4).

In his State of the Nation speech in January 1970, Ferdinand Marcos proposed legislation making family planning an official policy. The task of government, according to Ferdinand Marcos, was to educate the public on the urgent need to control population growth; disseminate knowledge about medically approved birth control techniques; and provide family planning services, particularly in rural areas and among the poor (Concepcion 1970).

In August 1971, Republic Act 6365 established the national population policy, which provided that "for the purpose of furthering national development, increasing the share of each Filipino in the fruits of economic progress and meeting the grave social and economic challenge of a high rate of population growth, a national program of family planning which respects the religious beliefs of the individual involved shall be undertaken" (SCRPPP 1978, p. 5). The act also adopted, as a matter of policy, the commission's 1969 recommendations, particularly the inclusion of broader population concerns other than fertility reduction. The act also created the government agency the POPCOM board under the Office of the President to carry out the purposes and objectives of the act.

In September 1972, Ferdinand Marcos declared martial law. Three months later, he issued a presidential decree to strengthen the family planning program. The presidential decree expanded the role of the POPCOM board and increased annual funding for the program from ₽4.5 million to ₽15 million.

Policy Articulation in Development Plans

The country's medium-term development plans also articulated population policy. Between 1970 and 1982, four such plans were formulated.

The Four-Year Development Plan (fiscal 1971–fiscal 1974) adopted by the National Economic Council in July 1970 was the first national development plan that included a chapter on population. Curiously, while it started by noting the worldwide concern about the problem of population growth, it did not explicitly state that the Philippines shared this concern. In other words, the language of the plan did not fully reflect the language found in the United Nations Declaration on Population nor the congressional resolution referred to earlier. A year earlier, the Catholic bishops had issued a pastoral letter publicly disagreeing with the government's intervention in couples' fertility decisions and objecting to the promotion of family limitation as a measure to reduce population growth. The plan had been developed under Placido L. Mapa, head of the National Economic Council, later the National Economic and Development Authority (NEDA), and a known supporter of conservative views on population and family planning as articulated by Cardinal Sin and the Catholic bishops.

By contrast, the Four-Year Development Plan (fiscal 1974–fiscal 1977), adopted by NEDA in 1973 under NEDA Director-General Gerardo P. Sicat, made strong statements regarding population growth reduction and family planning. In its "Overview" the plan stated that intensification of the family planning program was one of the major socioeconomic reforms that was instituted subsequent to the proclamation of martial law.

In September 1977, NEDA formulated and adopted the Five-Year Philippine Development Plan (calendar years 1978–82) under Sicat, who was also the minister of economic planning. The plan made a strong policy commitment to reducing the population growth rate and explicitly adopted family planning to this end. It aimed to reduce the rate of population growth from 2.5 percent in 1978 to 2.1 percent by 1987. It also set contraceptive prevalence targets of 27 percent in 1978 and 50 percent by 1987.

However, in May 1982, NEDA adopted the new Five-Year Philippine Development Plan (calendar years 1983–87) under Mapa, who again became head of NEDA.

Among the problems the plan recognized was population growth, but it indicated that population growth was something to be accommodated rather than influenced. Unlike the previous plans under Sicat, it did not contain population growth targets, much less fertility or contraceptive prevalence rate targets. The chapter on health and nutrition made no mention of family planning.

Thus, while the Sicat plans tended to closely reflect the view regarding the negative implications of rapid population growth contained in the legislation, the Mapa plans tended to view population growth as something to be accommodated. Moreover, the 1983–87 Mapa plan shifted the objective of population policy from fertility and population growth reduction to the achievement of individual and family welfare. Some observers have interpreted the plan's tendency to broaden the objectives of population policy, while desirable, as a way of quietly rejecting the fertility reduction objective.

As head of NEDA, Mapa was also the chair of the POPCOM board. A curious aspect of the Philippines' population policy and program was that the POPCOM board could be chaired by individuals who did not fully subscribe to all of the components of the program, in particular, the promotion of modern contraceptives. So while the official population policy was set out in legislation, actual implementation of all aspects of the family planning program often depended on who chaired the POPCOM board. Indeed, in 1983, the minister of the Department of Social Welfare and Development, who was more supportive of the family planning program, was appointed as the new chair of the POPCOM board to replace Mapa, and with an equally energetic executive director put the fertility reduction objective of family planning back into the policy agenda. POPCOM's aim was to achieve replacement fertility by 2000. These efforts were short-lived, however. The family planning program disappeared from the policy agenda in 1986, when President Corazón Aquino appointed a new chair of the POPCOM board, the secretary of Social Welfare and Development, Pardo de Tavera, a conservative like Mapa, who did not believe in promoting family planning that included modern contraceptives. This has been on ongoing pattern: when the chair is a conservative, the family planning program suffers a setback, illustrating the lack of continuity in policy implementation at the highest level.

Thus, while population policy under the Ferdinand Marcos administration as reflected in the constitution and various pieces of legislation had remained intact on paper through 1986, implementation of its main direct policy measure, the family planning program, shifted from vigorous to benign neglect depending on the head of the POPCOM board. The aggressive pursuit of family planning targets in 1983 was cut short by the People's Power Revolution. A significant shift in policy occurred with the installation of President Aquino, who was well known for her conservative views on population, views that were in line with the views of the Catholic Church hierarchy.

Role of Leaders of the Catholic Church Hierarchy
The policy articulation regarding the potentially negative effects of continued rapid population growth on development generally found support in discussions among senior government officials, population researchers, academics, and private sector representatives. However, as early as 1969, the Catholic bishops issued a statement on public policy regarding population growth (CBCP 1969). This statement first cast

doubt on the government's analysis regarding the existence of demographic problems, particularly with respect to their magnitude. The bishops argued further that should such a problem exist, then the government could undertake a number of social and development policies to address it, such as raising the minimum age of marriage and raising old-age pensions to minimize elderly people's dependence on their children. The bishops referred to such measures as macro measures of population control and agreed that it was within the competence of government to undertake such measures.

However, the bishops disagreed with respect to the government's role in intervening in couples' fertility decisions and emphasized couples' rights to determine the size of their families. The bishops also objected to the promotion of family planning as a measure to reduce population growth. They argued that such a measure would be effective in reducing population growth only if it "resolutely restricts its objectives to a reduced number of children as normative for the population, and eventually includes abortion and masked infanticide as necessary components of its program" (CBCP 1969, p. 325). Note that when Ferdinand Marcos first created the commission in 1969, CBCP representatives were included among the 22 board members. Apparently at that time, some working relationship or agreement existed between the government and the CBCP regarding the development of a family planning program. This relationship was severed when the CBCP requested to be removed from the board following what it considered as the government reneging on its promise not to include sterilization among family planning methods. Note that the commission had earlier recommended that abortion and sterilization should not be included as methods of family planning and that Ferdinand Marcos went along with this recommendation (Concepcion 1973).

In 1973, the Catholic hierarchy of the Philippines issued a pastoral letter on the population problem and family life. This echoed the theme regarding the lack of consensus among "reputable scientists" that resource shortages were caused primarily by the increase in population. According to the pastoral letter, the problem of shortages was caused principally by the inequitable distribution of resources among the world's population rather than an increase in the number of people competing for such resources. The letter expressed its strongest sentiments when it came to contraception:

> In our country there has been adopted as the principal solution to the population problem, massive conception control through the artificial contraceptive approach. This approach has followed a common pattern of development in countries where it has been espoused. The patterns show an escalation from the less radical to the more radical measures of sterilization and abortion. Only recently, the Department of Justice has removed all legal impediments to contraceptive sterilization by officially granting it legal clearance. Where formerly the population policy of the country explicitly gave the pledge not to encourage contraceptive sterilization, that reservation has now been dropped (CBCP 1973, p. 399).

The influence of the Catholic bishops appears to have been more political in nature than pastoral. The national demographic surveys of 1968, 1973, 1978, and 1983 showed high acceptance of modern family planning methods. The bishops' influence may have been increasing in the latter half of the 1970s, when the U.S. Agency for International Development (USAID) observed that the "unequivocal public statements by the President, First Lady and other high GOP [government of the Philippines] officials emphasizing GOP concern for the gravity of the population problem have been scarce, and mass media presentations on population issues less urgent and frequent. There are clear signs that high level GOP leaders, while strongly involved with, and committed to, population/family planning programs, perceive that public statements promoting modern methods of contraception including sterilization, could provoke overt Church resistance and erode needed Church support for the Ferdinand Marcos Government" (USAID 1979, p. 26). The apparent waning of political commitment to population policy and a family planning program by the Ferdinand Marcos administration (fewer public pronouncements, appointment of Mapa as chair of the POPCOM board in 1980) in the late 1970s and beginning of the 1980s appears to be related to the shifting political power of the leaders of the Catholic Church hierarchy on the one hand, and of the Ferdinand Marcos regime on the other. The political power of the Catholic Church reached its peak during the Aquino administration (1986–92). As a result, the family planning program and its fertility reduction objectives went into hiatus. Its implementation was later revived in 1988 under the Department of Health led by Dr. Alfredo Bengzon with the aim of promoting maternal and child health care, but explicitly rejecting demographic objectives (Bengzon 1992).

Family Planning Program Development

The family planning program underwent strategic and organizational changes to respond to findings about the program's impact and to resource availabilities.

Strategic Thrusts

The family planning program evolved from a clinic-based service delivery program during its early years (1968–73) to an outreach program that provided motivational activities and services beyond the clinics through a network of paid and volunteer workers in rural areas.

The Early Years, 1968–73

In 1968, the government created a small unit called the Project Office for Maternal and Child Health under the Department of Health. This unit was charged with overall responsibility for administering a national family planning program, marking the official entry of the Philippine government into family planning activities. The family planning program at that time involved the participation of voluntary family planning associations; national agencies such as the Department of Health; the University of the Philippines Population Institute; private institutions; and individual physicians who provided family planning services, training, or research in support of the program. USAID funding was instrumental in getting the program off the ground.

The basic strategy during the early years involved both the public and the private sectors in providing information and services pertaining to all family planning methods in established clinics. The key institutions that provided family planning and training were the Family Planning Organization of the Philippines, the Institute of Maternal and Child Health, the University of the Philippines College of Medicine, and the Department of Health. With respect to the latter, family planning services were added to its rural health units that were established in each municipality throughout the country. By 1973, 1,070 of its 1,400 rural health units were offering family planning services. Financial support was provided largely by the USAID through the Project Office for Maternal and Child Health until 1970, when the POPCOM board became the government's designated agency (SCRPPP 1978; USAID 1979).

Support to family planning service delivery included training in support of clinic activities provided by the Institute of Maternal and Child Health, the Family Planning Organization of the Philippines, the University of the Philippines College of Medicine, and the Department of Health; information, education, and communication conducted using the mass media and interpersonal communications by means of field motivators; and research and evaluation. In 1972, the Department of Education established the Population Education Program whose aim was to help students understand population processes and develop responsible attitudes and behavior in relation to family size (SCRPPP 1978).

Further policy support to family planning activities included enjoining all sectors to promote the concept of family planning and responsible parenthood (1972); directing the secretary of the Department of Public Information and the postmaster general to disseminate information on family planning (1972); and reducing the number of children for which additional tax exemptions could be claimed from an unlimited number to four (1973). The extent to which these policies had any impact on contraceptive knowledge and motivation to practice family planning is not clear.

At the start of the government's family planning activities in 1968, the contraceptive prevalence rate was 2.9 percent for modern methods and 12.5 percent for traditional methods (table 17.1), reflecting the efforts to promote family planning by voluntary organizations and the private sector. By 1973, the contraceptive prevalence rate had risen to 10.7 percent for modern methods and 6.7 percent for traditional methods.

The Transition Years, 1974–75

During the transition period, the government devised new strategies to deal with the growing number of family planning clients beyond the reach of clinics (SCRPPP 1978) and to expand the family planning program within the context of development (Concepcion 1977). To address the first concern, the role of nurses and midwives

TABLE 17.1 Trends in Contraceptive Use, Selected Years
percentage of currently married women aged 15–44

Survey	Modern methods	Traditional methods	Total
1968 national demographic survey	2.9	12.5	15.4
1973 national demographic survey	10.7	6.7	17.4
1978 Republic of the Philippines fertility survey	17.2	21.3	38.5
1983 national demographic survey	18.9	13.1	32.0

Source: National Statistics Office and ORC Macro 2004.

was expanded to include dispensing pills and inserting intrauterine devices, and appropriate training programs for these personnel were launched in 1974. In addition, the POPCOM board formally adopted sterilization as a family planning method and provided training in the procedure through POPCOM-accredited institutions.

Sterilization gained wide acceptance as a family planning method. Field personnel noted the great demand for tubal ligation, but not for vasectomy. Trained service providers for sterilization became available in hospitals and as mobile teams throughout the country. In 1976, the program allocated funds to reimburse providers, as well as field workers who referred clients to providers. The reimbursements were for medicines, other supplies, and transport costs. Based on data from the national demographic surveys, the prevalence rate for sterilization, which was only 1 percent in 1973, rose to 5 percent in 1978 and to 10 percent by 1983, when it accounted for 30 percent of the total contraceptive prevalence rate (Population Institute 1985).

To meet the objective of expanding the family planning program in a development context, in 1975, the POPCOM board formulated the total integrated development approach. This approach involved a shift from the clinic-based, doctor-centered, and contraceptive-oriented program to one that integrated family planning motivation and services at the community level with other development activities in rural areas. For the implementation of this approach, a new structure based on local governments was established to integrate programs, activities, and services at the provincial, municipal, and community levels, and the approach was piloted in seven provinces. In each province, the structure was headed by the provincial population officer in the office of the provincial governor. The officer was responsible for managing the program, including preparing provincial population plans. The key workers in the structure were the municipal population officers, whose primary functions included coordinating with workers in other agencies in the municipality to organize and integrate their agencies' population-related services. The municipal population officers were also responsible for organizing village development centers to act as resupply points and information centers in each village (SCRPPP 1978).

The concept of integrating family planning with development activities appears to have been influenced by the integration of population and development concepts discussed during the 1974 International Conference on Population and Development held in Bucharest (Concepcion 1977). Rafael Esmundo, POPCOM's executive director at that time, was an ardent advocate of this approach. For purposes of implementation, however, exactly how to go about integrating the various activities was not clear. In most cases, the concept of integration as applied in the field was more of a piggybacking, whereby, for example, while going about their usual work, agricultural extension workers would also advocate family planning. Similarly, family planning field workers were also expected to participate in community planning for nutrition, health, and other development activities and use these activities as an entry point for family planning activities. While the total integrated development approach was still being piloted in the seven provinces, the POPCOM board decided to implement a new project, the National Population and Family Planning Outreach Project (hereafter referred to as the Outreach Project), on a nationwide basis. From an operational point of view, fieldworkers found the total integrated development approach to be vague, leading to a lack of uniformity in implementation in the field (SRCPPP 1978).

During the transition period, the government introduced several more policies in support of the program. These included exempting contraceptives and other supplies necessary for the family planning program from customs duties; reducing the number of paid maternity leaves to four; requiring private companies to provide family planning services to their female employees; and removing the requirement for a prescription for oral contraceptives, thereby permitting wider distribution of pills by trained field workers through nonclinic outlets.

Beyond Clinics: The Outreach Project, 1976–86

In recognition that the clinic-based strategy limited the program's ability to reach more couples, the Outreach Project was launched in 1976 with the POPCOM board as the implementing agency. This recognition was based on data from the 1973 national demographic survey, which revealed that the contraceptive prevalence rate among couples dropped significantly beyond a 3-kilometer radius from a clinic and was also much lower in rural areas than urban areas (SCRPPP 1978). Moreover, service statistics compiled by the POPCOM board showed that the number of family planning acceptors had reached a plateau (table 17.2). Thus, the Outreach Project sought to provide family planning motivation activities and services to all couples regardless of their proximity to clinics through a network of paid outreach workers and volunteer village supply-point officers. The project became the core activity of the family planning program.

The Outreach Project used full-time outreach workers and village supply-point officers. To implement the Outreach Project, the POPCOM board entered into contracts with local governments and provided a full-time outreach worker for every 2,000 married couples of reproductive age. More than 3,000 outreach workers were trained as information workers, service providers, and community organizers. As service providers, they were expected to dispense pills; establish village service points; and distribute contraceptive supplies and information, education, and communication materials to the target population. By 1977, a total of 2,565 full-time outreach workers had been deployed and 15,597 village service points had been set up.

TABLE 17.2 Selected Family Planning Program Indicators, 1972–77

Indicator	1972	1973	1974	1975	1976	1977
Number of married women of reproductive age (thousands)	4,377.9	4,512.3	4,650.9	5,117.4	5,436.5	5,453.5
Family planning acceptors						
Number (thousands)	526.1	691.3	762.2	716.6	716.1	550.8[a]
Percentage of married women of reproductive age	12.0	15.3	16.4	14.0	13.2	10.1
Cumulative number of family planning clinics	1,490.0	2,042.0	2,192.0	2,719.0	2,794.0	2,956.0

Source: SCRPPP 1978.

a. Refers to the calendar year. All other entries refer to the fiscal year.

Policy support to the Outreach Project included a letter of instruction issued in 1976 that authorized governors and city mayors to gradually and progressively assume the responsibility of funding activities and projects related to population and family planning as agreed to by the POPCOM board and by local officials for their respective jurisdictions.

The implementation of the Outreach Project on a nationwide basis may have expanded the reach of the family planning program beyond clinics. However, it may also have shifted the focus of family planning implementation away from the Department of Health and the private sector, which provided clinical services to the POPCOM board through its secretariat, which implemented the Outreach Project with local government units. Instead of strengthening the integration of family planning with other health-related activities, the project made family planning look more like a separate vertical program implemented by the POPCOM board. Problems of coordination at the field level among outreach workers and clinical personnel in the rural health units were noted (SCRPPP 1978). Thus, the Outreach Project may have moved the program away from integration with the health sector and the concept of family welfare, which was needed as part of the overall effort at effective integration of population and development, and also as a way of dealing with critics, especially the leaders of the Catholic Church hierarchy. Moreover, the project's sustainability depended on local government financing, but this was not guaranteed, as local governments had limited financing capacities and little incentive to finance programs whose benefits accrued to the nation as a whole rather than only to their localities.

Organizational Structure

From the start, the family planning program was designed to be multisectoral and to involve multiple agencies. By 1978, about 40 agencies were participating in the program in such areas as clinic services; training; information, education, and communication; research; and evaluation. These agencies consisted of various government line agencies, regional and local government bodies, and the Population Center Foundation (founded in 1972 to forge a stronger partnership between the government and the private sector). The size and composition of the POPCOM board reflected the multi-agency character of the family planning program. In 1970, the board consisted of 21 members who included cabinet secretaries and representatives from the private sector and religious organizations. Its membership was reduced to 12 in 1971 and to 5 in 1972. Subsequent changes added more members, bringing the total number of board members to 10 by 1978.

The board was supported by the POPCOM secretariat, which was headed by an executive director. The secretariat expanded as the program expanded, so that by 1978, in addition to the Office of the Executive Director, the secretariat had six divisions (Planning; Clinic Service; Information, Education, and Communication; Training; Finance; and Administration). During 1970 to 1980, the secretariat had three executive directors, and leadership and staff also changed in all but the Information, Education, and Communication Division. This has been attributed in part to the relatively low compensation paid to secretariat staff members relative to that paid to the employees of other institutions involved in the program, such as the Population Center Foundation. Changes in the chair of the POPCOM board as well as the turnover of the executive director and key staff members of the POPCOM secretariat, affected the continuity of program implementation.

Financing and the Role of Foreign Donors

Initially, financial support for the program came mainly from foreign donors, especially the USAID. With its creation, however, the POPCOM board obtained its own budget, and gradually increased its contributions to the total costs of the program.

Until 1973, foreign donors contributed more than 60 percent of the total program financing. Beginning in 1974, the share of foreign assistance declined to about one-half of total expenditure by 1977 and to about one-third by 1982. Until 1972, the USAID provided virtually all the funds for the family planning program. From 1973, the USAID's share of total program financing gradually declined, accounting for only 31 percent in 1977 and 16 percent in 1980. This was due to the rising share of the government's contribution and contributions by other foreign donors. The next biggest source of foreign assistance for the family planning program during 1969 to 1977 was the United Nations Population Fund. The share of the latter's contribution reached 14.7 percent of total costs in 1976, but declined to 6.2 percent in 1977. Other foreign donors, such as the International Planned Parenthood Federation, the Ford Foundation, Pathfinder International, the Population Council, and the Asia Foundation, contributed, on average, about 10 to 15 percent of total program financing in during 1969 to 1977 (SCRPPP 1978).

Implementation of the Outreach Project, which started in 1976, necessitated increased participation by local governments, including making financial contributions to the family planning program. However, in 1978, the Special Committee to Review the Philippine Population Program found that most local government units did not have sufficient locally raised resources to support the family planning program. Indeed, most of them had to depend on assistance from the central government to implement the bare minimum of social and economic development projects.

While expenditures on the family planning program were increasing in current pesos, in real terms (1978 constant pesos) they were declining during the late 1970s and early 1980s (table 17.3). The impact of this decline is unclear. Most likely it limited further progress by the program at a time when needs were growing, that is, the number of married couples of reproductive age was increasing. In addition, the decline in real expenditures may have been an indication of waning commitment to the family planning program as also signaled by the less frequent public statements by the president and high-ranking officials regarding family planning.

Another aspect of financing was that the family planning program relied totally on donated contraceptives. The government never spent a single centavo to procure contraceptives for distribution to its public outlets. Some observers speculate that this was because donors, mainly the USAID, were willing and able to provide such commodities. Others suspect that the government felt that using government funds to procure contraceptives would further fuel the opposition to the family planning program by the leaders of the Catholic Church hierarchy.

TABLE 17.3 Family Planning Program Expenditures, 1972–1983

	Total expenditures		Percentage share of expenditures by source			
Year	Current (P millions)	Constant (1978 = 100)	Government of the Philippines	USAID	Other	Total
Fiscal year						
1972	54.4	126.2	15.1	71.1	13.8	100.0
1973	72.5	144.6	36.8	48.3	14.9	100.0
1974	113.8	180.1	51.3	30.3	18.4	100.0
1975	127.7	170.3	47.6	32.4	20.0	100.0
1976	113.9	140.2	49.5	26.2	24.3	100.0
1976 extension[a]	73.3	86.2	59.8	32.6	7.6	100.0
Calendar year						
1976[b]	130.2	153.3	55.3	29.8	14.9	100.0
1977	131.6	140.9	55.2	31.1	13.7	100.0
1978	131.3	133.3	74.2	21.6	4.2	100.0
1979	149.1	126.9	72.5	18.8	8.7	100.0
1980	163.7	117.9	79.0	15.9	5.1	100.0
1981	196.6	125.1	70.3	18.8	10.9	100.0
1982	196.2	113.3	67.4	24.1	8.5	100.0
1983	176.5	92.7	40.2	37.5	22.3	100.0
Total	1,702.6	1,643.8	59.8	28.1	12.1	100.0

Source: Herrin 1994.

a. Refers to July–December 1976.

b. Refers to calendar year 1976. Estimated by adding half of the expenditures for fiscal 1976 to the expenditures for 1976 extension.

Research and Evaluation

Basic and policy research supported program development. Occasional evaluation studies were also conducted, culminating in a special review of the program by a committee created by President Ferdinand Marcos in 1978.

Basic and Policy Research

Scholars in various academic and research institutions, including the University of the Philippines Population Institute, regularly conducted basic demographic research on levels and determinants of and trends in fertility, nuptiality, mortality, and migration. Analyses were based on individually collected data and on official statistics from vital registration and national surveys conducted by the National Statistics Office. Large multidisciplinary studies were also conducted, such as that on population, resources, the environment, and the future of the Philippines. This research program projected the physical, economic, and social conditions of the Philippines by 2000, including population projections and the implication of various population growth scenarios on economic and social development, and identified policy actions that could provide the best future.

A number of studies and surveys were also conducted specifically to inform policy and programmatic actions. These included the 1974 national acceptor survey and the 1978 and 1980 community outreach surveys, which provided information about the impact of program activities on family planning acceptance and contraceptive prevalence rates. A survey conducted in 1976 and 1977 sought to measure fertility declines and their determinants in the seven provinces where the total integrated development approach was piloted.

Special Committee to Review the Philippine Population Program
In January 1978, President Ferdinand Marcos created the Special Committee to Review the Philippine Population Program. The committee was tasked "to evaluate policies and programs related to population in the context of overall development goals of the country and shall further prepare, deliberate on and recommend program and policy directions in population for the future" (SCRPPP 1978, p. III). The committee's report, which consisted of findings and recommendations on a wide range of concerns from policy to program implementation, was approved and adopted by NEDA in August 1978.

The committee noted that while some efforts had been taken to link the broader Population Program (which included other aspects of population beyond family planning) with other economic and social dimensions of development, to a large extent, the program had focused almost solely on the family planning program. The committee therefore made the following recommendation:

> The Philippine Population Program should be designed on a broader scale and be fully integrated in the national development plans of the country. Economic, social and institutional policies should be evolved with a conscious consideration of their impact on demographic behavior and objectives. A total population policy should be designed to establish closer linkages between the demographic, more specifically, fertility aspects, and the manpower and welfare aspects of development. Fertility and family planning policies and programs should be formulated within the context of the family welfare objective (SCRPPP 1978, p. 122).

This recommendation had several aspects. The first was that consideration should be given to the demographic impact of development policies and programs. This required understanding the direct and indirect effects of development policies and programs on demographic behavior, and also some capacity to measure these direct and indirect effects for planning purposes. The second referred to what the committee meant by "total population policy" in the context of family welfare. Operationally, according to the committee, the state of well-being of the family as a whole and of the individuals that comprise the family consists of minimum requirements for a family's private consumption, essential services provided by and for the community at large, and employment yielding a sufficient level of income. Thus viewed from this broader concept of population policy as contrasted with a fertility reduction policy or family planning policy (that is, policies and programs to influence the action of couples to achieve their desired number and spacing of children), total population policy should have three integral components: "(1) a demographic policy influencing fertility, mortality, migration and social mobility; (2) a manpower policy defining the limits of the economically active age, the rate of labor force participation of the economically active population, length of the working day and the working week, professional training, job counseling, etc.; and (3) a welfare policy influencing wages and income, economic security, housing conditions, health and educational services, cultural amenities, etc." (SCRPPP 1978, p. 19). Family planning was seen as one way to raise family welfare in that a smaller family increased a family's chances of satisfying its various needs.

At the time the recommendation was made, neither the POPCOM board nor NEDA would have been ready to consider the demographic impacts of development programs or the integration of demographic, manpower, and welfare policies in the context of family welfare. However, in response to this recommendation, the Population/Development Planning and Research Project was prepared in 1980 through NEDA with support from the United Nations Population Fund. The project was aimed at improving the capacity of policy-making and planning bodies to integrate population and development planning along the lines of the committee's recommendations and in consonance with the general recommendations of the 1974 International Conference on Population and Development's World Plan of Action.

Evaluation of the Outreach Project

In 1978 and 1980, the POPCOM board undertook community outreach surveys through the University of the Philippines Population Institute with support from the USAID to evaluate the Outreach Project. Their findings revealed measurable progress in reaching a larger group of couples, as well as certain deficiencies that limited its potential impact.

Deficiencies noted in the 1980 survey included the following (Laing 1981). First, the potential of the village supply points for providing wider access to contraceptive supplies was limited, as fewer than half the married women living in supply point areas knew that such supply points existed and could provide them with pills and condoms. Later data—from the 1983 national demographic survey—showed that only 26 percent of current pill users and 40 percent of condom users obtained their supplies from outreach workers, while 54 percent of pill users and 30 percent of condom users obtained supplies from clinics.

Second, the information being provided to couples about the risks involved in using modern contraceptives lacked sufficient detail and the actual support services needed to maintain high-quality services were insufficient. This conclusion is inferred from data that a major reason for the nonuse of clinical methods was the fear of side effects. Among women who were currently using less effective methods, the percentage rejecting the pill, intrauterine device, and sterilization because of fear of side effects was 87 percent, 74 percent, and 61 percent, respectively.

Finally, the training of outreach workers (paid and volunteer) was inadequate, as revealed by their low, or even inappropriate, knowledge of the relative effectiveness of specific methods.

Despite these deficiencies, the surveys also indicated that some progress had been made. Based on a multivariate analysis of the 1980 survey data, Laing (1981) found that, controlling for socioeconomic variables and nonoutreach program variables, several indicators of outreach activities were significantly correlated with contraceptive prevalence rates at the village level, and that these indicators explained a substantial proportion of the variance in village-level prevalence rates.

An in-depth analysis of the 1980 community outreach survey data, however, suggested that the Outreach Project may have contributed less to raising overall contraceptive prevalence in the project areas and more to shifting contraceptive users from less effective to more effective methods (Herrin and Pullum 1981). The data on overall contraceptive prevalence rates based on all methods showed no significant change between 1978 and 1980; however, in the areas covered by the Outreach Project, the data indicated a substantial decline in family size preference as measured by the percentage of currently married, nonpregnant, fecund women who wanted no more children, particularly women with three or more children, and among women who wanted to stop childbearing, the use of more effective contraceptive methods had increased dramatically.

Although the shift from less effective to more effective methods was indeed a welcome development from the standpoint of project performance, for fertility decline to accelerate, overall contraceptive prevalence had to increase significantly, and preferably with the increase being attributable to the use of more effective methods. For an increase in prevalence rate, the Outreach Project had to increase its coverage nationwide and improve its effectiveness. Six years after its initial implementation, the project apparently had not had truly nationwide coverage: the POPCOM board estimated that in 1982, the Outreach Project covered only 62 percent of married couples of reproductive age outside of Metro Manila.

Reflections and Lessons for the Future

In reflecting upon the experience of the early years of the family planning program, one notes the policy inconsistency among national government agencies, the preoccupation with demographic objectives, and some unintended effects.

Policy Inconsistency

The Population Program began with strong policy commitment from the president and from legislators regarding the need to reduce the rapid population growth through a national family planning program that involved both the public and the private sectors and that respected couples' religious and moral convictions. However, other policy centers, specifically, the POPCOM board and the national planning agency (initially the National Economic Council and later NEDA), offered conflicting signals about the need for such a reduction depending on who was the head of the agency. During 1970 to 1982, the government had two sets of development plans that differed in terms of their emphasis on the role of population growth in development and the need for a strong family planning program. The same lack of policy consistency apparent at the national planning agency also appeared in the POPCOM board when the chair of the board steered the program in a direction that differed from official legislated policy. Thus, individuals with strong personal views on population and family planning could apparently influence the formulation of policies and plans without official guidance from higher-level authorities. This inconsistency at the highest level of policy making sent conflicting signals to those implementing the family planning program on the ground.

Similarly inconsistent or conflicting policy articulation is apparent later among NEDA (as reflected in its medium-term development plans) and the POPCOM board and the Department of Health (as reflected in their respective policy statements) on such matters as the need for the government to address the rapid growth of population, the need to implement a family planning program with a fertility reduction objective, the need for family planning to help couples achieve their desired fertility, and the need for family planning to promote maternal and child health (Herrin 2002). This situation did not augur well for a sustained program in later years.

This inconsistency in Philippine population policy can be understood in the context of the lack of a working consensus between government policy makers and politically influential leaders of the Catholic Church hierarchy regarding the promotion of contraceptives and sterilization. (They had reached consensus regarding outlawing abortion as a family planning method and including natural family planning methods among the government's program methods.) The major disruption to any potential consensus between the government and the Catholic bishops came when the government reneged on its promise not to include sterilization among its program methods. This created mistrust on the part of the Catholic bishops, who feared that down the road the government would approve abortion as a method. At the same time, even though the government's program methods included the rhythm and other so-called natural methods, the government program did not promote these as vigorously as "artificial" methods. Thus, an opportunity for the government to work closely with the Catholic Church hierarchy was not taken, but at the same time, the latter may not have been willing to engage in such a partnership to avoid the perception that it condoned artificial methods.

Preoccupation with Objectives of Family Planning

The early preoccupation with the issues surrounding rapid population growth naturally focused the objectives of the family planning program toward reducing fertility to moderate population growth. Moderating fertility, and thereby population growth, is a valid policy objective, but a family planning program can also help achieve other objectives, such as helping couples achieve their fertility goals and promoting maternal and child health. These other objectives, although mentioned in passing, were not given as much emphasis in the design of the program as the demographic objective. A hierarchy of objectives could be formulated that starts with helping couples achieve their desired family size as an end in itself. Data from the national demographic and other national surveys showed that many couples, particularly among the poor, had more children than they wanted. Moreover, many couples wanted to stop childbearing or to space births, but were not practicing family planning. Thus, a family planning program can be designed to help couples achieve their fertility goals, which has a direct effect on their well-being.

Births beyond the number of children desired are often high-risk births, for instance, births to young or old mothers, births at close intervals, and higher order births. Therefore, helping couples achieve their fertility goals through family planning can have a significant effect on maternal and child health. In addition, when couples are having more children than they desire, achieving their desired fertility would have the effect of reducing overall fertility, hence the demographic objective of national fertility reduction and population growth moderation would also be achieved.

A family planning program designed and promoted with this hierarchy of objectives in mind would be more consistent with the concept of integration espoused by the World Plan of Action. It is also more acceptable to a broader set of stakeholders, including those who oppose a family planning program. Thus, restating the hierarchy and interrelations of multiple objectives and designing the program to achieve these objectives might invite less opposition and more areas for achieving consensus. The objective of helping couples achieve their fertility goals is not likely to give rise to major disagreement. From a human rights perspective, achieving this objective requires that couples be able to make informed choices about available methods by being provided information about costs, safety, and effectiveness as well as having access to counseling by members of their religion. A collaboration or a division of labor between the government, the private sector, and religious organizations can then be made on the delivery of specific methods that couples choose.

Unintended Effects

Partly because of the opposition to the family planning program, particularly the promotion of contraceptives, by the Catholic bishops, and partly because of the availability of donated contraceptives, the Philippine government opted not to appropriate any funds to procure contraceptives. By not spending tax money to procure contraceptives, the government thought it could partly deflect overt criticism by the Catholic bishops.

The nature of the donated contraceptives, however, was that they should be distributed to clients for free. The more widespread the distribution, the more unlikely it was that the private sector would expand its own market. This approach had the unintended effect of continuing heavy reliance on the government for contraceptive supplies, which, in turn, made the government increasingly vulnerable to opposition by the Catholic bishops. Had the government procured its supplies of contraceptives for free distribution to the poor while allowing the private sector to expand supplies to service the nonpoor, the private sector might have expanded significantly more than it did. An expanded, decentralized, private sector would have been less vulnerable to the political influence of the Catholic bishops and could have helped sustain service delivery.

The Outreach Project, although it was intended to expand the reach of the program beyond clinics, was designed in such a way that it unintentionally took primary responsibility for family planning motivation and service delivery from the Department of Health. As a result, the program missed an opportunity to integrate family planning with health and family welfare activities. Such an integration could have created another dimension for closer cooperation between the government and the Catholic bishops.

References

Bengzon, Alfredo R. A. 1992. "Health Policy Reforms: Seeing and Doing, and Moving Onto Center Stage." *Philippine Economic Journal* XXXI (72): 62–68.

CBCP (Catholic Bishops Conference of the Philippines). 1969. "Statement of the Catholic Bishops on Public Policy Regarding Population Growth Control." In *Pastoral Letters, 1945–1995,* ed. Pedro C. Quitorio III, 322–27. Intramuros Manila: CBCP

———. 1973. "Pastoral Letter of the Catholic Hierarchy of the Philippines on the Population Problem and Family Life." In *Pastoral Letters, 1945–1995,* ed. Pedro C. Quitorio III, 396–400. Intramuros Manila: CBCP.

Concepcion, Mercedes B. 1970. *The Philippines.* Country Profiles Series. New York: Population Council.

———. 1973. "Philippine Population Policy and Program." In *The Filipino Family in the Seventies: An Ecumenical Perspective,* ed. Vitaliano R. Gorospe and Richard L. Deats, 51–60. Quezon City, Philippines: New Day Publishers.

———. 1977. "Philippines." In *Family Planning in the Developing World: A Review of Programs,* ed. Walter B. Watson, 19–20. New York: Population Council.

Herrin, Alejandro N. 1994, "Philippine Demographic Development and Public Policies: 1970–1985." In *Population, Human Resources and Development,* vol. 1, ed. A. N. Herrin, 507–30. Quezon City, Philippines: University of the Philippines Press.

———. 2002. "Population Policy in the Philippines, 1969–2002." Discussion Paper Series 2002–08, Philippine Institute for Development Studies, Makati, Metro Manila.

Herrin, Alejandro N., and Thomas W. Pullum. 1981. *Family Planning in the Philippines: A Preliminary Assessment of the Impact of Population Planning II.* Report prepared for the U.S. Agency for International Development, Manila.

Laing, John E. 1981. *Family Planning Outreach in the Philippines: Final Report of the Community Outreach Surveys.* Quezon City, Philippines: University of the Philippines, Population Institute.

National Statistics Office and ORC Macro. 2004. *National Demographic and Health Survey, 2003.* Calverton, MD: National Statistics Office and ORC Macro.

Population Institute. 1985. *Philippine Population Data: An Update.* Quezon City, Philippines: University of the Philippines, Population Institute.

SCRPPP (Special Committee to Review the Philippine Population Program). 1978. *Final Report of the Special Committee to Review the Philippine Population Program (SCRPPP).* Manila: National Economic and Development Authority.

USAID (U.S. Agency for International Development). 1979. "Back-up Papers for the Multi-Year Population Strategy Statement." Evaluation Report. USAID Mission to the Philippines, Manila.

V South Asia

18 Emergence of the Indian National Family Planning Program

OSCAR HARKAVY AND KRISHNA ROY

India has a long history of Malthusian concern about the effects of population pressure on its food supply and other resources. Thomas Malthus was a professor of political economy at the East India Company's college in England from 1805 to 1834. He was convinced that India's high rate of population growth was the prime cause of the periodic famines that afflicted that country. As noted by Caldwell and Caldwell (1986, p. 4), Malthus and his successors "insured that generations of British officials and scholars in India saw that country's society in Malthusian terms."

For many years, Indian nationals were also disconcerted by the serious consequences of their country's population growth. In 1916, for example, an Indian scholar, Pyare Kishan Wattal, published *The Population Problem in India* (Wattal 1916), portraying dire consequences of the population growth India was enduring. In 1928, a neo-Malthusian league was organized in Madras. Five years previously, India's first birth control clinic had been opened in Poona (Visaria and Jain 1976), but was restricted by Gandhian opposition to artificial methods of birth control. According to the 1931 population census, between 1921 and 1931, India's population had increased by more than 10 percent, or 27.7 million people.

A series of events preceding independent India's First Five-Year Plan (1952–57) pointed to the urgency of controlling population growth. The Bengal Famine Inquiry Committee, set up to examine the 1940 famine and its possible roots in rapid population growth, noted with alarm that India's population would increase by 100 million between 1945 and 1960 and recommended setting up a network of birth control clinics. The Health Survey and Development Committee (popularly known as the Bhore Committee), established in 1943, also called for a national family planning program to improve the population's health status. The secretary of the Bengal Famine Inquiry Committee, R. A. Gopalswami, became director of the 1951 census. He projected a 1981 population of 520 million (the actual figure was 690 million)

The authors are grateful for comments by Jack Kantner, Timothy King, Gadde Narayana, Ronald Ridker, Warren C. Robinson, and John A. Ross.

and feared that population pressure on the food supply would result in a famine causing even more devastation and deaths than the Bengal famine. In 1951, Gopalswami urged Prime Minister Jawaharlal Nehru to support a nationwide vasectomy program (Caldwell and Caldwell 1986).

The findings of the Bengal Famine Inquiry Committee and the Health Survey and Development Committee motivated the government of India to adopt the National Programme of Family Planning in 1947. In 1950, the government appointed the Population Policy Committee, chaired by the minister of health, and created the Family Planning Cell in the Office of the Director General of Health Services.

India's First Five-Year Plan allocated Rs 6.5 million (US$1.44 million) to the Ministry of Health for research on population issues and on the acceptability of natural family planning and other contraceptive methods. Only Rs 1.45 million (US$320,000) were used to support family planning clinics (Visaria and Jain 1976). With this modest initiative, India became the first country in the world to set up an official program to control its population growth.

In comparison with neighboring Pakistan and other developing countries, India's rate of population growth was not particularly high. Its overall annual rate of population increase was about 2.2 percent in 1961 and 2.5 percent in 1971, with substantial differences from region to region. Relatively high mortality, together with a high prevalence of widowhood and a cultural taboo on remarriage by widows, prevented extremely high levels of population growth. Nonetheless, more than a million people were added to India's population each month. Furthermore, 2.4 percent of the world's area, which contained about 15 percent of the world's population, accounted for a population density of 300 or more people per square kilometer (Visaria and Jain 1976). Govind Narain, Secretary of the Ministry of Health's Family Planning and Urban Development Department in the late 1960s, expressed the prevailing government outlook: "The high growth rate of this large population . . . poses tremendous socio-economic problems not only for the maintenance of minimal standards of living but also for raising them. Already a vast development by way of large increases in agricultural and industrial production has been neutralized by population growth. . . . The manifold expansion of employment, housing, educational and other facilities has been almost entirely swallowed by the fast growing population" (Narain 1968, p. 1).

Box 18.1 presents a timeline of events that triggered attempts at establishing family planning programs in India.

First Phase of the Family Planning Program

Caught between the pressing urgency of controlling population growth and the overwhelming influence of Gandhian heritage on the majority of Nehru's cabinet, especially the health minister, it was a Herculian task for the architects of independent India's First Five-Year Plan to reconcile the two opposite positions and still design a rational and effective family planning program.

BOX 18.1 Timeline of Major Events

1916: Pyare Kishan Wattal publishes *The Population Problem in India*, warning of the dire consequences of uncontrolled population growth.

1921: Decennial population censuses indicate the beginning of continual and rapid population growth, alarming politicians and intellectuals.

1923: India's first birth control clinic opens in Poona.

1928: A neo-Malthusian league is established in Madras symbolizing an organized start of population control measures using artificial methods.

1937: Lieutenant Colonel B. L. Raina, the Ministry of Health's first director of family planning, sets up a maternal and child health and family planning center named Help Our Mothers Society that offers free medical services.

1940: A government commission, set up to examine the causes and consequences of the Bengal famine in the early 1940s, warn of an unprecedented projected increase of population by 100 million between 1945 and 1960.

1943: The Health Survey and Development Committee (popularly known as the Bhore Committee) is established and calls for a national family planning program to improve the population's health status.

1947: The government adopts the National Programme of Family Planning.

1949: The Family Planning Association of India is established under the leadership of Lady Rama Rau and oversees the distribution to clinics of family planning funds allocated to the Ministry of Health during the First Five-Year Plan.

1950: The government appoints the Population Policy Committee, chaired by the minister of health.

The government creates the Family Planning Cell in the Office of the Director General of Health Services.

1951: R. A. Gopalswami, director of the 1951 population census, projects a 1981 population of 520 million (the actual figure was 690 million). He urges Prime Minister Jawaharlal Nehru to support a nationwide vasectomy program.

Minister of Health Rajkumari Amrit Kaur requests a World Health Organization mission to advise on promoting the rhythm method.

1952–57: The First Five-Year Plan, which includes a chapter on population, allocates Rs 6.5 million to the Ministry of Health for research on population issues and on the acceptability of natural family planning and other contraceptive methods and adopts a clinic-based approach.

1955: The Ford Foundation arranges for a consultancy to advise on efforts to extend family planning beyond natural family planning.

1961: An estimated 4,000 birth control clinics offer contraceptives.

1956–61: The Second Five-Year Plan commences and extends the clinic-based approach.

1961–66: India's Third Five-Year Plan calls for a 10-fold increase in funds for family planning over the amount allocated in the preceding plan.

1962: The futility of the clinic-based approach is demonstrated by the unabated population growth uncovered by the 1961 population census.

The government sets the goal of reducing the crude birthrate from 41 live births per 1,000 population to 25 by 1970.

Studies by the Gandhigram Institute for Rural Development and Family Planning further confirm the failure of the clinic-based approach and recommend an extension approach.

(Continued)

BOX 18.1 Timeline of Major Events (Continued)

1963:	An extended family planning campaign is started, involving extension educators, assistant surgeons, family welfare workers, auxiliary nurse-midwives, and contraceptive depot holders (those responsible for storing and dispensing contraceptives) at the village level.
1965:	The Indian Medical Council approves the intrauterine device.
1966:	The target of a crude birthrate of 25 live births per 1,000 population was to be reached as quickly as possible instead of waiting until 1970.
1966–67:	All-India targets for contraceptive use, together with demographic goals for drastic reduction in population growth, that led to the so-called HITTS (Health Department operated, incentive-based, target-oriented, time-bound, and sterilization-focused) model in 1962 proved futile within a short period.
Late 1960s:	The Ministry of Health is renamed the Ministry of Health and Family Planning and includes a Department of Family Planning. The position of secretary of state for family planning is created.
1965:	The Central Family Planning Institute is established. With the collaborative involvement of the National Institute of Health Administration and Education, established in the early 1960s, and the Central Family Planning Institute, 19 intensive family planning districts patterned after intensive agricultural districts are set up. An intensive program for training family planning administrators in the United States is set up, jointly sponsored by the government and the Ford Foundation.
1968:	A crude birthrate target of 23 live births per 1,000 population by 1978–79 is set.
1969:	The All-India Hospital Postpartum Programme is created.
1970–73:	During the Fifth Five-Year Plan, the Hospital Postpartum Programme serves 1.2 million obstetric and abortion patients and more than 18 percent accept a birth control method.
1970–77:	Vasectomies, together with substantial monetary and in-kind incentives, become the defining feature of the family planning initiative. Vasectomy camps become a major instrument for achieving large number of acceptors.
1971:	Secretary of State Dr. S. Chandrasekhar successfully lobbies Parliament to legalize abortion.
1971:	The Medical Termination of Pregnancy Act is passed, legalizing abortion.
1972–73:	Some 23,000 abortions are performed annually in authorized hospitals and clinics.
1972:	The Family Planning Foundation is established and starts funding high-quality social science research relevant to the national family planning program.
1974:	The Family Planning Foundation funds a major volume that influences the Indian delegation to the 1974 World Population Conference.
1975:	The Hospital Postpartum Programme enrolls 255 hospitals. Between 1956 and 1975, more than 20 million births are averted. The birthrate of 42 live births per 1,000 population in 1960–61 declined to 35 in 1974–75. Prime Minister Indira Gandhi declares an emergency because of an economic crisis and proposes a 20-point program not including population control; however, her son, Sanjay Gandhi, promotes his own four-point program for population control. States raise their sterilization targets and introduce coercive methods.

BOX 18.1 (*Continued*)

Under the intense coercive campaign, sterilizations conducted during the previous 12 months escalate to 8.26 million.

1976: A national population policy is formulated and adopted by Parliament that calls for a frontal attack on population problems.

1977: The National Institute of Health Administration and Education and the Central Family Planning Institute merge to form the National Institute of Health and Family Welfare.

The 19 intensive family planning districts are scaled down to 4.

The national population policy legitimizes the excesses of the sterilization campaign and coercive measures and finally results in the collapse of Indira Gandhi's government.

A revised population policy is inaugurated.

Family planning is renamed as family welfare to promote education and motivation highlighting birth spacing rather than lowering fertility.

Sterilization targets are drastically reduced.

The government raises the minimum marriage age to 18 for girls and 21 for boys.

Gandhian Ideology and Population Policy

While Prime Minister Nehru and his Planning Commission saw the need to control population growth, they were frustrated by the Gandhian legacy of dependence on natural methods of birth control, especially self-restraint. The minister of health, Rajkumari Amrit Kaur, a loyal disciple of the late Mahatma Gandhi, was a staunch opponent of efforts to launch a national family planning program employing anything but natural methods of contraception. In 1951, she requested a World Health Organization (WHO) mission to advise on promoting the rhythm method. The WHO dispatched Dr. Abraham Stone, director of the Margaret Sanger Birth Control Clinic in New York, to undertake this assignment (Harkavy 1995).

Confined by the terms of his mission, Stone took the advice of a physician in Delhi and devised a necklace consisting of 28 beads intended to allow women to keep track of their menstrual cycles. The beads were red for fertile days, green for non-fertile days, and orange for days of menstrual flow. The necklace was to be custom designed for each woman in accordance with her own menstrual cycle to enable her to follow the rhythm method. She was to move the beads from one side to the other, beginning with the first day of menses (Raina 1988). This scheme proved to be a fiasco—some of the necklaces ended up adorning the horns of cows—and natural methods of family planning never became a significant method of birth control in India.

In addition to its impracticality, the natural family planning initiative failed to recognize that family planning is not only a function of health and education, but of a number of social and cultural factors that drive the motivation for having children, especially sons, in tradition-bound countries such as India.

Artificial Contraception through a Clinic-Based Approach

Prime Minister Nehru and his Planning Commission insisted on moving forward with an effective family planning program. He enlisted Douglas Ensminger, the Ford

Foundation's representative in India, in furthering this effort. In 1955, Ensminger arranged a consultancy by Dr. Leona Baumgartner, New York City's commissioner of health, and Frank Notestein, director of the Princeton Office of Population Research (Baumgartner and Notestein, 1955). The report of their mission persuaded Rajkumari Kaur to support the creation of a national family planning board to oversee a nationwide effort that would extend beyond natural family planning (Ensminger 1971).

A nationwide effort to control population was a daunting prospect. To quote Dipak Bhatia, a senior family planning official: "The sheer size of this country, with its 560,000 villages and 3,000 cities and towns is . . . part of the problem. The persons who seek to put across massive programs of development are faced with gigantic barriers that include wide-spread illiteracy, inadequate transportation, diversity of cultures and languages, and a frustrating lack of channels of mass communication to the rural areas where 80 per cent of the population lives" (Bhatia 1969, p. 68).

A growing number of birth control clinics sponsored by the Indian elite were part of the Indian landscape, particularly in the cities. In 1949, the Family Planning Association of India was established under the leadership of Lady Rama Rau, a redoubtable figure in the early years of the international planned parenthood movement. The association oversaw the distribution to clinics of most of the family planning funds allocated to the Ministry of Health in the First Five-Year Plan. By 1961, India had an estimated 4,000 birth control clinics that offered the contraceptives available at that time: condoms, diaphragms, and vaginal foaming tablets. Family planning strategists agreed, however, that simply opening clinics and waiting for clients was a weak response to burgeoning population growth. Nonetheless, the clinic approach was extended during the Second Five-Year Plan (1956–61).

Second Phase of the Family Planning Effort

Massive attempts to limit population growth, which were mounted even during the pre-independence period and gathered further momentum during the First Five-Year Plan through concerted efforts at establishing a nationwide network of family planning clinics, did not demonstrate a significant impact on reducing population growth.

Outreach and Goal Setting: Main Strategy of Second Phase
The 1961 population census revealed the futility of the clinic approach, as population growth had continued unabated and the fertility level had actually increased. To address this challenge, in 1962 the government established the goal of reducing the crude birthrate from 41 live births per 1,000 population to 25 by 1970. Reducing fertility became the overarching objective of all population planning for the next 20 years.

Unfortunately, the setting of a target for a drastically lower birthrate over a specified period of time was accompanied by a relatively weak attempt to popularize family planning through education and communication. Significantly, however, the clinic-based strategy was replaced by an extension approach whereby family planning workers were asked to make house-to-house visits to motivate couples to accept family planning methods (Srinivasan 2006).

Two pioneers spearheaded the evolution of India's birth control effort from a clinic-based approach to a population-based, public health outreach approach. One was Lieutenant Colonel B. L. Raina, the Ministry of Health's first director of family planning. Raina had been a medical officer in the Indian army and had a long-standing interest in birth control. In 1937, he had set up a maternal and child health and family planning center named Help Our Mothers Society (Matra Sewa Sang) that offered free services by doctors, nurses, and social workers. Margaret Sanger was one of the center's board members.

The second pioneer was Dr. Moye Freymann, an American public health physician who joined the Ford Foundation's staff in India in 1957. Freymann, a Johns Hopkins Medical School graduate with a doctorate in the social sciences from Harvard, originally engaged in promoting action research on sanitation and latrine building. He quickly became frustrated by the rigidity and lack of innovation of the government's public health bureaucracy, but he found that the Institute of Rural Health at Gandhigram in the south of India was open to innovative experimentation. Thus, Freymann and Raina turned to the institute for pilot efforts in relation to population-based family planning.

The institute's strategy was to respond to villagers' perceived high-priority needs and then to introduce health and family planning services as they gained the villagers' confidence. The institute, which later changed its name to the Gandhigram Institute of Rural Development and Family Planning, reported a major early success when the birthrate in its pilot area, which had a population of about 100,000, fell from 43 live births per 1,000 population in 1959 to 28 in 1968 (McCarthy 1985). Note, however, that later analysis of these data by the institute suggests that an increase in the age of marriage in the pilot area was more important than the family planning program in bringing down the birthrate (Visaria and Jain 1976).

An important part of the institute's efforts was a series of short-term studies on program implementation and factors affecting contraceptive acceptance, anticipating the massive worldwide operations research effort subsequently supported by the U.S. Agency for International Development (USAID). The institute's studies confirmed doubts about the effectiveness of clinic-based programs and pointed toward an extension approach, which the government adopted in the mid-1960s. Unfortunately, the government, when planning its large-scale family planning campaign, did not generally take into account the results of the institute's work that looked at the adaptability of service delivery accompanied by operational research offering lessons for program success and failure.

The Extended Family Planning Program

India's Third Five-Year Plan (1961–66) called for a 10-fold increase in funds earmarked for family planning over the amount allocated in the preceding plan. Starting in 1963, the clinic-based program was replaced with a "reorganized" or "extended" family planning campaign. An army of family planning workers was deployed throughout the countryside and included state and district family planning officers who supervised extension educators, assistant surgeons, family welfare workers, auxiliary nurse-midwives, and volunteer contraceptive depot holders at the village level. Depot holders were responsible for overseeing storage and dispensing of contraceptives. The objective of this campaign was to meet the government's goal of reducing the birthrate from 41 live births per 1,000 population to 25.

Having a sufficient number of adequately trained personnel—roughly 150,000 people—for this ambitious scheme remained a daunting challenge. As of 1968, 75 percent of the allocated positions were filled, but only 25 percent of the staff had appropriate training. The shortage of physicians, especially women doctors and auxiliary nurse–midwives, was particularly severe. The government devised various monetary incentive schemes to encourage medical personnel to participate, for example, offering stipends of Rs 100 per month to female medical students who agreed to serve with the family planning program upon graduation. In addition, several government-sponsored centers, such as the Central Family Planning Institute in New Delhi, were charged with organizing regional training programs (Narain 1968).

The extended family planning program adopted a number of features that remained more or less constant during subsequent decades. The government provided almost all the funding for programs administered by each state. The central government set targets for contraceptive acceptors by type of method and applied these more or less mechanically to states, districts, subdistricts, and eventually to individual family planning workers.

In 1966–67, the all-India target was 2.33 million for intrauterine device (IUD) insertions, 1.38 million for sterilizations, and 1.83 for condoms (Raina 1966). Targets were scheduled, unrealistically, to rise each year, and by 1970–71, they were set at 19.69 million for IUDs, 4.51 million for sterilizations, and 4.66 million for condoms (Raina 1966). Demographic goals were set for every state and district, and achievement of the goals became the responsibility of each district. These targets were to be achieved during specified time periods: "targeted and time-bound" appeared often in official pronouncements. The targets were to be followed regardless of the enormous differences in the social, cultural, and physical environments found in the various regions of India. According to Srinivasan (2006 p. 10) "The program became entrenched in a HITTS model, i.e., Health Department operated, Incentive-based, Target-oriented, Time-bound, and Sterilization-focused programme."

Changes in Government Organization

The government tried to strengthen its organizational structure to implement this ambitious program. In the late 1960s, the Ministry of Health was renamed the Ministry of Health and Family Planning and a separate Department of Family Planning was set up within the ministry. General S. P. Bhatia first held this position, followed by Lieutenant Colonel Dipak Bhatia. Both were committed and energetic army physicians who found themselves continually butting heads with the entrenched bureaucracy.

Continuing the organizational restructuring at the top levels of government, Prime Minister Indira Gandhi appointed S. Chandrasekhar to the newly created position of secretary of state for health and family planning. A demographer with a doctorate from New York University, Chandrasekhar had written several popular books on population issues and had become a passionate champion of population control. As secretary, he spearheaded a major campaign promoting birth control and successfully lobbied Parliament to legalize abortion in 1971. He was an enthusiastic proponent of the IUD, which the Indian Medical Council had approved in 1965. He is perhaps best remembered for his plan to give a transistor radio to any man willing to undergo a vasectomy.

Experiments with Alternative Approaches

Following their work with the Gandhigram Institute, Freymann and Raina collaborated with allies in the government to improve the effectiveness of the massive government effort. With US$26 million in rupees from the government and US$12 million from the Ford Foundation, a collaborative ambitious plan was devised calling for the establishment of 19 intensive family planning districts to be supported by two new institutions—the National Institute of Health Administration and Education (NIHAE) and the Central Family Planning Institute—established in 1965.

The intensive family planning districts were patterned after intensive agricultural districts, whereby U.S. agricultural extension officials were assigned to help individual farmers improve their production through demonstration projects in each Indian state. Similarly, the intensive family planning districts were to serve as demonstration projects in each of the 15 states into which India was divided at the time and in four large cities.

Serving as a staff college for the intensive district scheme, the NIHAE, designed by Freymann, was to offer short in-service training programs for family planning administrators and, eventually, graduate programs in health education and administration, even conferring doctoral degrees. Broad instruction in public health administration was to be made relevant to family planning by using examples from this field in course work.

To supplement the NIHAE's training for family planning administrators, the Ford Foundation provided fellowships for some two dozen Indian family planning officers at schools of public health in the United States. In the early 1960s, none of these schools offered a curriculum in family planning administration whereas some faculty members at Harvard and the University of North Carolina did have experience with family planning programs in Puerto Rico and on native American reservations in the United States. Accordingly, the Indian fellows were sent to the latter institutions. At the same time, the Ford Foundation's New York–based Population Program made sizable grants to these schools and to the University of Michigan to help strengthen their family planning curricula, and in the 1960s and 1970s they became major centers for training family planning officers from around the developing world.

Freymann confessed that he had a hidden motive in sending Indian officials to U.S. public health schools. He hoped that officials trained abroad would fully appreciate a population-based, outreach approach to family planning and not revert to the earlier clinic-based strategy (Freymann interview with Oscar Harkavy 1990).

The NIHAE's companion institution, the Central Family Planning Institute, was to become the technical branch of the overall family planning program, conducting a variety of training and research programs ranging from demography to clinical testing of contraceptives.

Unfortunately, the NIHAE and the Central Family Planning Institute never managed to take firm root in the government bureaucracy and were eventually merged into the National Institute of Health and Family Welfare in 1977. The plan for 19 intensive districts ran into opposition from Ministry of Health officials and was scaled back to four districts. Even this modest version was never put into operation because of government opposition. Thus, hopes that the intensive-district demonstration projects would allow flexible experimentation with service delivery approaches and so inform the nationwide program were dashed. Rather than encouraging experimental pilot projects directed at specific subpopulations, typical of successful family planning programs in places like the Republic of Korea, the Indian effort "too early became standardized . . . applied uniformly on a national basis, often regardless of local readiness, local conditions, availability of qualified personnel, or the need to learn and to adjust to local and distinctive conditions" (Freedman 1987, p. 63).

Third Phase of the Family Planning Program

The massive effort initiated by the government's Department of Family Planning and state health departments in 1961 showed few signs of success. Population growth rates were not declining, as confirmed by the 1971 census (Srinivasan 2006), resulting in extensive frustration in government circles.

Vasectomy Camps: 1970–77—Attempts at Coercive Approach

After his assignment as Registrar General of Census in 1951, R. A. Gopalswami, while serving as Chief Secretary of Madras Presidency, had calculated that if 7 vasectomies per 1,000 population were performed each year for 10 years, all fourth and higher order births would be avoided, reducing the birthrate to 25 births per 1,000 population. His work encouraged the use of incentives for those accepting vasectomies, and also created great expectations about the value of target setting.

Indeed, vasectomies, together with substantial monetary and in-kind incentives to undergo them, became one of the defining features of the Indian family planning initiative. Female sterilization (tubectomy) was also part of the effort, but was not as prominently featured as its male counterpart. The so-called vasectomy camps became a major instrument for achieving large numbers of acceptors in short periods of time.

Typically, the camps were mobile field hospitals set up at primary health centers. One enthusiastic physician established a busy vasectomy facility at the main Bombay railway station. Physicians and paramedics were temporarily assigned to the camps to perform sterilizations and also to insert IUDs. The opening of a camp was preceded by an aggressive publicity campaign. In addition to those undergoing sterilization, candidates were brought to the camps by promoters, and medical personnel performing the services were all rewarded with monetary incentives of varying amounts. Government officials participated in many of these camps, lending a coercive element to the process.

In 1970, the most spectacular vasectomy camp was organized in the Ernaculum district of Kerala. S. Krishnakumar, the district collector (chief government administrator), launched a massive publicity campaign prior to a one-month vasectomy camp. He organized a march by thousands of men carrying family planning banners to the town hall, where the vasectomies were performed. Incentive payments included a bonus of Rs 31, one week's worth of food for the patient's family, 8 kilograms of food grain contributed by CARE, and participation in a raffle with prizes ranging from Rs 5 to Rs 200. The total incentive package amounted to about one month's income for the typical acceptor. A second one-month camp took place the following year. At the two camps together, some 78,000 men and women were sterilized.

During the period of aggressive vasectomy campaigns, India led the world in the number of sterilizations performed, both vasectomies and tubectomies. During his assignment as Home Secretary (1971–73), Narain estimated this number as exceeding 4.6 million, almost half the total performed worldwide.

Coercion and "The Emergency"

In 1975, Prime Minister Indira Gandhi declared an emergency because of an economic crisis brought on by crop failure and doubled oil prices. She proposed a 20-point program to deal with the crisis that, surprisingly, failed to mention control of population growth. Sanjay Gandhi, her son and heir apparent, however, promoted his own four-point program, which gave top priority to population control. Accordingly, he set about persuading politicians throughout the country to adopt harsh measures to bring down the birthrate. Sterilization was the method of choice, inspired by the success of the vasectomy camps with their packages of incentives and active involvement by local government officials.

Consequences of The Emergency

States raised their sterilization targets and introduced coercive measures to meet these targets. For example, in Bihar, public food rations were to be withdrawn from couples with more than three children. In Uttar Pradesh, teachers (excepting those unmarried and childless) were required to undergo sterilization or lose a month's pay. A law was passed in Maharashtra requiring sterilization for couples with more than three children. In addition to these official actions, local civil servants, such as police officers, railroad ticket collectors, and those who ran government fair price shops, demanded that eligible male members of every family undergo vasectomy on pain of arrest or loss of services. While such coercive measures were adopted to curry favor with Sanjay Gandhi, few were actually implemented (Gwatkin 1979).

The government's commissioner of family planning assumed enormous powers, as did family planning officials at the state level. The number of sterilizations conducted during the 12 months beginning in April 1975 escalated to 8.26 million, "more than the total number done in the previous five years and more than the number done in any other country in the world until that time" (Srinivasan 2006, p. 10).

Reversal of Coercive Population Control Measures

The excesses of Sanjay's Gandhi's sterilization campaign and the coercive measures that accompanied it created a tremendous backlash that resulted in the collapse of Indira Gandhi's government in January 1977. Even though the government's family planning program was not halted, politicians were reluctant to be associated with it, and the program remained extremely weak during the subsequent decade.

Fresh Start at Democratic Approach to Family Planning

A revised population policy was inaugurated in 1977. Family planning was renamed as family welfare and sterilization targets were reduced significantly. The new policy was designed to promote education and motivation and was directed primarily at spacing births rather than lowering fertility.

The Gandhigram Institute's studies had established that later age of marriage, reinforced by more female education and employment, was a more potent cause of lower fertility than the adoption of prevalent contraceptive methods. The government acted on this information by raising the official minimum age of marriage to 18 for girls and 21 for boys. Politicians and policy makers had also learned the hard lesson that couples opted for sterilization so late in their reproductive lives that the procedure barely made a dent in population growth.

The All-India Hospital Postpartum Programme, begun in 1969, was an attractive addition to the government's program. It was based on a plan originated by Dr. Howard Taylor, professor of obstetrics at the Columbia College of Physicians and Surgeons, and Bernard Berelson, president of the Population Council. As Taylor and Berelson recognized, women who have recently delivered or aborted are particularly willing to accept a birth control method (Ross and Mauldin 1988). By 1975, 255 hospitals had enrolled in the postpartum program. During 1970 to 1973, these hospitals served some 1.2 million obstetric and abortion patients, more than 18 percent of whom accepted a birth control method while in the hospital. According to follow-up data, another 5 percent accepted a method within three months of their discharge (Visaria and Jain 1976).

Although hospital-based programs had appealing features, their scope was limited, as an extremely small percentage of births took place in hospitals in India, even in the cities; such facilities were not available in most rural areas. Hospital-based programs could at best reach urban elites, who generally did not need incentives for practicing family planning.

Highlights of India's Family Planning Effort

Never before had a country of India's size and diversity attempted such a bold experiment as India did so soon after an exhausting period of independence from British rule and so early during its ambitious economic development efforts.

Bold Experiment

By its nature, such an audacious experiment in an untraversed field as family planning as part of the economic development process was bound to face many setbacks, even in the midst of successes. Nonetheless, the vision, insight, and conviction of the architects of India's development guided the process whereby population trends slowly came under the control of policies and programs. Despite their negative experience during the colonial period, India's political leaders were not slow in asking for international assistance to support their family planning efforts.

Early in his term, Prime Minister Nehru and his Planning Commission recognized the urgent need to control population growth and to permit the use of artificial methods of birth control, a drastic diversion from the Gandhian legacy that had guided the path to an independent India. A cornerstone of the early efforts at family planning was the courage of elected leaders to make far-reaching decisions, even on matters affecting the most intimate aspects of people's lives. Without experience from other countries to draw on, policy makers were prepared to take decisions and to change course and seek advice and assistance when necessary.

Although by no means an unmitigated success, the Indian program left an indelible mark on the history of early family planning efforts in the 20th century. The government's Department of Family Planning estimated that more than 20 million births were averted between 1956 and 1975. Calculations based on the number of births averted concluded that the annual birthrate fell from about 42 live births per 1,000 population in 1960–61 to about 38 in 1970–71 and about 35 in 1974–75. Incomplete vital statistics make these birthrate calculations approximate at best.

Furthermore, "It is quite difficult to isolate the effect of the family planning program on the birthrate of a country or to establish a causal relationship between program efforts and a decline in the birthrate even when adequate data on the many interrelated factors affecting the birthrate are available" (Visaria and Jain 1976, p. 41).

Social Setting

From the earliest days of family planning until the present, the acceptance of family planning between the south and north of India has diverged sharply. The so-called four poor-performance states of Bihar, Madhya Pradesh, Rajasthan, and Uttar Pradesh in the northern "Hindi belt" are notable for their poverty and for their slow progress in relation to all elements of development, not just family planning.

Literacy is a reliable predictor of development success. In 1971, for example, the literacy rate in such states as Bihar and Rajasthan was about 18 to 20 percent, in contrast to some 60 percent in Kerala, a high-performance state in the southwest. While overall literacy has increased markedly since the 1950s, population growth has caused the absolute number of illiterate people to increase. For example, the number of illiterate people increased by about 16 percent during 1961 to 1971 (Visaria and Jain 1976). Perhaps even more significant than overall literacy, women's literacy is a crucial precondition for family planning acceptance. In the Hindi belt, however, female literacy averaged less than 10 percent. The two most critical issues that were responsible for poor family planning performance in India, and indeed, in most of the early East and South Asian efforts, were illiteracy among women and women's total economic and emotional dependency on their husbands, fathers, and other elderly male members of the family.

As of 1974–75, the proportion of married couples with three or more children adopting birth control methods ranged between 5 and 10 percent in such states as Bihar, Rajasthan, and Uttar Pradesh, compared with 20 to 49 percent in such relatively literate states as Gujarat, Karnataka, and Maharashtra.

The Indian experience offers a clear demonstration of an analysis by Freedman and Berelson (1976) of the joint effects of the strength of a family planning program and the social setting. The major components of the social setting are literacy and education, especially of women; the level of families' economic well-being; the accessibility of health facilities, including family planning facilities; and child survival levels. Strong program efforts in a high social setting produce good results in terms of the percentage of couples using contraception. Weak program efforts in a low social setting produce disappointing results. Moreover, a high social setting helps achieve a strong program effort and vice versa. This is demonstrated in table 18.1.

TABLE 18.1 Percentage of Couples Protected in Indian States, by Social Setting and Program Effort, 1972–73

Program effort	Social setting						Mean range
	High		Middle		Low		
Strong	Punjab and Haryana	23.0	Orissa	17.2	—		**17.5**
			Andhra Pradesh	16.6			11.6–23.0
	Kerala	19.2	Mysore	11.6			
	Mean	**21.1**	Mean	**15.1**			
Moderate	Maharashtra	23.4	—		Madhya Pradesh	13.5	**16.1**
	Gujarat	17.9					7.8–23.4
	Tamil Nadu	17.7			Bihar	7.8	
	Mean	**19.7**			Mean	**10.7**	
Weak	West Bengal	11.6	Assam	8.1	Uttar Pradesh	7.7	**8.4**
			Jammu and Kashmir	7.6	Rajasthan	6.8	6.8–11.6
	Mean	**11.6**	Mean	**7.9**	Mean	**7.3**	
Mean	**18.8**		**12.2**		**9.0**		**14.0**
Range	11.6–23.4		7.6–17.2		6.8–13.5		6.8–23.4

Source: Freedman and Berelson, 1976, 27.

Note: — = not available.

Resources spent on women's literacy and education, on agricultural extension services in rural environments, on other income-earning capability in urban situations, and on raising women's ability to earn income over which they have control empowers them to successfully negotiate and control the size of their families and the spacing of their pregnancies. These are the essential ingredients of a high social setting—a prerequisite for sustainable development resulting in small family size (Roy 1993).

Methods of Birth Control

India's evolving family planning program employed a variety of contraceptive methods in addition to sterilization. In their earliest days, foaming vaginal contraceptive tablets of dubious effectiveness, diaphragms, and condoms were dispensed at private and government clinics. In the 1950s, a widely repeated rumor alleged that some village women had mistakenly swallowed the vaginal pills and started to foam at the mouth, thereby discouraging their use.

Condoms continued as an important part of the contraceptive mix. Social marketing of condoms, subsequently taken up throughout the developing world, originated in India, the brainchild of Peter King, a Ford Foundation consultant who served as a visiting professor at the Calcutta Institute of Management. Under King's marketing plan, condoms provided free by the USAID were distributed by large corporations with operations in India, such as Lipton Tea and Hindustan Lever. Named Nirodh (meaning protection in Hindi), the neatly packaged condoms were sold at low prices to minimally cover distribution costs to retailers, who resold them to consumers at three for 15 paise (about US$0.001 each). However, as the family planning program developed, a number of condom distribution channels were used such as family planning centers, hospitals, and clinics that made them available without charge. In addition, India began to manufacture its own condoms through a public sector company, M/S Hindustan Latex Limited (Narain 1968). Unfortunately, condoms were widely associated with illegitimate and extramarital sex, discouraging their use within marriage.

Beginning in 1966, the plastic IUD or Lippes Loop, popularly known as the "loop" became a major method of birth control in India, though the term IUD was avoided, because it was the common acronym for intrauterine death in the Indian medical vocabulary. The Population Council was largely responsible for reviving the IUD as a mainstream contraceptive method after earlier versions made of steel had fallen into disrepute. In 1962, the council sponsored an international conference on the IUD that prominent Indian physicians attended. Drs. Sheldon Segal of the Population Council and Anna Southam of the Columbia College of Physicians and Surgeons, posted to India as consultants to the Ford Foundation in the early 1960s, actively encouraged their Indian colleagues to conduct small-scale clinical trials of the IUD. However, Dr. Shushila Nayyar, the Indian Health Minister, vigorously opposed adoption of the method because of her concerns about its safety. It took a visit by Alan Guttmacher, the famed Johns Hopkins obstetrician and president of Planned Parenthood of America, to convince Nayyar that the method was safe. In 1965, the Indian Council of Medical Research approved inclusion of the IUD in the national family planning program (McCarthy 1985).

As reported by Freymann, Indian family planning officials were overenthusiastic in promoting the IUD (Freymann interview with Oscar Harkavy 1990). A crash program of insertion was mounted before instructional manuals had been prepared and service providers had been sufficiently trained. In addition, patient counseling was largely neglected. While more than 800,000 IUDs were inserted in 1965–66, followed by nearly 1 million in 1966–67, rumors about harmful side effects spread rapidly and the IUD fell into disrepute. Indeed, in the immediately following years, more devices were removed than inserted. The collapse of the IUD initiative was believed to be a major factor in the disenchantment with the overall government family planning initiative that took over in the early 1970s.

The contraceptive pill was never a major ingredient of the Indian program. The medical establishment had doubts about its safety and questioned whether illiterate women could follow a prescribed schedule for its use. Furthermore, pills are associated with illness, while pregnancy and the birth of a child are joyful occasions that could never be associated with illness in the traditional Indian mindset. The recurrent cost of pills and the need for medical follow-up were further reasons given for official skepticism. Several locally manufactured "birth control" pills were available, but these were based on native plants and were not subjected to rigorous testing in relation to their efficacy or safety. One motivation for the remarkably successful effort by Segal and Southam to help build a network of world-class reproductive scientists in India was to create indigenous capacity to evaluate contraceptives.

Abortion, theoretically illegal until 1971, was not one of the government's birth control methods, but estimates indicate that up to 5 million illegal abortions were performed annually prior to passage of the Medical Termination of Pregnancy Act in 1971. This legislation legalized abortion subject to a variety of restrictions. Some 23,000 abortions were performed in authorized hospitals and clinics during 1972 to 1973 (Visaria and Jain 1976).

Contraceptive use surveys were rare in the early years of India's family planning effort. In the 1960s and 1970s, surveys conducted by the government's Department of Family Planning, the Office of the Registrar General, and the independent Operations Research Group differed considerably with respect to their findings. A 1970 Operations Research Group survey found that 13.6 percent of couples nationwide were practicing family planning, of which only 9.7 percent were using methods provided by the official program: sterilization (6.3 percent), condoms (2.6 percent), IUDs (0.7 percent), and other conventional methods (0.1 percent). Another 4 percent of respondents reported their use of withdrawal and abstinence (Visaria and Jain 1976). Because sterilization, usually adopted by older couples at the end of their childbearing years, was the favored method, the effect of the total family planning effort on fertility was less than would have been the case if spacing methods by younger, fecund couples had been more popular.

Publicity Campaigns

From the early days of the family planning program, the provision of contraceptives was accompanied by publicity campaigns to encourage their use. Notable among these efforts was the red triangle and "four faces." The red triangle—an equilateral triangle, apex pointed down—was painted on billboards, rocks, and the sides of buildings throughout India and became universally identified as the family planning symbol. Together with the triangle was the slogan "Have only two or three children, that's enough." The red triangle was often painted against a bright yellow background that showed the smiling faces of a father, mother, son, and daughter—the four faces. This initiative was originated by T. K. Tyagi, assistant commissioner for media in the Department of Family Planning, and Frank Wilder, the Ford Foundation's consultant on communication for family planning.

Tyagi gained fame for his elephant, called Lal Tikon (red triangle). Raina (1988, 205–6) who continued his keen interest in the evolution of the family planning program, paid tribute to Tyagi as "quite a unique person, dedicated to the red triangle" and described the genesis of Lal Tikon as follows. When he met an unemployed elephant keeper, Tyagi motivated a small group of supporters to raise money and designed a badge featuring an elephant and red triangle to be worn by the sponsors. With their financial support, the elephant decked with red triangle, moved from place to place distributing flyers and condoms. Tyagi's last tribute to Lal Tikon was, at his death, to have Lal Tikon badges showered on his body at the funeral march accompanied by his favorite family planning song.

To supplement the red triangle campaign, the family planning message was delivered through the mass media, including radio and television; puppet shows; and folk songs. Traveling troupes of actors and singers spread the message in the countryside (Narain 1968). The Indian public is used to getting important health messages through puppet shows, folk songs, popular dramas, and the like, and thus, Tyagi's strategy was not foreign to traditional families. What was foreign was the idea that the family should limit itself to one son and one daughter. While one daughter may have seemed plausible, given the need to provide dowries early in their lives, just one son was regarded as woefully inadequate to ensure enough field labor, proper old-age economic security, and, more important, preservation of the family name. Considering the high levels of infant mortality, especially in rural areas, a family of two seemed absurd. No local staff members involved in the program, let alone foreign technical assistance personnel, appeared to have anticipated such opposition to their propaganda.

Impact Measurement and Feedback

In a field so little explored as birth control in a country of India's diversity and size, impact measurement and, more important, feedback from the target population, were indispensable. Unfortunately, such exercises were scarce and weak.

Beginning in the early 1960s, a variety of research centers in India engaged in systematic attempts to measure family planning knowledge, attitudes, and practice. As in other developing countries, India's surveys revealed increasing knowledge of family planning on the part of respondents, even a heartening increase in those reporting themselves to be positively motivated to limit their family size, but a disheartening proportion who were actually using effective birth control methods. Despite the chasm between the number of respondents declaring their wish to limit their family size and those actually practicing birth control, family planning officials believed that the results, which documented favorable attitudes toward family planning by large proportions of the general public, encouraged politicians to increase financial support for government birth control programs.

As part of its family planning efforts, the government supported a variety of demographic and communication action research projects coordinated by the Central Family Planning Institute, a government-financed autonomous body. The Demographic Training and Research Center, established by the United Nations (later renamed as the International Institute for Population Studies) was a notable center for such research, as well as for training in demography (Narain 1968, p. 9).

Throughout the 1960s and 1970s, Indian social scientists at universities and free-standing research institutes were reluctant, for the most part, to engage in research on family planning. The work at the Gandhigram Institute was a notable exception. Senior social scientists interviewed in 1971 reported that family planning operations were in the hands of physicians and that policy was set by senior civil servants, neither of which were particularly interested in contributions by social scientists. Ashok Mitra, head of the Planning Commission and himself a distinguished social scientist, ruefully noted that the bureaucracy viewed academics as troublemakers. For their part, academic social scientists avoided research on the national family planning program, leaving it to those officially responsible for implementing family planning programs and employed by the Ministry of Health and Family Planning.

Social Science Research

Social science contributions to population issues were substantially enhanced by the formation of The Population Foundation of India (formerly known as Family Planning Foundation) was established in 1970 by a dedicated group of industrialists and population activists led J. R. D. Tata, who guided it as the founding chair until his death in 1993. As early as 1951, Tata, India's leading industrialist, had proposed a nongovernmental population institute. His vision came to fruition two decades later, with himself as chair and J. C. Kavoori, a former professor of social work, as director. Tata failed to convince other wealthy individuals to support the Family Planning Foundation, and became its principal benefactor, contributing a three-to-one match of the Ford Foundation's initial US$100,000 grant.

The Population Foundation of India funded a number of high-quality social science research studies directly relevant to the national family planning program, including an essay on the consequences of population growth by Ashok Mitra and an examination of family planning strategies by M. N. Srinivas, India's leading anthropologist. The Planning foundation also funded in the early part of 1970s a major volume titled *Population in India's Development*—a compilation of several essays on population and its impact on development. The latter influenced the Indian delegation to the 1974 World Population Conference in Bucharest, at which India's spokesperson famously declared that "development is the best contraceptive." This declaration implied growing disenchantment with the government's approach to family planning, which relied on top-down imposition of targets and incentives for sterilization. Realization of the failure of the policy approach led to incorporating family planning in maternal and child health initiatives, which lent it legitimacy and popularity. Renaming the Ministry of Health and Family Planning as the Ministry of Health and Family Welfare formalized this strategic transition (personal correspondence with Ronald Ridker 2006).

Foreign Assistance

In the early years of India's family planning program, foreign technical assistance was perceived by the leaders as replacing the political colonialism from which India had just rid itself with technical colonialism in family planning. Neither of these two styles of colonialism were sufficiently respectful of the traditional culture that governed the lives of the majority of Indians, 80 percent of whom lived in rural villages. Nor were they willing to let Indians assume ownership of even their own initiatives. The following subsections discuss the major providers of foreign assistance.

The Ford Foundation

In the earliest days of the Indian family planning effort, the Ford Foundation took the lead in assisting, if not shaping, the emerging enterprise. Much of this can be attributed to the close association of their representative, Ensminger, with Prime Minister Nehru, who encouraged the foundation to take a leading role. Furthermore, Ensminger's personal style of recruiting large numbers of American experts to offer technical assistance to their Indian counterparts on a host of initiatives accentuated the foundation's prominence in the early days of India's population activities (Ensminger 1971).

While Freymann, King, Segal, Southam, and Wilder made significant contributions, as described earlier, many other technical assistance people whom Ensminger brought to India found themselves less useful. The collapse of the intensive family planning scheme in the late 1960s left foreign experts recruited to work in those districts without Indian counterparts. Ironically, some of the latter were abroad on Ford Foundation fellowships. The NIHAE and the Central Family Planning Institute lacked sufficient office space in their early days, which caused foundation advisers assigned to help these institutions to spend most of their time at the foundation's New Delhi headquarters rather than in productive contact with Indian colleagues. Furthermore, the prominent role of foreign advisers in devising a variety of initiatives tended to discourage Indian ownership of some such projects.

The USAID

The USAID initiated its assistance to India's family planning program in 1968. Historic monsoon failures in 1965–66 and 1967–68 raised fears of massive starvation in the following decade. A 1966 mission from USAID headquarters recommended the termination of three health projects supported by the agency and a focus instead on family planning. In 1968, the USAID initiated a US$7.7 million assistance package for family welfare planning, part of which consisted of local currency, controlled by the USAID, that the government had earmarked to match U.S. emergency food relief (designated as Public Law 480 rupees).

Reimart Ravenholt, the dynamic director of the USAID's Office of Population, doubted that loans and Public Law 480 rupees were an effective means of assistance. Accordingly, he urged his agency to approve a US$50 million outright grant to the government for vehicles, contraceptives, and general support for the government's family planning program. He was eventually successful in engineering US$20 million to build primary health centers and to finance a doubling of the number of auxiliary nurse-midwives employed by the family planning program. As a result, the USAID became India's largest family planning donor. The deployment of 74 American advisers was included in this plan. While the USAID surpassed the Ford Foundation in the number of technical assistance personnel assigned to family planning in India, the actual number was considerably less than 74. As recounted by John Lewis, the USAID's mission director in India, "Washington put us under pressure to push resources, and then extract program changes in exchange" (Minkler 1975, p. 245).

In 1973, relations between the governments of India and the United States cooled, caused, among other things, by a perceived U.S. tilt toward Pakistan. Consequently, the USAID was abruptly ordered to quit family planning assistance in India. Prime Minister Indira Gandhi had embarked on a program of national self-reliance that affected the Ford Foundation as well. K. K. Das, secretary of the Ministry of Health and Family Planning, broke off arrangements with foundation-supported consultants to the ministry and refused to meet with foundation officials.

Other Donors

A partnership between the World Bank's International Development Association and the Swedish International Development Cooperation Agency became the second largest donor in 1973, when it spent US$32 million on ambitious demonstration projects in the states of Karnataka and Uttar Pradesh. The objective was to test alternatives to the government's family planning programs, particularly "by linking . . . family planning services to a supplementary nutrition program, by concentrating on recently delivered mothers, by making greater use of mobile teams for motivation and service, and by providing better training and supervision"(Visaria and Jain 1976, p. 34).

Over the years, the United Nations Population Fund and the Danish, Japanese, and Norwegian assistance agencies donated smaller sums for a variety of family planning–related activities. The effect of all such investments was proportionate to the extent to which the donors understood the traditional values and cultural traits of the Indian population.

Lessons Learned

India mounted a massive nationwide birth control campaign with insufficient regard to the enormous variations in social settings across the country's regions. Although the government was flexible enough to move from the clinic-based approach with which it began in the early 1950s to a public health–based outreach program beginning in the early 1960s, the model adopted was applied, for the most part, on a one-size-fits-all basis. Experimentation with a variety of approaches adapted to specific populations rarely occurred. Furthermore, hundreds of thousands of family planning workers were recruited without sufficient training or supervision. In rural areas, workers faced formidable obstacles in traveling to villages to which they were assigned. A 5-mile trek on foot was not unusual. Many workers went unpaid for long periods because of difficulties in reaching them. Freedman (1987) notably contrasted the Indian experience with the more successful models used in the Republic of Korea, which featured small-scale experiments and adaptation by national programs based on lessons learned. In all fairness, however, India's size and social complexity made the family planning task much more daunting than in Southeast Asia.

Two hallmarks of the Indian program have come under critical scrutiny. One was the use of centrally decreed, time-bound targets for the acceptance of each major birth control method offered by the government and the application of such targets to family planning workers throughout the bureaucratic chain of command. Target setting had several problems. More often than not, local family planning workers found targets completely unrealistic and simply ignored them. Targets were most easily applied to sterilization, leading to a focus on couples who wished to end their childbearing, with less effect on overall fertility than spacing methods used by younger couples at the height of their childbearing years. As most international assistance agencies subsequently switched from supporting demographically driven national efforts to curb population growth to focusing on the reproductive health and welfare of individual women and their families, the Indian model of the 1960s and 1970s has become the exemplar of what went wrong in nationwide family planning programs.

The second hallmark was the use of relatively large monetary or in-kind incentives to promote sterilization. Together with target setting, the early Indian program has been criticized in some quarters as at least quasi-coercive, becoming, for a time, openly coercive during the "emergency" of 1975–77. It is fair to say that coercive aspects of the Indian program (along with those in China and Indonesia) have given ammunition to donor agencies that have abandoned their efforts to reduce population growth, even in Sub-Saharan Africa, parts of the Middle East, and South Asia, where population pressure still has a profoundly negative effect on human welfare.

Finally, foreign, particularly American, technical assistance personnel played a major role in shaping India's emerging family planning program, many with insufficient understanding and appreciation of local conditions. A number of these individuals made crucial contributions; others became redundant as the program matured. Furthermore, foreign experts tended to get ahead of the program and to be perceived as owning the initiatives they were intended to assist. Consequently, the host country was reluctant to adopt such initiatives.

Partly as a result of this experience, the Ford Foundation sharply altered its approach to operations in the developing world. Harry Wilhelm, Ensminger's successor as the foundation's representative in India in 1970, changed course from direct support to family planning operations to grants to Indian institutions engaged in research and training. Under Ensminger, some 80 percent of Ford Foundation funds in support of family planning went to U.S technical assistance personnel, with the remaining 20 percent going to Indian institutions. Wilhelm reversed these ratios, and the Wilhelm model now typifies Ford Foundation practice in all its overseas development assistance.

By the 1980s, examples of successful programs could be found even though a majority of the population still lived in tradition-bound villages. One example was the Project for Community Action in Family Planning, which covered more than 154 villages in the state of Karnataka. As early as the mid-1980s, more than 43 percent of couples were using family planning in the project area, fully 14 percentage points more than the state average. This achievement was attributed to the project's significant improvement in the status of women, involving them and empowering them to bring about change in their communities. This is particularly notable considering how the deeply entrenched inferior status of women negates official efforts to decrease their fertility.

Despite its weaknesses, the Indian family planning initiative of the 1960s and 1970s had significant achievements. It enjoyed support at the highest levels of government, illustrating the importance of political will in furthering a national enterprise. Too many family planning efforts in other countries have been handicapped by the lack of such will. In those Indian states ranked high in social setting, the acceptance of modern contraceptive methods was substantial.

References

Bhatia, Dipak. 1969. "India: A Gigantic Task." In *Family Planning Programs: An International Survey*, ed. B. Berelson, 73–88. New York: Basic Books.

Baumgartner, Leona, and Frank W. Notestein. 1955. *Suggestions for a Practical Program of Family Planning and Child Care*. Population Council Report, New York.

Caldwell, John, and Pat Caldwell. 1986. *Limiting Population Growth and the Ford Foundation Contribution*. London: Frances Pinter.

Ensminger, Douglas. 1971. "The Ford Foundation's Relations with the Planning Commission." Oral history. Ford Foundation Archives, New York.

Freedman, Ronald. 1987. "The Contribution of Social Science Research to Population Policy and Family Planning Program Effectiveness." *Studies in Family Planning* 18 (2): 57–82.

Freedman, Ronald, and Bernard Berelson. 1976. "The Record of Family Planning Programs." *Studies in Family Planning* 7 (1): 1–40.

Gwatkin, Davidson R. 1979. "Political Will and Family Planning: The Implications of India's Emergency Experience." *Population and Development Review* 5 (2): 32, 44–45.

Harkavy, Oscar. 1995. "India Faces Its Population Problems." In *Curbing Population Growth: An Insider's Perspective on the Population Movement*, 129–61. New York: Plenum Press.

McCarthy, Kathleen D. 1985. *The Ford Foundation's Population Programs in India, Pakistan and Bangladesh, 1959–1981*. Archive Report 011011. New York: Ford Foundation.

Minkler, Meredith. 1975. "Role Conflict and Role Shock: American and Indian Perspectives on the Role of U.S. Family Planning Advisors in India." Unpublished doctoral dissertation, University of California (Berkeley).

Narain, Govind. 1968. "India: The Family Planning Program since 1965." *Studies in Family Planning* 1 (35): 1, 5, 7–9.

Raina, B. L. 1966. "India." In *Family Planning and Population Programs,* ed. Bernard Berelson, Richmond K. Anderson, Oscar Harkavy, John Maier, W. Parker Mauldin, and Sheldon Segal, 111–42. Chicago: University of Chicago Press.

———. 1988. "A Quest for a Small Family." Unpublished manuscript.

Ross, John, and W. Parker Mauldin, eds. 1988. *Berelson on Population.* New York: Springer-Verlag.

Roy, Krishna. 1993. "Critical Links: Women, Population, Environment, and Sustainable Development." In *Proceedings of the Inter-Regional Workshop on the Role of Women in Environmentally Sound and Sustainable Development,* 83–93. New York: United Nations Institute for Training and Research on Women.

Srinivasan, K. 1995. *Regulating Reproduction in India's Population: Efforts, Results and Recommendations.* New Delhi: Sage.

———. 2006. "Population and Family Planning Programmes in India: A Review and Recommendations." Lecture at the Fifth Dr. C. Chandrasekaran Memorial Lecture Series, February 3, Indian Institute of Population Studies, Deonar, Mumbai.

Visaria, Pravin, and Anrudh K. Jain. 1976. *India.* Country Profiles Series. New York: Population Council.

Wattal, Pyare Kishan. 1916. *The Population Problem in India: A Census Study.* Bombay: Bennett, Coleman and Company.

19

Family Planning Programs and Policies in Bangladesh and Pakistan

WARREN C. ROBINSON

Bangladesh and Pakistan began their national existence in 1947 as two *wings* of the same country—East and West Pakistan—when the previously undivided union of British India achieved independence. The two wings inherited an administrative and governance structure from the colonial period, but quickly developed their own political and economic systems and began to shape their own development plans and programs. The two wings were bound together by their common religion, Islam, but language and other cultural differences created internal tensions from the outset. Nonetheless, East and West Pakistan shared common social and economic development until 1970, when a political dispute erupted into civil war, leading to the intervention by India and the creation of the new state of Bangladesh in 1971.

Pakistan (both wings) was a poor, mostly rural and agricultural country, with low levels of per capita income, poor social infrastructure, and virtually no industrial capacity. Lahore, in West Pakistan, had been the cultural center of the Punjab in prepartition India, but most of its supporting region was now in India. East Pakistan was cut off from its geographic capital, Calcutta, now in India. Both wings lay on the periphery of the Indian subcontinent and had functioned as frontier areas, supplying raw materials to the economic centers in north and central India, in turn drawing on these centers for most manufactured goods and technical services. This economic marginality was reflected in Pakistan's social and demographic characteristics: in 1947, Pakistan averaged lower literacy levels and higher mortality than India, as well as higher fertility levels and lower levels of contraceptive practice.

Formal economic planning was launched in Pakistan in 1955 with the First Five-Year Plan (1955–59). The Second Five-Year Plan (1960–64) argued that the prevailing rapid rate of population growth posed a threat to the nation's economic future and allocated a modest sum for policy and program interventions through the Ministry of Health. At that time, Pakistan was receiving substantial technical assistance from the Ford Foundation, the Harvard Development Advisory Service, and other international

This chapter draws heavily on a somewhat more detailed treatment of the same topic published in Sathar and Phillips (2001) by the author.

donor groups, and awareness and concern about the population explosion were growing among such groups. The Population Council, another international group, had by this time begun demographic research, particularly on fertility and growth.

By the Third Five-Year Plan (1965–69), population policy had became a major objective and a priority program, and President Mohammed Ayub Khan had become a firm supporter of population limitation. A detailed operational scheme was developed for both wings, top-flight civil service administrators were assigned to the task, and the program moved into high gear. Donor groups, including by then the U.S. Agency for International Development (USAID), quickly became deeply involved in financial and technical aspects of the program, but direction of the program was distinctly Pakistani. The director of the program, Enver Adil, was fond of saying that he took orders only from the president, and most who knew him believed this to be true. He certainly did not take orders from donors.

Conservative Islamic groups were troubled by the notion of family planning, and although this never seems to have seriously hindered any program activities, it was a constant background factor that probably influenced some policy decisions. Such antiprogram sentiment was probably greater in West Pakistan than in East Pakistan, but the issue was not part of the continuing quarrels that lead to the break between the two wings in 1971.

The two wings thus had a common population policy and program structure for the crucial initial years of 1965–70. Differences in practice did emerge, but the approach followed was, generally speaking, the same, and so was the experience flowing from these efforts. Yet neither wing had much to show for its efforts by the end of the plan period. Contraceptive practice had not risen appreciably, and fertility had not fallen. The creation of Bangladesh did not change this picture. Family planning continued to be a policy and program in both countries, but the programs languished. Both countries seemed to provide excellent case studies of why family planning programs in poor developing nations were a hopeless or foolish idea.

In their eagerness to explain this failure, most commentators failed to note that by the mid-1980s, the situation was changing, and Bangladesh and Pakistan had begun to follow sharply divergent demographic paths. In Bangladesh, contraceptive prevalence rose and fertility fell, slowly but steadily, whereas in Pakistan, contraceptive prevalence remained static at low levels and fertility actually appeared to be rising. Box 19.1 provides a timeline of major events in relation to family planning in the two countries.

Pakistan

In the period immediately after Pakistan achieved independence, nearly all important government activities and agencies came into being in the west wing, centered around Karachi. Lahore, a larger and more cosmopolitan city, was deliberately bypassed as the capital for fear that the Punjabi element in the political and economic leadership would dominate the country. Karachi had been a relatively minor port in British India, but now became the capital.

BOX 19.1 Timeline of Policy and Program Developments in Bangladesh and Pakistan

1947:	Pakistan achieves independence, with two "wings," East Pakistan and West Pakistan, separated by India.
1960:	The Second Five-Year Plan (1960–64) creates a family planning project.
	The Ford Foundation, the Population Council, and the Swedish International Development Cooperation Agency all begin technical assistance and demonstration projects.
1965:	The Third Five-Year Plan (1965–69) creates the National Family Planning Board.
	Enver Adil is named commissioner for family planning. The program enjoys strong political support and becomes nationwide within a year.
1968–69:	The first national survey, the impact survey, reveals a lack of program achievement.
	Adil is replaced as the program's director.
1970:	The continuous motivation scheme is launched.
	Political support for the program weakens.
1971:	Civil war breaks out in East Pakistan over disputed elections, India intervenes, and Bangladesh is born.
1973–75:	The USAID-directed inundation contraceptive delivery scheme is launched in Pakistan in support of the continuous motivation scheme.
	Bangladesh reorganizes its family planning program under the Ministry of Health and Family Planning with strong political support.
1975:	The Pakistan fertility survey shows a slight increase in fertility.
	In Bangladesh, nongovernmental organizations take the lead in raising the contraceptive prevalence rate and surveys show a fertility decline.
1978–2000:	The Pakistan program undergoes several reorganizations, engages in a social marketing scheme (1986), briefly attains ministerial status (1990), and establishes a better database for evaluation by means of numerous surveys. The contraceptive prevalence rate rises, and fertility falls.

Program and Policy, 1965–69

The Pakistan government launched the family planning program in 1965, an era of strong commitment to development planning by developing country governments, generous international and private donor support for such efforts, and boundless enthusiasm and optimism for the tasks that lay ahead. Only a few dissenters questioned whether a development plan based on a macroeconomic model and representing a bundle of projects was the correct approach to transforming a stagnant, traditional economy such as that of Pakistan (Lewis 1969). Ansley Coale and Edgar Hoover had shown how the population factor could be made part of such planning, and their model had been applied to Pakistan (Hoover and Perlman 1967).

Thus, the family planning program initiative had top-level political and administrative support, was based on the best available technical advice, and was motivated by the belief that the country's rapid population growth posed a serious threat to its future. This represented a conventional wisdom not seriously challenged from any quarter. Family planning was, to be sure, a new initiative and a bit of a gamble, but donors and government alike viewed it as a vital program, well worth trying. Other large-scale interventions in the health area had worked, such as malaria and smallpox eradication, so why not family planning? The view was that family planning required a sound plan, strong leadership, and adequate resources.

Let us recall what family planning meant in 1965. The important new developments in contraceptive technology—the pill and the intrauterine device (IUD)—were new and more than a little controversial. There was much talk at that time about the cafeteria approach to family planning, meaning that the client would have a choice of several methods of birth control, and five methods were listed as officially available: (a) surgical contraception (or sterilization), both female and male; (b) the IUD; (c) the pill; (d) female barrier and spermicidal methods; and (e) the condom. The first two were considered in Pakistan and elsewhere to be clinical methods requiring an appropriate medical setting for proper use, and their availability was generally limited to clinics in urban areas. The IUD was, moreover, still a relatively new method. In 1965, responsible medical opinion in Pakistan and elsewhere was opposed to using paramedics or fieldworkers to insert IUDs, even had such workers been available. The pill was still first generation, and side effects were common. The minidosage varieties had not yet been developed, and many trained medical people were extremely suspicious of this powerful, new, hormonal intervention. The traditional barrier methods had proven difficult for village women, who lacked privacy and a sound knowledge of their own anatomy, to use effectively, and hence were never popular. This situation meant that in 1965, the Pakistan program offered most rural couples the condom. Strongly motivated couples could obtain an IUD or the pill, but follow-up for complications or resupply was unreliable. Surgical contraception required an even greater effort by the client and involved genuine health risks for many.

All the foregoing considerations had to do with creating a supply network. In 1965, most outside observers agreed that a latent demand for contraceptives existed. Early field trials and action research projects in Comilla in East Pakistan and Lulliani in West Pakistan, where well-designed experimental programs achieved respectable levels of contraceptive practice among rural women, provided modest support for this contention. This database was admittedly thin, but it was all that was available. The year 1965 was also long before the revolutions in survey data collection techniques, data processing, and nearly instantaneous publication of results. Independent evaluation of a program took special effort and considerable time and money.

Main Features of the 1965 Program

The family planning scheme under the Third Five-Year Plan called for the creation of a new administrative entity, the Family Planning Council, and outlined a detailed program whereby 20 million couples in 36 districts of West Pakistan and 16 districts of East Pakistan would be reached, the goal being to reduce fertility by 20 percent by 1970. The scheme operated mostly through the existing political and administrative structure of government—provinces, districts, and *thanas* (*talukhas* in East Pakistan, both being roughly the equivalent of a county), and village union councils—by attaching family planning staff at each level or adding family planning to staff functions. The scheme aimed at nationwide coverage, and, for the most part, represented an effort to distribute conventional contraceptives through village midwives and other local agents. Clients desiring clinical methods were to be referred to clinics, most of which were established in existing urban hospitals and rural health centers, but the scheme was explicitly not clinic oriented. Day-to-day supervision and control was decentralized, and the key people were district executive officers and *thana* family planning supervisors. Publicity was a province-level responsibility, and only evaluation, research, and training were central government functions (Robinson 1966).

The time schedule for launching the plan was extremely ambitious, but it was met. Expatriate staff members from the Population Council, the Ford Foundation, the USAID, the Swedish International Development Cooperation Agency (SIDA) and other donors did much of the early training of staff members. By 1966, the scheme was under way, and apparently making real headway. The program was one of the first generation of such government family planning efforts, along with those in Egypt, India, Taiwan (China), and one or two other places. A steady stream of visitors came from other countries to see what many were calling a model program. Articles were written explaining why Pakistan had succeeded in relation to family planning and India had failed (Finkle 1971). A substantial volume of good quality research was generated, and Wishik developed the famous couple-years-of-protection measure as an evaluation tool for the Pakistan program (Wishik and Chen 1973). Pakistan proved a fertile training ground, and its "graduates" become the cadre for numerous international family planning organizations.

Outcome of the First Program

The service statistics generated by the program indicated that success was indeed being achieved, that is, supplies were being distributed, and the volume of couple years of protection rose steadily; however, no independent surveys of prevalence or fertility were undertaken to validate these apparent achievements, and concern and doubt about the actual results slowly grew. Finally, in 1968–69, the program itself sponsored a national impact survey in both wings of the country that showed conclusively that the contraceptive prevalence rate was only 6 percent of currently married women and that fertility was unchanged. The good news was that most women had heard of family planning, knew of at least one method, and approved of the idea. The bad news was that few were currently using any method. The contraceptive prevalence rate (CPR) was only slightly higher in urban areas, which was still more discouraging.

The program did seem to have achieved modestly more success in East Pakistan than in West Pakistan. In particular, the use of clinical methods was twice as high, and even though the program never emphasized surgical contraception, it proved a more popular method in East Pakistan than in West Pakistan.

In 1969, the program's top leadership was replaced, and much soul searching occurred. The 1965–70 debacle had effectively discredited the program in the eyes of all other government ministries and had demoralized the family planning staff members and many of the donors. The new secretary correctly decided that using village midwives as part-time fieldworkers had not worked well and announced a new approach, the continuous motivation scheme, whereby full-time male-female teams (who were both college graduates and, typically, it was hoped, married couples) would be permanently assigned to a given area and make continuous rounds of all prospective clients to motivate them to use family planning and to provide contraceptive supplies. Most other aspects of the program were left much as before. The scheme had barely got under way when civil war broke out in East Pakistan, then a full-scale war with India. The hostilities resulted in almost complete suspension of all program activities in both wings of the country, and in 1971, the two wings became separate countries.

The Program after 1972

Political changes followed from the events of 1971–72. Khan was ousted from power in Pakistan. The new leadership was indifferent to the program, but the population policy remained in place, as did much of the continuous motivation scheme organization.

The USAID, especially the dynamic Reimart T. Ravenholt, head of its Office of Population, was reluctant to accept that the previous effort had really failed, and instead argued that it simply had not been pushed hard enough and for long enough. The result was the ill-fated inundation scheme. The logic of the inundation approach was that the 1965–70 plan had simply failed to do what it set out to do: make contraceptives instantly available to all prospective clients throughout the country, and if this could yet be accomplished, success might still follow. What was required was more outlets and more supplies, the scheme was to be expanded, and the country truly inundated with contraceptives. The failure of this dogged return to a lost cause is well known. Millions of condoms and pill cycles were imported and distributed, but actual prevalence and fertility remained virtually static. The 1974–75 Pakistan fertility survey, part of the world fertility survey, showed a total fertility rate of nearly 7.0 births per woman, up slightly from the estimate of the 1968–69 impact survey. The CPR remained at less than 10 percent, with only modest interprovincial and rural-urban differences (Robinson 1978).

The scheme was shifted briefly to the control of the Ministry of Health in 1978 from the Family Planning Directorate and shifted yet again to the Ministry of Planning and Development in 1981, where it became part of the Population Welfare Division, and a new strategy emerged. The newly created Population Welfare Division was charged with operating a network of multipurpose family welfare centers that would be responsible for family planning motivation and for distributing supplies, but would also be involved in maternal and child health, nutrition education, female employment training, and other "good works." The Ministry of Health continued to be responsible for clinical methods of contraception, as most clinics were based around urban hospitals and health centers. This new strategy and framework followed the recommendations of a working group of some two dozen leading experts from inside and outside the country. The scheme, hopefully referred to as a "new beginning," stressed holistic, multisectoral approaches to be undertaken "patiently" and in ways "consistent with existing socio-cultural and ideological" frameworks. This new approach seems to have reflected the population and development paradigm then popular in international donor circles. The new beginning also gave somewhat greater formal recognition to the role of nongovernmental organizations (NGOs) by creating an NGO coordinating committee in 1985 and to the private sector by creating a contraceptive social marketing program to subsidize sales in the private sector in 1986 (Robinson 1987).

The Family Welfare Division was given independent ministerial status in 1990, but this move and various other organizational changes in the 1980s and 1990s did not make any fundamental changes to the program's approach or structure. The number of family welfare centers has been increased over time, as has the number of fieldworkers based in them. The contraceptive social marketing program has finally begun playing a major role, and relations between the government and NGOs appear to have improved. Recently, however, the politicalization of some Islam-based NGOs has created new problems about working with them. The program has reverted to a lower profile and is defensive about conservative criticisms because of generally increased religious tensions.

Political support for the program has waxed and waned since 1972, ranging from distinct coolness during General Muhammad Zia-ul-Haq's regime (1977–88) to warm endorsement by Nawaz Sharif (1991–92) and ambivalence by Benazir Bhutto (1988–91, 1993–96). Foreign donor financial and technical support, which played such an important role in the first 10 years of the program, continued, but on a much reduced scale. Assistance from the USAID in particular ebbed and flowed, driven by larger political events such as the Soviet invasion of Afghanistan, the question of Pakistan's possession of nuclear weapons, and relations with India (Conly and Rosen 1996), and more recently, events following the terrorist attacks on the United States on September 11, 2001, and U.S. involvement in Afghanistan and Iraq.

The Role of Foreign Donors

Pakistan's program was one of the first large-scale national programs, which came into being well ahead of the creation of the United Nations Population Fund and the involvement of the World Bank and other major multilateral donor groups in family planning. The USAID was deeply involved, and in reality was probably a step or two ahead of its own legal authorization. The technical and financial assistance rendered by the family planning program in the early 1960s was done under the rubric of health, as the USAID's Office of Population was not set up until 1967. The USAID quickly came to play a major role in Pakistan, and for the most part has been an important player since that time. Other important groups in the early days were the Ford Foundation, the Population Council, and SIDA.

Pakistan and the USAID enjoyed a close relationship for many decades, especially in relation to family planning. The USAID paid for nearly all nonlocal costs (and some local costs as well) of the first and second programs and maintained a large resident advisory staff. It is not an exaggeration to say that Pakistan served as a training ground for the USAID's later efforts in other countries. Similarly, the programmatic approach followed in Pakistan became, by default, the model for other countries. Indeed, the USAID seems to have adopted and institutionalized several important elements of its Pakistan experience.

First, it fell into routinely following a supply-oriented approach. This is illustrated by the inundation scheme (Donaldson 1990), the determined effort in the 1970s to make the continuous motivation scheme succeed. With hindsight, this can be viewed as simply a stubborn aberration, a mistake by the USAID's top leadership that was doggedly executed by a loyal field staff, but this would be an incorrect interpretation. The inundation scheme was the purest and best example of the USAID's underlying philosophy and strategy for achieving population control. In a notably clear statement, Ravenholt (1969a, p. 124) wrote, "The main element initially in any population planning and control program should be the extension of family planning information and means to all elements of the population." The need for fertility control was obvious to the program managers, so they believed it must have been equally obvious to prospective clients. For the next two to three decades, this unspoken assumption guided much of the USAID's programming (Ravenholt 1969b).

Second, the USAID acquired a preference for national, or at least extremely large-scale, programs and projects. Some of this was purely pragmatic: spending small sums of money can sometimes be just as difficult as spending large sums, and the USAID typically spent large sums. At the same time, managing and overseeing many small projects is far more difficult and time-consuming than looking after a few large ones. Although expedient, the large-scale approach is not always productive, as limited absorptive capacity often makes large-scale donor efforts self-defeating. The inundation model's preference for large-scale initiatives no doubt informed and helped mislead USAID population strategy all the way through the big-country strategy of the 1990s.

Third, the USAID also learned to like dealing with separate population and family planning structures set apart from the regular, traditional administrative structures. It favored new structures that it could guide even if this meant bypassing useful existing structures and creating overlaps. Pressure on missions by Washington for results was a constant factor, and a new agency or interministerial council gave the USAID something to show for its efforts.

Finally, the Pakistan program never saw the importance of the private sector—both NGOs and the private commercial sector—and for most of its history the USAID's population efforts have taken the same route, and the USAID typically did not work outside official agencies. Sometimes this was at the request of host country governments, while in other cases USAID auditors insisted on dealing only with groups that could satisfy cumbersome financial reporting procedures that were beyond the capacity of many local NGOs. In all fairness, one should note that USAID missions in some countries did find innovative ways to fund local NGOs with some success. Indeed, Bangladesh was one such exception.

When the USAID did bring the international NGO and private voluntary organization community into USAID operations, it was as contractors administering ongoing USAID projects and following strict rules that often negated what should have been the advantages of their nongovernmental status. Similarly, for many years the USAID's efforts in the private commercial sector ignored existing markets and suppliers in favor of newly created, subsidized, social marketing schemes to distribute commodities or to undertake education and service provision in the workplace.

In sum, the USAID had a powerful effect on Pakistan's early efforts at family planning, but the shared experience probably had an even more profound effect on the USAID's population strategy and programming for the next several decades.

The Ford Foundation, the Population Council, and SIDA provided important technical assistance, training, research, and support for institution building, working directly with the government during the 1960s. The Ford Foundation played a more important role in program and service delivery of technical and advisory assistance, while the Population Council concentrated more on building up statistical demographic databases and creating local research capacity for exploiting such data. Both used short-term and long-term training devices and facilitated the flow of research from the program into international scholarly circles. SIDA (and some other donors) followed the lead of the Ford Foundation and the Population Council, with perhaps a more deliberate effort to blend programmatic services with research and training. Cooperation among these donors was good, and all favored the creation of small demonstration projects whereby service delivery approaches could be tested, evaluated, and reported upon. The action research projects in Comilla in East Pakistan and in Lulliani in West Pakistan were the best, but not the only, examples of this approach.

The use of small-scale research projects leading to national program applications (Notestein 1968) became a standard model for the Population Council for years to come, and, to some extent, is still in use today. The Ford Foundation later took a different route. Within a decade of its experiences in Pakistan (and in India; see chapter 18), it de-emphasized direct field research and program involvement, substituting a greater emphasis on long-term training, institution building, and work with smaller-scale nongovernmental groups (Harkavy, Saunders, and Southam 1968). SIDA all but gave up supporting family planning programs to work on women's empowerment (education, employment, and cooperatives) and other types of interventions. Presumably, the Pakistan experience demonstrated to these donors that, in a country lacking the vast resources needed to support national programs, their comparative advantage lay in focused training, research, and private sector development. Pakistan was a learning experience for all concerned.

Current and Future Prospects

Numerous national contraceptive prevalence and fertility surveys have been conducted in Pakistan in the past 30 years, including those in 1968–69, 1975, 1979, 1984–85, 1990–91, 1994–95, 2001, and 2003. These surveys indicated no appreciable change in the CPR through the 1980s; however, a breakthrough did finally occur, and the 1995 survey showed a CPR of 24 percent, more than double the rate in 1990. The most recent survey (in 2003) reported that the CPR was 32 percent, that 80 of the respondents knew of several modern contraceptive methods, and that unmet need accounted for 33 percent of respondents.

Another encouraging sign in the 2003 data is that clear differentials have developed among regions and socioeconomic strata of the population. In the largest cities, the CPR is 36 percent and the overall urban CPR is 32 percent. In Punjab, the most economically and socially advanced of Pakistan's four provinces, the CPR is 20 percent, compared with 15 percent for the Northwest Frontier and Sindh and 4 percent for Balochistan. Those respondents with a secondary school or higher level of education have a CPR of 40 percent, and even primary school attendance resulted in a CPR of 26 percent, higher than the national average (Ministry of Population Welfare 1996). Thus, contraception appears to be beginning to take hold as indicated by a decline in fertility: the most recent estimate puts the total fertility rate at below 5.0 births per woman. Pakistan finally appears to be turning the corner (Conly and Rosen 1996; Sathar 1993; Sathar and Casterline 1998; World Bank 1994).

Bangladesh

Bangladesh's war for independence cost it heavily in terms of human lives and physical infrastructure. As noted by Cleland and others (1994, p. 107), "The devastation of the war was particularly debilitating to the health and social services sectors of the government. The bureaucracy had collapsed, universities and training institutes were decimated, and many of the critically needed health facilities were destroyed. Basic communication was disrupted, further straining capacities to organize effective government . . . [and] mechanisms for coordinating complex tasks at the periphery, where family planning services would have their effect, simply did not exist."

Bangladesh's first president, Sheihk Mujib Rahman Khan (1971–75), was ambivalent about family planning, but his successors, General Ziaur Rahman (1975–81) and General H. M. Ershad (1982–90), were enthusiastic supporters. The First Five-Year Plan (1973–77) of the new nation gave high priority to population, and the government moved quickly to replace lost staff members and to rebuild its organization and facilities. The reconstituted program was placed under the auspices of the Ministry of Health and Family Planning, thereby eliminating the previous separate Family Planning Council framework. The plan also sketched out an ambitious multisectoral approach that allocated some family planning functions and responsibilities to eight different ministries. By 1975, the program was up and running again.

For a time, Bangladesh's program seemed to follow a course similar to that of Pakistan, and during 1975 to 1985, progress was slow at best. The existence of overlapping, parallel structures engaged in family planning in several ministries led to bureaucratic in-fighting over budgets. The health bureaucracy seemed particularly resistant to new methods or field structures being proposed by donors and already in use by NGOs. It continued the old procedures and operating rules laid down in 1965 without questioning their usefulness in the 1980s. Nevertheless, modest increases in the CPR did occur, from 8 percent in 1975, to 13 percent in 1979, to 18 percent in 1981, and to 19 percent in 1983 (Cleland and others 1994). (Bangladesh has had a highly reliable series of fertility and contraceptive prevalence surveys covering the 1980s and 1990s.)

Curiously, as Bangladesh's success started to become clear, the program came under virulent attack from several quarters. Some critics alleged that family planning was a coercive scheme that was forced on the helpless peasants of Bangladesh by outsiders, that is, foreigners (Warwick 1982), and was based on the continued use of incentive payments, referred to as bribes by critics, and on the important role played by surgical contraception, referred to as castration by critics. Furthermore, the militant international women's movement found the male-dominated family planning program in Bangladesh a particularly inviting target (Hartmann and Standing 1985), as did the equally militant religious groups opposed to any kind of birth limitation (O'Reilly 1985). For a time in the early 1980s, the program was very much on the defensive, particularly in international donor circles.

At the same time, several important positive elements gradually helped strengthen the program and point it in the right direction. Well before independence, Dhaka had a major international epidemiological research center then called the Pakistan-Southeast Asia Treaty Organization Cholera Research Laboratory. This laboratory operated an epidemiological surveillance area in Matlab thana in the rural area south of Dhaka that collected birth, death, and morbidity statistics. After independence, the laboratory was reconstituted as the International Center for Diarrhoeal Disease Research, and beginning in 1975, used the test area and field staff in place for a series of carefully designed epidemiological interventions and experiments, including family planning. With support from the Population Council and the USAID, these studies generated an enormous volume of high-quality research, nearly all of it highly pertinent to program improvement. This research showed conclusively that when services were delivered in a high-quality fashion, contraceptive prevalence in rural settings rose sharply and fertility fell. From 1983 onward, this work was extended to several other rural areas in Bangladesh to see if the same approach and procedures would work when applied to regular government facilities whose staff members had been retrained to deliver higher-quality services. (This was the so-called Extension Project, which continues in a different form today.) The answer to this new hypothetical question was a resounding yes. When properly delivered, family planning services seemed to find clients nearly everywhere in Bangladesh.

The second favorable, if exogenous, factor for the Bangladesh program was the presence of a large number of NGOs operating in rural areas. Some 7,000 such organizations were registered with the Ministry of Social Welfare and were engaged in everything from agricultural improvement to women's education and employment. Some 400 were involved in family planning and maternal and child health activities, typically with links to and support from international donor organizations such as Pathfinder International, the Asia Foundation, and the Ford Foundation. Other larger rural development groups, such as the Bangladesh Rural Advancement Committee and the Grameen Bank, also came over time to include family planning and other social welfare components in their programs (Cleland and others 1994). Most of these NGOs undertook family planning activities in conjunction with programs aimed at empowering women through education, employment, and income-generation schemes.

The result was that by the mid-1980s, a significant and increasingly visible non-governmental family planning success story was emerging in Bangladesh. This came to represent as much as one-quarter of the CPR and was highly cost-effective. As noted earlier, many of these NGOs aimed at bettering the situation of women in general, and the success of these other programs interacted symbiotically with contraceptive delivery efforts. To this was added the highly effective social marketing program for contraceptives, which distributed condoms and pills through thousands of private sector outlets. Although sanctioned by the government, the social marketing program was completely independent in terms of its operations and came to represent another one-quarter of the total CPR.

The initial reaction of Ministry of Health officials to these nonofficial success stories was to ignore them, or even to attempt to discredit them, as their success represented an implicit criticism of the official program. By the mid-1980s, this behind-the-scenes struggle reached crisis point and the ministry made a bid to take over all NGO operations and regularize them. This would have meant that all budget and administrative control would have been in the hands of the ministry. The NGOs, with strong donor support, resisted this move. The donors, who were paying for the overwhelming share of all development activities in Bangladesh, had for some time been unhappy with the progress of the official program. At one point, the donor consultative group, chaired by the United Nations Development Programme, had even commissioned its own review of the situation, which produced a set of sweeping proposals for change, the so-called donors' plan of 1983. Some of these proposals would have moved the official program in the directions that the NGOs were already taking.

The rising importance of the nonofficial components in the total program mix also meant that by the late 1980s the CPR had begun to rise more sharply, reaching 25 percent in 1986, 30 percent in 1989, and 40 percent by 1991, as indicated mostly by locally conducted surveys. Success is hard to fight, and ministry officials came to see that cooperating and building on the approaches and structures that were leading to such irrefutable results were in everyone's best interests.

Fertility has, of course, also changed substantially. A definitive recent review of the data states, "The decline probably started in the late 1970s and accelerated in the mid-1980s . . . . In 1975 the total fertility rate was about seven births per woman. By 1988, it had fallen to five births per woman, equivalent to a 30 percent drop . . . [and] fertility in 1990 was almost certainly well below five births" (Cleland and others 1994, p. 131). This review also notes that the decline in fertility was pervasive, affecting nearly all socioeconomic strata and all geographical regions of the country.

Lessons to Be Learned

The two countries went separate ways, but important lessons can be learned from the experience of each one. Both ended up being reasonably successful in relation to their policies and programs, but the east wing did so much more quickly than the west.

Lessons Learned from Pakistan's Failure

The real lessons can be learned from Pakistan's program as it was implemented in 1965 before Bangladesh split off from the country. These are as follows:

- The program was overambitious. Putting a new program in place nationwide was an administrative tour de force, but a logistical nightmare. Beginning with those districts centered around a large urban location and then moving outward in a phased way so as to reach most districts by the end of five years might have been manageable, but Adil rejected the gradualist approach as being politically unacceptable.

- The decision to make family planning a new administrative program run from the center put it at odds with the existing health programs, which were provincially administered. This decision gave family planning a priority status, allowing it to bypass the existing health bureaucracies. This was understandable in the context, as at that time Pakistan's Ministry of Health was full of former Indian army doctors who barely believed in public health, much less family planning, and bypassing them must have seemed easier than fighting with them. However, it meant that the program was, from the outset, explicitly and deliberately not a health-related endeavor. The program limited itself to mostly nonclinical methods, as it had little control over the facilities that supplied clinical methods. The situation also created enduring enmity between the two programs, making it harder to bring new methods on line as they were developed and to meet clients' actual demands, which were (and continue to be) mainly for long-term, if not terminal, methods of contraception.

- The program paid inadequate attention to information, education, and communication. Even in 1965, radio was a major medium of communication in Pakistan, and television had appeared on the scene before the end of the First Five-Year Plan. Too much attention was concentrated on brochures and posters, which impressed visitors, but were meaningless to illiterate rural women. This followed partly from an unstated decision that the program should keep a relatively low profile.

- The program paid insufficient attention to evaluation and detailed monitoring of results. The rapid feedback now possible with techniques of demographic health surveys was obviously not available, but even small-scale local surveys could have been undertaken to provide a reality check on service statistics and the optimism of program advisers and officials. The National Research Institute for Family Planning, attached to the program's central secretariat, was intended to perform such tasks, but because of weak leadership and inadequate staffing, never became a real resource. Numerous training and research centers were also established at the provincial level, but these also quickly lost their edge. Ironically, a contributing factor to staff weakness was a continuing drain of key personnel into jobs with international agencies as these groups moved into family planning globally.

- The program did not make use of the private sector to any significant extent. Many private physicians knew nothing about the program, and those who knew about it realized it was not a medical program, and hence were deeply suspicious of it. The NGOs also were not made full partners, nor did the program draw on their experience for program tactics. The government tended to believe that only it could take on the really big jobs and that the private sector would merely get in the way.

- The program was linked to the political governance apparatus—union councils, districts, and so on—which meant that it faced the inevitable pressure to meet the normal demands of political patronage and largesse. Moreover, identifying the program with the political power structure can be a mistake in situations in which the power structure is suspect in the eyes of the masses. Strong political support can be a two-edged sword.

Lessons Learned from Bangladesh's Success

As late as the early 1980s, the programs in both countries still seemed mired in the same bureaucratic and administrative morass, but several structural changes seem to have led Bangladesh to its early success. These include the following:

- The program had become a health program, and this was important, as the health bureaucracy was no longer threatened by the program, but came to accept it as legitimate. As the health system grew, so did the family planning network, and vice versa.

- The program was actively debated, and a growing body of local research became available about what worked and what did not work. Over time, this resulted in the program becoming less of a monolithic supply network and adopting more of a pragmatic, program-focused, problem-solving approach. The discussions were public and led to family planning becoming more generally accepted, even in rural areas.

- The NGOs grew and prospered and became the cutting-edge for program improvement. The government, albeit reluctantly, came to accept this and to learn from them.

- The international donor community, both bilateral and multilateral, was allowed to play an important role, providing technical assistance as well as financial support. This provided another force for change and for critical review of the program.

Bangladesh now faces some uncertainty about completing its success story. Concern is growing in some quarters that the decline in fertility may be slowing and that it is threatening to stall well above replacement levels (Bongaarts 2005). Contraceptive knowledge and practice are widespread, and whether the issue is a stubborn preference for more than two children by many couples or a problem with matching the available mix of methods with consumer desires is not clear.

References

Bongaarts, John. 2005. "Are Family Planning Programs Plateauing?" Research Division Working Paper, Population Council, New York.

Cleland, John, James F. Phillips, Sajeda Amin, and G. M. Kamal. 1994. *The Determinants of Reproductive Change in Bangladesh: Success in a Challenging Environment*. Regional and Sector Studies. Washington, DC: World Bank.

Conly, Shanti R., and James E. Rosen. 1996. *Pakistan's Population Program: The Challenge Ahead*. Country Study Series 3. Washington, DC: Population Action International.

Donaldson, Peter. 1990. *Nature against Us: The United States and the World Population Crisis.* Chapel Hill, NC: University of North Carolina Press.

Finkle, Jason. 1971. "Policies, Development Strategies and Family Planning Programmes in India and Pakistan." *Journal of Comparative Administration* 3: 135–52.

Harkavy, Oscar, Lyle Saunders, and Anna Southam. 1968. "An Overview of the Ford Foundation's Strategy for Population Work." *Demography* 5 (2): 541–52.

Hartmann, Betsy, and Hilary Standing. 1985. *Food, Saris, and Sterilization.* London: The Bangladesh Action Group.

Hoover, Edgar M., and Mark Perlman. 1967. "Measuring the Effects of Population Control on Economic Development." *Pakistan Development Review* 6 (4): 541–66.

Lewis, Stephen R., Jr. 1969. *Economic Policy and Industrial Growth in Pakistan.* London: George Allen and Unwin.

Ministry of Population Welfare (with the Population Council). 1996. *Pakistan Contraceptive Prevalence Survey, 1994–95, Basic Findings.* Islamabad: Government of Pakistan.

Notestein, F. W. 1968. "The Population Council and the Demographic Crisis of the Less Developed World." *Demography* 5 (2): 553–60.

O'Reilly, W. M. 1985. *The Deadly Neo-Colonialism.* Washington, DC: Human Life International.

Ravenholt, R. H. 1969a. "AID's Family Planning Strategy." *Science* 163 (January): 124–25.

———. 1969b. "The A.I.D. Population and Family Planning Program: Goals, Scope and Progress." *Demography* 3 (2): 561–73.

Robinson, Warren C. 1966, "Family Planning in Pakistan's Third Five-Year Plan." *Pakistan Development Review* 6 (2): 255–81.

———. 1978. "Family Planning in Pakistan, 1955–1977: A Review." *Pakistan Development Review* 17 (2): 233–47.

———. 1987. "The 'New Beginning' in Pakistan's Family Planning Programme." *Pakistan Development Review* 26 (1): 107–18.

———. 2001. "Common Beginnings but Different Outcomes: The Family Planning Programmes of Pakistan and Bangladesh." In *Fertility Transitions in South Asia*, ed. Zeba Sathar and James Phillips, 347–63. Oxford, U.K.: Oxford University Press.

Sathar, Zeba. 1993. "The Much Awaited Fertility Decline in Pakistan: Wishful Thinking or Reality?" *International Family Planning Perspectives* 19 (4): 142–46.

Sathar, Zeba, and John B. Casterline. 1998. "The Onset of Fertility Transition in Pakistan." *Population and Development Review* 24 (4): 773–96.

Sathar, Zeba, and James Phillips. eds. 2001. *Fertility Transition in South Asia.* Oxford: Oxford University Press.

Warwick, Donald P. 1982. *Bitter Pills.* New York: Cambridge University Press.

Wishik, Samuel, and Kwan-Hwa Chen. 1973. *Couple-Years of Protection: A Measure of Family Planning Program Output.* Family Planning and Population Program Manuals 7. New York: Columbia University, International Institute for the Study of Human Reproduction.

World Bank. 1994. *Staff Appraisal Report, Islamic Republic of Pakistan, Social Action Program Project.* Report 12588-PAK. Washington, DC: South Asia Region, Country Department III, Population and Human Resources Division.

20 Early Family Planning Efforts in Sri Lanka

NICHOLAS H. WRIGHT

Just as in the West, early family planning efforts in Ceylon sprang from the feminist movement, a concern for child health, and also from eugenics.[1] In 1932, Dr. Mary Rutnam, concerned by a tide of undernourished babies at the milk feeding center of the Ceylon Social Service League, advocated the promotion of family planning knowledge. However, the Ceylon Medical Council rejected her suggestion to include birth control and eugenics in the curriculum of the Ceylon Medical School. In 1937, Rutnam opened a family planning clinic in Colombo in the premises of the Ceylon Social Service League, but with Ceylon as the United Kingdom's forward base against Japanese expansion into the Indian Ocean, the army commandeered the clinic's space in 1939, and private family planning activity was put aside until 1949, the year after Ceylon became independent.

In that year, E. C. Fernando was a member of the Ceylonese delegation attending a seminar for Eastern women in Stockholm designed to present the Swedish approach to economic development, that is, a "middle way" that was neither capitalist nor state socialist. Elise Ottesen-Jensen, a pioneer family planning leader, addressed the seminar, and privately advocated setting up a family planning association in Ceylon so as to better attract support. Shortly after, another family planning pioneer, Dr. Abraham Stone, visited Ceylon at the request of Minister of Agriculture Dudley Senanayake. Stone had been in India teaching the rhythm method at Mysore in 1951 on a visit sponsored by the World Health Organization. In 1952, Stone returned to Ceylon a second time in company with Margaret Sanger en route to a conference in Bombay. On that occasion, he also strongly urged that a family

This account is dedicated to the fond memory of E. C. (Sylvia) Fernando, a founding member of the Ceylon Family Planning Association with whom I sometimes disagreed, but who always fought fairly, and who was always concerned with the status of Sri Lankan women from the beginning; Goesta Nycander, my Swedish colleague, in whose home I listened on the radio to the landing of Apollo 11 on the moon in 1969, and who did not hesitate to look with clear eyes at the field results of training activities by the joint Sweden-Ceylon program, and, as necessary, criticize them; and Dr. Soma Weeratunga, director of health services after 1970, and later Sri Lankan ambassador to the former Soviet Union, who understood that a world of need existed outside his consulting room in Kandy, and who went into the field to help change the performance of Ministry of Health field staff members. These people were committed to better health for Sri Lankan families of every ethnic group and political persuasion. Their strong, early voices deserve to be remembered.

planning association be formed. This was accomplished in January 1953, and an association with the International Planned Parenthood Federation followed in 1954. Dr. Clarence Gamble, founder of the Pathfinder Fund, donated early supplies of contraceptive foam tablets and also paid for three workers at the first clinic at De Soysa Maternity Hospital in Colombo. By 1958, the Ceylon Family Planning Association (FPA) was running 23 clinics in Colombo and other urban locations around the country and was providing some training and orientation and contraceptive supplies to government and private physicians willing to provide services at government institutions or their offices. In 1958, the FPA started to receive an annual grant from the government of SL Rs 75,000. In addition, the government provided space and staff to run several of the clinics. By 1966, the FPA had 109 family planning clinics, most of them in urban areas (Abhayaratne and Jayewardene 1968).

The Government and Population Policy, 1949–59

Unlike most developing countries, Ceylon had a well-established tradition of censuses going back to 1871. In addition, registration of vital statistics was substantially complete by independence in 1948. The government had not failed to notice the surge in population growth following an unprecedented 30 percent decline in mortality from 1946 to 1947. Arguments over the causes of the rapid decline in mortality went on for years, and ranged from the control of malaria by spraying DDT to the rapid expansion of maternal and child health services, including infant feeding, under a national health service modeled on that of the United Kingdom (Meegama 1967; Newman 1965). The analysis was complicated by a slight rise in mortality among all age groups that had occurred in 1943–45, perhaps because of nutritional privation that was relieved by the resumption of normal food imports after the end of the war (Frederiksen 1961). At that time, Ceylon was not food self-sufficient.

The first government official to speak openly of the new demographic situation, and not only in Ceylon, was S. W. R. D. Bandaranaike, the minister of health in the first postindependence government. At the Second World Health Assembly, held in June 1949 in Rome, he declared:

> Another subject I should like to see some consideration of is one on which we have been discretely silent. There is a growing need for the consideration of the problem of birth control on an international plane. Do you realize that the very health work we are doing is making that problem increasingly urgent? Without asking for a decision in this Assembly, I do suggest that a beginning be made in the preparation of the necessary statistics and data with the help of the appropriate specialized agencies of the United Nations, so that later on, even next year, we can consider this problem which is becoming a most urgent one in the World today (Bandaranaike 1963, p. 176).

In 1969, the author interviewed Dr. W. G. Wickremasinghe, director of health services in 1949 and who had accompanied Bandaranaike to Rome. Wickremasinghe said that Bandaranaike's remarks were unexpected, extemporaneous, and possibly a reaction to a recently issued royal commission report on the British population. He noted that the U.S. delegates in Rome were furious at the speech. Wickremasinghe supported Bandaranaike at a key committee meeting at which he specifically promoted a view of maternal and child health (MCH) that held that family size should be restricted to four children on medical grounds. Even that more limited approach failed to move forward (personal communication with W. G. Wickremasinghe, November 13, 1969).

On his return to Colombo, some evidence suggests that Bandaranaike pushed the Ministry of Health toward better performance and showed interest in having existing family planning methods taught and provided to women in the postpartum setting, but no general government support for that position was forthcoming during his term of office. Sir John Kotelawa, Ceylon's third prime minister (1952–56), told the author in 1969 that Bandaranaike's 1949 remarks were "anomalous" and that in the early 1950s, the government was not interested in population matters (personal communication with John Kotelawa, December 13, 1969).

In 1956, however, Bandaranaike returned to the government as prime minister. Anecdotal evidence suggests that family planning was still very much on his mind. In 1958, for example, he spoke about fertility control for upward of two hours in a private interview in Colombo with the visiting director general of the World Health Organization, Dr. Maurice Candau, a Catholic and an outspoken opponent of family planning (personal communication with J. Padley, November 10, 1969). Later that year, following discussions with the Swedish ambassador to Ceylon, Alvah Myrdal, the government signed a bilateral agreement with the Swedish government to support pilot family planning activities. At about the same time, the Swedish government became involved in fertility control efforts in Pakistan. These were the first two instances of bilateral assistance for family planning.

Box 20.1 sets out the timeline of main events in relation to family planning in the country.

In 1959, the National Planning Council issued its 10-Year Development Plan, (mid-1959–mid-1969) which included an extensive statement noting that rapid population growth was a barrier to economic development. A sophisticated document for its time, the report ruled out a Malthusian solution, asking whether "the course of the birthrate could be influenced by a deliberate effort on the part of social policy, which excludes at the same time all forms of compulsion?" The discussion concludes that "although there are other factors outside the field of conscious decision which affect fertility among married couples, it is a fact that the conscious decision to limit births has elsewhere played a crucial part in the reduction in family size. The question that arises is whether such decisions can be actively influenced by policy. The answer would appear [to be] in the affirmative" (National Planning Council 1959, p. 16).

Political Background

Before 1948, policies under the British colonial government had for several generations favored the Ceylon Tamil minority. The resentment caused by this, as well as the failure to use the language of the majority of the country's population in government and the courts after independence, was especially strong among elements of

BOX 20.1 Timeline of Major Events

1932: The first private family planning initiatives take place.

1949: Bandaranaike addresses the World Health Assembly in Rome.

1958: The Sweden-Ceylon Family Planning Project is initiated.

1959: The National Planning Council's 10-Year Development Plan (mid-1959–mid-1969) includes a statement on control of fertility.

1963: The Population Council funds population studies by the University of Ceylon and the FPA.

1965: Following the elections, the government decides to formulate a national population policy.

1966: The Ford Foundation provides support for evaluating the National Family Planning Program.

1968: The Family Planning Bureau is set up.

1969: Early evidence indicates that the integration of family planning with MCH in the field program is not proceeding as anticipated.

1970: Program activities slow down before the election, leading to a fall in the number of acceptors.

The government shows reluctance to consider the possibility of organizing a postpartum family planning program in hospitals.

Leaving the door to continued assistance open, the Population Council withdraws its evaluation adviser.

The United Nations Population Fund sends its first needs assessment mission.

1971: A survey of the behavior of public midwives in the field reveals serious weaknesses in the national plan.

1972: The government abandons demographic targets.

The Family Health Bureau replaces the Family Planning Bureau.

1973: The United Nations Population Fund begins to support the program, including providing support for hospitals to perform voluntary sterilizations.

1976: Program activities slow down as another election approaches.

1977: The new government resolves to increase the availability of family planning through the curative sector.

The number of voluntary sterilizations rises rapidly as a result of publicity and allowances to medical personnel and acceptors of tubal ligation and vasectomy.

1980: The United Nations Population Fund sends a second needs assessment mission.

1987: A prevalence survey shows that 62 percent of married women of reproductive age are practicing a method of family planning, with 30 percent of them protected by tubal ligation or vasectomy. Thirty-nine percent of all married women of reproductive age are using a modern method of contraception.

2006: The net reproduction rate is two.

the majority Sinhalese population. Ethnic issues became part of the national political stage during the 1956 elections, when Bandaranaike became prime minister. Sinhalese became the official language under the Official Language Act of 1956, thereby stirring unrest among the Ceylon Tamils. Provisions were made for use of the Tamil language in specified parts of the country where Ceylon Tamils were in the majority, and other ethnic issues were also addressed in a 1957 agreement, but that accord was repudiated in 1958 under extreme pressure from right-wing Sinhalese elements, including a significant number of Buddhist monks.

That same year saw the eruption of savage riots. The government's declaration of a state of emergency temporarily cooled things down, but it had clearly lost control of the situation. In this difficult political environment, and possibly because of personal animosities within the cabinet, Bandaranaike was assassinated in 1959. The evidence suggested that some elements of the Buddhist *sangha* (Buddhist clergy or monks) had been involved (Manor 1989). Other exclusionary measures designed to favor the Sinhalese followed over the years, as did periodic violence between Tamils and Sinhalese.

While Sinhalese nationalism was the most important factor in this unrest rather than the tenets of Hinayana Buddhism, there was always the sense in Ceylon that its version of Hinayana Buddhism was a special and purer form of that ancient religion (Ryan 1954; World Fellowship of Buddhists 1969). At the same time, one knowledgeable observer also attributes the feelings that were exploited politically in 1956 to the pressure created by the failure of economic development to keep pace with modern needs and to a high rate of population increase (Vittachi 1958).

These ethnic feelings were still raw in the 1960s and led directly to widely expressed concerns among nationalistic Sinhalese and segments of the *sangha*, which the government and independent commentators rarely addressed, that family planning threatened the existence of the Sinhalese race. That the usually unpublished data on fertility and family planning acceptance by ethnic group suggested no such thing was irrelevant to such fears, and was almost totally ignored. Much less strident opposition also came from a Catholic minority that included both Sinhalese and other ethnic groups. For all these reasons, many in the government wanted a low-profile family planning program.

Although far less commented upon, another major demographic issue also agitated Sinhalese nationalists. Resident in Ceylon, although stateless because they had left India without papers of any kind, were an estimated 1 million Indian Tamils and their progeny, who had been brought to Ceylon by the British in the 19th and early 20th centuries to work in the tea industry. After considerable negotiation, in 1964, Prime Minister Sirimavo Bandaranaike, widow of S. W. R. D. Bandaranaike, signed the so-called Sirima-Shastri Agreement with Prime Minister Lal Shastri of India, whereby during the next 10 to 20 years India would accept repatriation of 525,000 of the Indian Tamils and Ceylon would give citizenship to 325,000. The balance was handled later in a 1974 agreement between Bandaranaike and Indira Ghandi. Such a massive prospective migration no doubt removed some of the urgency posed by rapid population growth in the 1960s.

The Sweden-Ceylon Family Planning Project

Under the 1958 agreement, whose implementation was delayed for several months by civil unrest, the governments of Ceylon and Sweden agreed to cooperate to promote and facilitate a pilot project involving community family planning that would take place in two or more rural areas in Ceylon, with the aim of extending such activities nationwide depending on the results (Wahren 1968). In collaboration with the Ministry of Health and the FPA, officials selected two areas. The first was in Bandaragama, close to Colombo, whose population of 7,000 consisted predominantly of Sinhalese Buddhists engaged in cultivating rice, rubber, and coconuts, about 20 percent of whom were illiterate. The other area selected was in Diyagama, an upcountry tea estate area with a population of about 7,000 Indian Tamils, mostly Hindus, who worked in the tea industry, about 75 percent of whom were illiterate.

Activities centered on village subdivisions, the smallest administrative unit in the National Health Service. Censuses were taken, as were knowledge and attitude surveys among fertile couples. Family welfare centers were opened that provided prenatal and postnatal care and well child clinics. Family planning methods were made available free of charge, including vaginal foam tablets, condoms, and instruction in the rhythm method. A limited amount of advice and services was also provided to infertile couples, an activity thought to play an important psychological role in relation to the acceptance of fertility control services. Even though the project had a resident Swedish adviser from the beginning, assisted as necessary by visiting consultants, it sought to base its activities as much as possible on existing Ceylonese health personnel. Training activities included both medical and paramedical staff members and included staff members within and outside the project areas. In 1962–63, the project expanded to two new and larger areas, Point Pedro, with a Ceylon Tamil population on the Jaffna peninsula, and Polonnaruwa-Matale, which had an ethnically mixed but predominantly Sinhalese population (Greenberg 1962; Kinch 1966).

By May 1965, a report provided to the Swedish International Development Cooperation Agency claimed that the crude birthrate had declined in the Bandaragama project area, with the most notable decline in births occurring among women "around the age of 35" (Tornberg 1965). The same report also noted that 76 percent of 771 project families canvassed viewed family planning positively by 1964, an increase from 65 percent of 679 families in 1961. (In 1959, 52 percent of 539 families had viewed family planning positively.) Although no data were reported on the prevalence of contraceptive use, the condom was said to be the most popular method. The new, plastic intrauterine device (IUD) had been introduced in 1964, and by the end of that year, 263 had been inserted. This number had increased to 2,009 by mid-1967, clearly indicating that clinic activities were attracting acceptors from outside the immediate target area (Aramugam 1968). A more formal analysis of demographic changes in the Bandaragama and Diyagama areas was undertaken, but because of incomplete birth registration, extensive migration, and other data problems, the small observed changes during 1963 to 1965 could not be attributed to family planning program activity (Hyrenius and Ahs 1968).

Early Demographic Analysis, 1963–68

In 1963, with support from the Population Council to the University of Ceylon, and in collaboration with the FPA, a series of demographic studies was undertaken and completed in 1967–68 (Abhayaratne and Jayewardene 1967, 1968). In addition to a complete review of historical vital data, the authors undertook a village survey that showed a small majority of respondents professing knowledge of family planning, but, surprisingly, only about one-third approving of the use of such methods. A strong reason for opposition was the concern that use was "against religion," presumably mostly on the part of Catholics and conservative Buddhists. What proportion of respondents had ever used or were then using a method of contraception is difficult to ascertain from the published data, but traditional methods such as withdrawal and rhythm were well represented, as was the condom. The proportion of those who had ever used contraception and who also reported a tubal ligation was between 1 and 3 percent depending on the region (Abhayaratne and Jayewardene 1967).

Beginnings of the National Family Planning Program, 1965–69

Soon after the elections of March 1965, the cabinet of the new government, headed by Senanayake, now the prime minister, decided to extend family planning nation-wide and to renew the agreement with the Swedish government for three years to August 1968. The agreement emphasized continued cooperation in relation to train-ing activities for the National Family Planning Program, primarily in Bandaragama and Point Pedro, and supply of required contraceptives.

In February 1966, the minister of health appointed an advisory committee to develop a detailed plan of operation. The committee issued its report in August 1966 and declared that the program would be a routine activity of the Department of Health Services and would be integrated with its MCH services (Advisory Committee 1966). The introduction of services was to be staggered by region over the following three years. The target was a slow reduction in the birthrate from 33 live births per 1,000 population to 25 in 8 to 10 years. Assuming a constant crude death rate, the crude rate of population increase was expected to be 1.6 per-cent by 1976. The report estimated that 550,000 couples, or about 55,000 per year, should be motivated to practice family planning by 1976, thereby averting 110,000 births. Another preliminary analysis circulating at the time estimated that 176,200 births would have to be prevented to reach the overall goal, which in turn would require 881,300 users, or contraceptive use by about 45 percent of couples by 1976 (Kinch n.d.). Both sets of calculations estimated that roughly five current users would prevent one birth, but neither considered various method mixes and their implied use-effectiveness rates. Indeed, at that time, reliable local field data for examining this issue were not available.

The arbitrary official acceptor target for different methods was 60 percent for IUDs, 25 percent for the contraceptive pill, 5 percent for sterilization, and 10 percent for other methods. IUD insertions were to be free of charge. Oral contraceptives were to cost SL Rs 1.50 per monthly packet, and condoms and foam tablets were to cost SL Rs 0.05 each (Advisory Committee 1966). The necessary instructions to health personnel were issued in November 1966, more than a year after the cabinet deci-sion to launch a family planning program (Ministry of Health 1966).

Although the immediate training and retraining needs of health personnel were daunting, grounds for optimism were strong. Ceylon had public health and curative health systems that had been free for more than 15 years. These services had played a significant role in reducing the incidence and severity of malaria, bringing down infant and maternal mortality rates by means of improved prenatal and obstetric care (about 65 percent of births occurred in a hospital by 1965), and lowering child mortality through immunizations and child feeding programs. Unlike in almost all other Asian countries, these efforts penetrated deeply and seemingly effectively into remote rural areas, where 75 percent of Ceylonese lived. In addition, education had been free through the tertiary level since shortly after World War II, and rice, a basic foodstuff, was heavily subsidized. At the same time, these benefits burdened government budgets, especially after the Korean War economic boom ended, reducing rubber exports. Ceylon's economy, based primarily on exports of tea, rubber and coconut, faltered. Nevertheless, the benefits were politically untouchable. By the end of the 1950s and into the 1960s, Ceylon's population was enjoying one of the highest levels of human development in Asia.

The second most senior position in the Ministry of Health after the minister was the permanent secretary of health, with the third being the director of health services. The latter chaired an advisory committee on family planning that was responsible for making policy recommendations. The next most senior positions were four deputy directors, one each for public health services, medical services, laboratory services, and administration. The deputy director of public health services had an assistant director responsible for MCH who was charged with integrating family planning services into the MCH system. Fifteen superintendents of health services (SHS) located around the country managed both preventive and curative (hospital and health center) services in their respective areas and reported directly to the director of health services in Colombo.

In all 95 districts across the country, excluding several urban areas controlled by local governments, the medical officers of health (MOOH) were responsible for MCH, school health programs, malaria and filariasis eradication, and environmental sanitation (including safe water and human waste disposal). In terms of population, the districts ranged from 80,000 to 200,000 people. The MOOH were typically young physicians performing their compulsory two-year government service in return for having their education paid for. As might have been expected from the traditional medical school curriculum in Ceylon at that time, their primary concern was curative rather than preventive work.

Serving under the MOOH were about 2,000 public health midwives (PHMs), or about 20 per district, each serving a population of about 5,000, including about 700 couples of reproductive age. Roughly 85 percent of the PHMs were under 40 years old, married, and with children. The newest cohorts of PHMs had 10 years of formal education (rather than 8 as in the past), plus a year of theoretical and practical training at a special training hospital and 6 months of field experience under supervision. A PHM's area could vary from 1 to 10 square miles, which she would cover on foot, or perhaps by bicycle. Of the approximately 175 annual births in her subdistrict, she would deliver about 20 to 25 of them at home. The remainder were delivered in hospitals or in smaller maternity hospitals. The PHM was expected to assist and advise all pregnant women in her area both before and after delivery, wherever that delivery might occur. On certain days, she was expected to assist the medical officer of health and the public health nurses at MCH outpatient clinics. Family planning was now added to the PHMs' duties following nine days of specialized training.

The public health field structure also included about 1,000 public health inspectors (PHI), each covering an area equivalent to about two or four PHM subdistricts. The original plans for the National Family Planning Program envisaged a motivational role for the public health inspectors, especially among men, thereby complementing the work of health educators in each SHS. By the late 1960s, about 60 percent of the public health inspectors had received training in family planning.

Even though initial efforts were concentrated on integrating family planning into the MCH field infrastructure, hospitals clearly also had a role to play, especially in delivering sterilization services. Ceylon had 11 provincial hospitals with specialized obstetric and gynecology services; 2 specialized maternity hospitals; 12 smaller hospitals with obstetric specialists; and almost 300 still smaller, or peripheral, hospitals and maternity homes, some staffed by physicians. Few developing countries could approach the coverage provided by these curative services. By the mid-1960s, 65 percent of births in Ceylon were already taking place in government hospitals, and close to 20 percent more occurred under the supervision of a PHM, usually at home.

As internal momentum slowly built toward formally beginning the National Family Planning Program, an October 1966 visit from a staff member of the Ford Foundation in Bangkok led to an agreement with the government that, through a grant to the Population Council, an adviser on evaluation would be placed to the Ministry of Health and the Ministry of Planning and Economic Affairs. The author was nominated by the Population Council, accepted by the Government, and began his appointment in Ceylon in October 1967. The agreement also provided for short-term foreign study and training for Ministry of Health staff members and for funds for equipment, supplies, and research.

Evaluation and Program Performance, 1967–69

An immediate issue, and one members of the government raised in late 1967 and 1968, was the observation that the crude birthrate had declined by 12.2 percent between 1953 and 1963, and therefore perhaps the 1976 target might be reached without pushing family planning (or political luck) unnecessarily. The underlying problem—which emerged repeatedly in private conversations and sometimes in hysterically virulent form in widely read newspapers from at least 1965 on as plans for a national family planning program took shape and continued up to the 1970 elections—was deep-seated ethnic fears about the continued political dominance of the Sinhalese majority, which at that time accounted for about 70 percent of the total population.

A quick perusal of Ceylonese data suggested that, independent of any actual fertility decline within marriage, at least two powerful demographic forces were at

TABLE 20.1 Percentage of Women Aged 15–49 Currently Married and Ever Married, 1953 and 1963

Age (years)	Currently married		Ever married	
	1953	1963	1953	1963
15–19	23.7	15.0	24.3	15.3
20–24	65.8	57.4	67.5	58.5
25–29	84.4	80.9	87.2	82.7
30–34	87.7	89.1	92.5	92.2
35–39	86.5	89.9	94.6	95.1
40–44	80.7	86.1	95.0	95.8
45–49	66.9	81.7	95.6	96.1

Source: Department of Census and Statistics data.

work during 1953 to 1963. The first was a striking delay in the age of marriage, dramatized in the falling proportions of women married when younger than 25 (table 20.1). In addition, because of a severe malaria epidemic in the mid-1930s that saw more deaths than births during 1934 to 1935, Ceylon had a relative shortage of young women of reproductive age during 1953 to 1963.

Between 1953 and 1963, the crude birthrate declined by 12.2 percent from 39.4 live births per 1,000 population to 34.6. Controlling for the delay in the age of marriage (by that time almost all births in Ceylon were to married couples) reduced the decline to only 5.3 percent. Controlling also for the change in age distribution among women aged 15 to 49 almost completely explained the observed 1953–63 decline; *that is, had the proportions of women married and their age distribution not changed after 1953, the crude birthrate would not have declined* (Wright 1968).

Marital fertility rates over the period were calculated and showed, as might have been expected, that among women aged 20 to 39, who accounted for 90 percent of all births, the change in fertility had been marginal. The message was clear: no overall reduction in fertility within marriage had taken place between 1953 and 1963. While further decline in the proportion of women currently married was a matter for speculation, the difficulties that young men faced in finding employment and the squeeze effect, that is, the expected relative shortage of women available to marry men five years older (the societal preference), made further decline in the crude birthrate likely. However, because of the rapid decline in mortality that had occurred by 1947, the number of women of reproductive age was likely to rise rapidly from the late 1960s and make the announced crude birthrate target for 1976 more difficult to achieve. While the likely balance of these competing effects after 1963 could not be predicted with confidence, it seemed prudent to aim for more marital fertility decline to meet the desired target birthrate.

With the approval of the Ministry of Health, and in collaboration with the Department of Census and Statistics, a family planning statistics feedback system was prepared for implementation in 1968. Three evaluation and research assistants hired under the Ford Foundation grant to the Population Council began visiting MOOH

TABLE 20.2 New Family Planning Acceptors by Method, 1966–69

Year	Total[a]	IUD	Pill	Other and traditional[b]	Sterilization[c]
1966[d]	15,000	10,000	1,000	1,000	3,000
1967[e]	36,695	18,506	8,892	5,601	3,616
1968[f]	48,164	20,615	16,014	6,325	5,210
1969[g]	60,000	20,000	28,000	6,000	6,000

Source: See table footnotes.

a. Totals include FPA figures for 1967–69.

b. Figures include condoms, foam tablets, diaphragm and jelly, and the rhythm method.

c. Sterilization was almost exclusively female. Sterilization figures for 1968 and estimates for 1969 were obtained from special questionnaires.

d. Figures are crude estimates.

e. Figures are derived from a special questionnaire.

f. The figures are higher than officially reported because of unreported sterilizations and are derived from the Ministry of Health's Family Planning Service Statistics.

g. The estimates for 1969 are based on official returns through June 1969, rapid feedback reports through October 1969, and special questionnaires to pick up unreported sterilizations. The official total for 1969 was 47,768 acceptors (UNFPA 1980).

districts and hospitals to introduce the new reporting forms. During the course of their visits, the assistants noticed that MOOH and other public health staff members were often on leave or had recently been transferred and not replaced. Many other staff members claimed to lack special training for the new family planning activity. The assistants also began to help conduct continuation rate studies after acceptance so that use effectiveness could be established.

The data taken from the service statistics system in the early years of the National Family Planning Program were not reassuring (table 20.2).

It was clear before the end of 1968 that because of the shortfall of acceptors recruited to that point, and with use-effectiveness rates lower than expected, especially among oral contraceptive acceptors, the previously set acceptor target would not achieve the desired birthrate by 1976. A subcommittee of the Family Planning Advisory Committee recommended the more realistic goal of 1 million acceptors by the end of 1975. As about 100,000 had already been recruited and 200,000 to 250,000 more could be expected from the private sector, the subcommittee thought that 700,000 more acceptors were needed in the public sector from 1969 through early 1975, or about 110,000 per year. These were then broken down by MOOH area and accepted by the government (Evaluation Subcommittee 1968).

In addition, many clinics were not reporting family planning activities at all, and how many of the 375 family planning clinics in hospitals and health centers were actually functioning was hard to determine. The reporting of sterilizations from hospitals was also incomplete and irregular, and special surveys were necessary to capture those figures more reliably. A rapid feedback system did not improve the picture. The notional targets of 1966 were not being met. Based on five follow-up surveys done by the Evaluation Unit in 1969, estimates indicated that only 99,000 of an estimated 160,000 new acceptors in 1966–69 were still using the original method by the end of 1969, or about 5.5 percent of married couples where the wife was aged 15 to 49. This was well short of the numbers necessary to reach the (implied) 1976 target of 45 percent (Wright 1970b).

Especially disappointing was the reality that the use of oral contraceptives had not expanded more rapidly, although the number of acceptors rose most rapidly for that method between 1968 and 1969. Given the presence of 2,000 PHMs, the number of new acceptors suggested a recruitment level of less than two per month per PHM. This occurred despite the April 1968 policy change to reduce barriers to pill acceptance: the price had been halved (to SL Rs 0.75 per cycle) and the process of acceptance had been "de-medicalized" by allowing PHMs to prescribe and dispense the pill without an initial medical examination by a medical officer of health (Director of Health Services 1968). However, pill continuation rates in the field remained alarmingly low in 1969, suggesting major problems in ongoing field supervision and resupply that the new policy failed to rectify (Wright and Perera 1973).

Because the official provisional crude birthrate in 1968 was 32 live births per 1,000 population and was higher than in 1967, leading to official concern, a new analysis of the 1963–68 period was undertaken to assess the effects of demographic factors and marital fertility. The analysis revealed that delay in the age of marriage continued to intensify during the period, while at the same time, the number of women of reproductive age was increasing. The overall direction of both these factors combined was negative, but could not explain all the observed decline in the crude birthrate since 1963, suggesting the likelihood of some marital fertility decline. Estimates of marital age-specific fertility rates over the period suggested declines in all age groups among women aged 15 to 49 except for the youngest women. The decline among women over 30 was clearly higher than for those under 30 (Wright 1970a). A later analysis of fertility during 1963 to 1969 suggested that demographic factors accounted for 80 percent of the observed decline in the crude birthrate (Fernando 1972).

Given the lack of political support at virtually every level as the 1970 elections approached, program activity slipped well below expectations, and perhaps even went into reverse in 1969. A detailed administrative report on a sample of 21 of the 95 MOOH areas carried out in late 1969 sheds some light on the overall situation (Wijesooriya 1971). The 21 areas represented a population of about 2.5 million. Except for the PHMs, for which 5 percent of positions were vacant and of which 25 percent were untrained in family planning, vacancies were few and training in family planning was substantially complete. Given the 102 approved family planning clinics in the 21 MOOH areas and their scheduled frequency of operation, the expectation of one clinic session per week for every 35,000 to 40,000 people would have been reasonable. While no figure was supplied, the report states that "the impression gained was that a considerable number of clinic sessions are missed. The main reason appeared to be non-availability of medical officers due to their being on leave or away on other urgent duties"(Wijesooriya 1971, p. 19). Field distribution of oral contraceptives took place in only 17 of the areas, and not continuously in all of those areas. Various reasons were offered for this state of affairs. Examination of stocks of oral contraceptives showed that seven areas had none and nine others had only a one-month supply or less. In addition, reports were not filed as requested in a significant minority of areas (Wijesooriya 1971). Even though the Ministry of Health attempted to remedy these pervasive and discouraging administrative and attitudinal problems, it appeared likely that the number of acceptors in 1970 would be less than in 1969.

Effects of the 1970 Elections

The May 1970 elections gave a powerful mandate to the left-leaning nationalist party headed by Sirimavo Bandaranaike. The government took time to get organized, and it soon became clear that the government would not abandon family planning; however, it would no longer set demographic targets, and the Family Planning Bureau, created in 1968 to integrate family planning into the existing mix of more traditional MCH services, was re-named the Maternal and Child Health Bureau, and later the Family Health Bureau. A new leadership team was put in place that was strongly committed to MCH and to making the field program perform more efficiently and effectively. Field visits and inspections increased, and identified deficiencies were punished on occasion by on-the-spot fines and transfers (personal communication with M. Stiernborg, October 2006).

The final results of a large study of PHMs in the field were presented to the new government in 1970 and published the next year (Nycander 1971). The main objectives of the study were to observe and assess the working behavior of the PHMs as they visited mothers for family planning motivation and follow-up, to see whether this working behavior conformed to an expected and operationally defined standard, to ascertain whether the training the PHMs had received was adequate for their situation in the field, and to look at other factors in addition to training that might affect the performance of the PHMs and which of these might be improved upon by new policy decisions and more efficient administration of the program. Trained social workers undertook the observations in typical field settings. Despite sampling issues in the design of the study and the civil disturbances of 1971, which allowed for only partial follow-up, the PHMs emerged as appreciated and respected in their areas. They were familiar with their clients and capable of gaining their confidence. They were positive toward family planning, but tended to be confused as to what was expected of them and, more critically, of how active they should be as motivators.

A disheartening finding was that, contrary to expectations, the PHMs seldom carried contraceptive pills into the field so that clients could begin taking them immediately or former acceptors could continue taking them. Nor did they carry sample IUDs so that prospective clients might see what they looked like. The information they gave was often incomplete, and they were not equipped to counter reports—real or rumored—of side effects. They rarely checked potential acceptors for contraindications to the pill. Clearly, they did not regard family planning to be as important as their more traditional activities. Knowledgeable observers felt that some of the problem lay with the MOOH offices, where young physicians, often with little inclination toward undertaking preventive activities, were confused, if not intimidated, by national fears, a hyperbolic press, and sometimes outright political interference in their work (Nycander 1971).

At the same time, it did not seem to be just family planning that was being affected by the increasingly problematic preventive sector of Ceylon's health system. A national nutrition survey sponsored by the Ministry of Health, CARE, and the U.S. Centers for Disease Control in 1975–76 showed that 6.6 percent of Sri Lankan children under six were acutely malnourished. In one district, the proportion approached 9.0 percent. The survey also revealed that 27 percent of pregnant mothers were anemic (Potts 1978). As late as 1981–82, the family health impact survey documented levels of basic childhood immunization that the government must have viewed as disappointing (Family Health Bureau 1984). Further survey work in the 1980s addressed the care mothers received during pregnancy. While tetanus toxoid immunization was widespread, the surveys identified a significant group of mothers who had not been immunized (UNICEF 1986). Whereas most mothers had attended a prenatal clinic, many of the basic clinic functions, such as checking blood pressure and testing urine for sugar, had not been done. Finally, PHMs had made home visits only to approximately half the pregnant mothers in their subdistricts, more often those not living in abject poverty. Furthermore, those visits that were made did not seem to have any effect on increasing clinic visits, on advancing immunization with tetanus toxoid, or on shifting mothers away from untrained midwives. Thus, it would seem that knowledge and information on health practices, including family planning, were more often obtained from sources other than the PHM. It was also reported that about one-third of the mothers in the survey did not feed their first milk (colostrum) to their infants (UNICEF 1986). A World Health Organization (1978) report had also noted these difficulties and weaknesses and supported the conclusion that earlier optimism in relation to the prospects for integrating family planning into a supposedly effective preventive MCH service was not well grounded.

In 1970, a United Nations mission visited Ceylon and drew up a plan of operation for several family health projects. The World Health Organization was to be the executing agency for three projects funded by the United Nations Population Fund, one of them intended specifically to strengthen and upgrade medical institutions in relation to the delivery of clinical and contraceptive services (Ministry of Plan Implementation and Research Triangle Institute n.d.). This work had begun by 1973. In addition to expanding and improving the delivery of sterilization at the larger teaching and provincial hospitals, new facilities were created at smaller hospitals and nonspecialist medical officers were trained in sterilization (Family Health Bureau 1984).

Table 20.3 clearly shows that the 1970 elections had a negative effect on program performance. More important, evidence indicates that by 1973 the curative sector, arguably the most functional sector in the Ceylonese health system, had begun to support the National Family Planning Program more fully by making provision for voluntary female (inpatient) and male (outpatient) sterilization. During the same time, IUD and contraceptive pill acceptors increased modestly, plateaued, and then declined. The program continued to follow election cycles, with another downturn in 1976, a year before the right-center government under Prime Minister J. R. Jayawardene was elected.

TABLE 20.3 Number of New Family Planning Acceptors by Method, 1970–85

Year	Total	IUD	Pill	Injection	Traditional[a]	Other	Sterilization Male	Female
1970	55,269	15,799	26,889	0	6,924	686	4,971[b]	
1971	49,323	11,446	25,828	0	7,306	408	245	4,090
1972	71,137	18,599	32,300	0	9,662	—	498	9,078
1973	82,020	27,558	34,214	0	—	—	1,850	18,398
1974	107,851	29,693	35,924	0	—	—	7,292	34,942
1975	109,639	32,755	37,720	0	—	—	6,034	33,130
1976	88,215	27,030	25,597	0	—	—	2,924	32,664
1977	67,889	21,321	27,514	0	—	—	1,302	17,752
1978	79,226	23,085	31,146	3,046	—	—	2,325	19,264
1979	92,156	20,187	30,394	5,932	—	—	5,640	30,003
1980	171,159	19,232	29,296	9,705	—	—	51,284	61,642
1981	121,797	14,833	22,189	8,142	—	—	30,333	46,300
1982	114,481	16,115	26,231	10,211	—	—	13,048	48,876
1983	173,197	16,328	33,821	11,271	—	—	44,979	64,798
1984	160,023	16,140	32,895	9,660	—	—	37,542	63,786
1985	122,758	12,588	31,990	16,375	—	—	16,724	45,081

Source: Family Health Bureau, Evaluation Unit data. Data for 1981 are taken from Ministry of Health 1985, table 7.3 Total pill figures for 1974 and 1975 are estimated.

Note: — = not available. The data do not take into account a private sector social marketing program begun in 1973 by Population Services International for the distribution of oral contraceptives and condoms. If one assumes that 100 condoms or 13 oral pill packets sold each equal one acceptor, then by 1975 and 1976, approximately 40,000 acceptors—and about 60,000 in 1977—could be added (Potts 1978). This program was transferred to the FPA before 1980.

a. Figures include condoms and foam tablets. Acceptor data for these methods from the Family Health Bureau are not available after 1972.

b. Source did not distinguish between male and female sterilizations.

Sterilization, 1977–85

After a recovery period of two years following the 1977 elections, the number of sterilizations performed, especially of vasectomies, increased by an order of magnitude in response to an incentive scheme for both providers and acceptors. Table 20.4 shows that the popular response was remarkable, although the yield per month at the highest acceptor allowance level (SL Rs 500) diminished over time. Surveys in Colombo suggested that the higher levels of allowances brought forward a group of men for vasectomy who belonged to a lower economic group and who had already achieved a large family size (de Silva and others 1988).

The following conditions had to be satisfied before sterilization would be done. Men undergoing vasectomy had to be less than 50 years old and women undergoing tubal ligation had to be younger than 45 on the date of surgery. They had to be legally married or in a common law marriage and have at least two living children on the date of surgery. A system of counseling was put in place to ensure informed

TABLE 20.4 Trends in Voluntary Sterilization by Type of Allowance, 1978–85

Type of allowance and amount	Total number of sterilizations	Average number of sterilizations per month
None, January 1978–April 1979	29,929	1,871
Allowance to medical teams, May–December 1979[a]	27,670	3,459
Allowance to medical teams plus additional out-of-pocket expenses to acceptors		
SL Rs 100, Jan.–Sept. 1980	46,178	5,130
SL Rs 500, Oct. 1980–Feb. 1981	103,557	20,712
SL Rs 200, March 1981–Dec. 1981	39,819	3,982
SL Rs 300, Jan. 1982–May 1983[b]	87,259	5,133
SL Rs 500, June 1983–Dec. 1983	84,442	12,063
SL Rs 500, Jan. 1984–Dec. 1984	101,328	8,444
SL Rs 500, Jan. 1985–Dec. 1985	61,805	5,150

Source: Adapted from Family Health Bureau 1984; Ministry of Plan Implementation 1983.

a. A team performing a tubectomy was entitled to SL Rs 65 divided among the team per case above a stipulated number per month. For vasectomies, the team received SL Rs 33.50 for each case above a minimum of five per month. From June 1, 1983, surgical teams received payment for all cases performed.

b. Figures are provisional data.

consent (Ministry of Plan Implementation 1983). The author examined the incentive scheme in 1983 and again in 1985 to ensure that it was indeed voluntary, and in 1985 also assessed its medical quality. On neither occasion did he find evidence of compulsion. All the female acceptors interviewed, some still in the hospital after surgery, praised the government for making the service so easy to obtain. Many had close female relatives who had had the surgery. One woman, when asked if she understood that the method was permanent, hesitated, and then said, in translation, "That is what I was told, and I certainly hope so." The compensation received seemed not unreasonable given the documented range of personal expenses. Despite the absence of any reports of serious complications or deaths within 48 hours of surgery, the performance of surgery in some of the smaller hospitals and in mobile vasectomy clinics suggested the need for a directed, active surveillance effort (Wright 1984, 1985).

The new government elected in 1977 was more committed to family health programs, including family planning, than any previous government, as expressed forcefully by J. R. Jayawardene, the new prime minister, in a speech on taking office. A new Ministry of Plan Implementation that reported directly to the prime minister was put in charge of formulating and implementing national population policy. By 1980, at the time of the second United Nations Population Fund needs assessment mission, the commitment of the government to control population growth through the provision of family planning services was reiterated publicly, as was the determination to use financial incentives to encourage medical teams to perform sterilizations and to motivate patients by covering their incidental expenses, travel costs, and lost income resulting from acceptance of sterilization. Finally, the government planned to amend the tax laws to limit deductions for children (Ministry of Plan Implementation and Westinghouse Health Systems 1983). A seminar titled "Family Planning above Party Politics" was held on the occasion of the visit by the needs assessment mission (Ministry of Plan Implementation 1980). In pursuit of these policies, the government set up 25 district population committees, each led by the head of a district administration, whose members represented relevant ministries and departments and included field officers, to monitor population policy (Ministry of Plan Implementation and Westinghouse Institute for Resource Development 1988).

Completion of the Demographic Transition, 1966–the Present

The original demographic targets formulated in 1966 and abandoned in 1970–71 were not met in 1976. In 1976, the crude birthrate was 27.8 live births per 1,000 population, not 25.0; the crude death rate was 7.8 deaths per 1,000 population, not 9.0; and the crude rate of natural population increase was 2.0 percent, not 1.6 percent. The birthrate had declined slowly from 32.3 in 1966 to 27.8 in 1976, but as noted earlier, was influenced by the age at marriage, which kept increasing during the period.

Researchers carried out a number of cross-sectional studies to determine the prevalence of contraceptive use among married women of reproductive age (MWRA) from 1975 to 1987 (table 20.5). Because questionnaires differed in their questions

TABLE 20.5 Contraceptive Prevalence, Selected Years
percentage of married women or their spouses currently using each method

Year	All	Modern methods	Sterilization		Pill	IUD	Injectable	Traditional methods[a]
			Female	Male				
1975a	43	18	8	1	2	6	0	26
1975b	34	18	10	1	2	5	0	16
1977	41	20	12	2	2	4	0	21
1981	43	28	18	4	2	3	1	14
1982	58	29	22 [b]		3	3	1	29
1987 [c]	62	39	25	5	4	2	3	23

Source: Family Health Bureau 1984; Ministry of Plan Implementation and Westinghouse Health Systems 1983; Ministry of Plan Implementation and Westinghouse Institute for Resource Development 1988; Ross and others 1988.

Note: For 1975–1, 1981, and 1987, the married women considered are aged 15 to 49. For other years, they are aged 15 to 44.

a. Measurement of the principal traditional methods, rhythm, condom, and withdrawal, varied by survey, and this accounts for the inconsistent results in total traditional method use, and therefore in total use.

b. The figure is the total for females and males.

c. Two northern areas were not sampled because of civil conflict.

about traditional methods, the figures in the last column are erratic, and therefore the figures for total use are erratic. However, use of modern methods follows a regular trend, and does so for each individual method.

As noted earlier, the first estimate of the prevalence of contraceptive use carried out in late 1969 using program acceptor and follow-up survey data suggested a current modern-method user rate of 5 to 6 percent. Except for condom acceptors in the public sector, reliable data on the use of traditional methods such as rhythm or withdrawal were not available at that time (Wright 1970b). In 1987, less than 20 years later, Sri Lanka was clearly a contraceptive-using society, with 39 percent of MWRA using a modern method (30 percent of those by means of sterilization) and another 23 percent of MWRA using a traditional method. That fully 30 percent of MWRA or their spouses were protected by sterilization is consistent with service statistics data. The use of the pill and IUD remained low, reflecting the chronic problems with these methods in a weak field program, and perhaps also the widespread perception by Sri Lankan women, and one not adequately addressed, that pill use was associated with serious health risks (Thapa and others 1988). It also suggested that, at least for the pill, the reach of the social marketing program was perhaps less extensive than it had been in the mid-1970s.

Even though the program failed to reach its acceptor and demographic targets by 1976, the evidence suggests a decline in marital fertility during the prior 10-year period. Induced abortion, illegal during this period, and later, is likely to have increased as the economic pressure for smaller families intensified and approval of family planning increased (Potts 1978). No direct information is available on this issue, but hospital morbidity and mortality data may be indicative. For example, hospitalization for complications attributed to induced abortion increased by more than 30 percent between 1970 and 1985. Fortunately, hospital mortality associated with these cases decreased over the period (Ministry of Health 1985). Abhayaratne and Jayawardene (1967) point out that use of the traditional methods may have been far more extensive than thought. To the extent that this is true, they may have played an important role in keeping the historic crude birthrates lower than might have been expected, and also contributed to the early marital fertility decline in the late 1960s and early 1970s (Caldwell and others 1987).

The 2006 Population Reference Bureau (2006) reports Sri Lanka's crude birthrate as 19 live births per 1,000 population, the crude death rate as 6 deaths per 1,000 population, and the population growth rate at 13 births per 1,000 population or 1.3 percent. The total fertility rate is two births per woman, slightly below replacement level. Of MWRA aged 15 to 49, an estimated 70 percent are using a family planning method and 50 percent are using a modern method. Infant mortality is 11.2 deaths per 1,000 live births and life expectancy at birth is 73 years. The estimated population is 19.9 million, almost double that in the 1963 census. Had not large numbers of Indian Tamils been repatriated in the years after 1964 and had not many Sri Lankan Tamils left after 1983 to escape ethnic conflict, the total population would have been significantly higher.

Lessons Learned

Although many of Ceylon's political leaders voiced concerns about rapid population growth early on and the first bilateral family planning pilot project in a developing country began¹ in 1958 with Swedish assistance, the movement to a national population policy was slow, reluctant, and hardly an example of continuous revolutionary progress. Even with strong popular approval of family planning and, by Asian standards, an exceptionally privileged developmental setting, as demonstrated by the provision of a broadly based, free education system open to both men and women; a national health system; and subsidized food, the prevailing ethnic politics made the work of extending family planning contentious. Because the many hysterical pronouncements on family planning and the feared extinction of the Sinhalese race were almost never contradicted at any official level, clear decision making and progress in extending family planning in the field was often paralyzed from 1965 to the mid-1970s.

Saying that family planning would be integrated into an existing MCH field network was all very well, but unfortunately, the system was not working efficiently, not even for long-accepted and less contentious MCH activities. Family planning presented special problems, because ethnic politics were in conflict, because professional leadership in the field was only weakly committed to prevention, and because services were excessively medicalized. The difficulty of orienting physicians traditionally trained as problem solvers for individual patients toward medicine addressed toward mass prevention in human populations was not unique to Sri Lanka. This field problem persisted into the 1980s.

The extensive use of traditional methods was not fully appreciated, and, if political considerations had permitted, they probably should have been promoted more strongly.

With almost 70 percent of births occurring in a hospital by 1965, a postpartum family planning program would have been effective both in delivering services and, in the prevailing political environment, in keeping the service safely within the walls of the hospital. This promising strategy was derailed by the 1970 election cycle.

Program efforts finally started to move forward decisively in 1977–80, when the government decided to promote voluntary sterilization by means of better services and allowances to surgical staff members and to acceptors. In this way, at last, the curative sector of the Ministry of Health was fully mobilized to support the program. In addition, strong efforts were made to place family planning above ethnic politics.

Along with the deteriorating economic environment after the 1950s, the failure of the family planning program to move forward as many thought it might have put tremendous pressure on families. The level of induced abortion almost certainly rose as family size preferences began to change and families struggled to deal with unwanted pregnancies during 1965 to 1985.

Note

1. Ceylon officially changed its name to Sri Lanka in 1972.

References

Abhayaratne, O. E. R., and C. H. S. Jayewardene. 1967. *Fertility Trends in Ceylon*. Colombo: Colombo Apothecaries Company, Ltd.

———. 1968. *Family Planning in Ceylon*. Colombo: Colombo Apothecaries Company, Ltd.

Advisory Committee. 1966. "Plan and Programme for National Family Planning Project," unpublished report, Advisory Committee, Colombo.

Aramugam, L. G. 1968. "The Introduction of Intra-Uterine Contraceptives in a Rural Area: Bandaragama." Address to the Association of Obstetricians and Gynecologists of Ceylon, February 21, Colombo.

Bandaranaike, S. W. R. D. 1963. *Speeches and Writings*. Colombo: Government Publishing House.

Caldwell, Jack, K. W. H. Gamminiraten, P. Caldwell, B. Caldwell, N. Weeraratne, and P. Silva. 1987. "The Role of Traditional Fertility Regulation in Sri Lanka." *Studies in Family Planning* 18 (1): 1–21.

De Silva, V., S. Thapa, L. R. Wiilens, M. G. Farr, K. Jayanaghe, and M. J. Mahan. 1988. "Compensatory Payments and Vasectomy Acceptance in Urban Sri Lanka." *Journal of Biosocial Science* 20 (2): 143–56.

Director of Health Services. 1968. Circular My No. PB44/66 to the Superintendents of Health Services (SHS), April 7, 1968.

Evaluation Subcommittee. 1968. "Targets for Ceylon's National Family Planning Program," Report to the Family Planning Advisory Committee, unpublished report, Evaluation Subcommittee, Colombo.

Family Health Bureau. 1984. *Family Health Impact Survey, Sri Lanka, 1981–2*." Colombo: Ministry of Health.

Fernando, Dallas F. S. 1972. "Recent Fertility Decline in Ceylon." *Population Studies* 26 (3): 445–53.

Frederiksen, Harald 1961. "Determinants and Consequences of Mortality Trends in Ceylon." *Public Health Reports* 76 (August): 659–63.

Greenberg, D. S. 1962. "Birth Control: Swedish Government Has Ambitious Program to Offer Help to Underdeveloped Nations." *Science,* September 28. Reprinted in *Population Bulletin* 19 (1): 19–23.

Hyrenius, Hannes, and Ulla Ahs. 1968. *The Sweden-Ceylon Family Planning Pilot Project*. Report 6. Goteborg, Sweden: University of Goteborg, Demographic Institute.

Kinch, Arne. N.d. (but probably end of 1965). "Provisional Scheme for a Nationwide Family Planning program in Ceylon: 1966–1976." Unpublished report, Colombo.

———. 1966. "Ceylon." In *Family Planning and Population Programs*, ed. Bernard Berelson, Richmond K. Anderson, Oscar Harkavy, John Maier, W. Parker Mauldin, and Sheldon Segal, 105–10. Chicago: University of Chicago Press.

Manor, James. 1989. *The Expedient Utopian: Bandaranaike and Ceylon*. Cambridge, U.K.: Cambridge University Press.

Meegama, S. A. 1967. "Malaria Eradication and Its Effect on Mortality Levels." *Population Studies* 21 (November): 207–37.

Ministry of Health. 1985. *Annual Health Bulletin, Sri Lanka*. Colombo: Ministry of Health.

Ministry of Plan Implementation. 1980. *Family Planning Above Party Politics: Proceedings of a Seminar on Population and Development*. Colombo: Ministry of Plan Implementation.

———. 1983. *Voluntary Sterilization Programme in Sri Lanka*. Colombo: Population Division.

Ministry of Plan Implementation and Research Triangle Institute. N.d. *A Study of the Cost Effectiveness of the National Family Planning Programme in Sri Lanka, 1975–1981*. Research Triangle Park, NC: Ministry of Plan Implementation, Population Division.

Ministry of Plan Implementation and Westinghouse Health Systems. 1983. *Sri Lanka Contraceptive Prevalence Survey Report, 1982*. Colombo: Ministry of Plan Implementation, Department of Census and Statistics.

Ministry of Plan Implementation and Westinghouse Institute for Resource Development. 1988. *Sri Lanka, Demographic and Health Survey, 1987*. Colombo: Ministry of Plan Implementation, Department of Census and Statistics.

National Planning Council. 1959. *The Ten Year Plan*. Colombo: Government Press.

Newman, Peter. 1965. *Malaria Eradication and Population Growth, with Special Reference to Ceylon and British Guiana*. Research Series 10. Ann Arbor: University of Michigan, School of Public Health.

Nycander, Gunnel. 1971. "Family Planning in the Field: Standardized Observations of Field Midwives' Working Behavior and Analysis of Factors Affecting the Quality and Outcome of the Ceylonese Field Programme." Report prepared for the Swedish International Development Cooperation Agency, Colombo.

Population Reference Bureau. 2006. *Data Sheet*. Washington, DC: Population Reference Bureau.

Potts, Malcolm. 1978. *Review of Population and Family Planning Activities in Sri Lanka*. Colombo: Overseas Development Agency and Ministry of Plan Implementation.

Ross, John A., Marjorie Rich, Janet Molzan, and Michael Pensak. 1988. *Family Planning and Child Survival*. New York: Columbia University, Center for Population and Family Health.

Ryan, Bruce. 1954. "Hinayana Buddhism and Family Planning in Ceylon." In *The Interrelations of Demographic, Economic, and Social Problems*, 90–102. New York: Milbank Memorial Fund.

Thapa, S., M. Salgado, J. Fortney, Gary Grubb, and V. De Silva. 1988. "Women's Perceptions of the Pill's Potential Health Risks in Sri Lanka." *Asia-Pacific Population Journal* 2 (3): 39–56.

Tornberg, G. 1965. *Some Findings from a Family Planning Pilot Project in One Rural Area*. Report prepared for the Swedish International Development Cooperation Agency.

UNFPA (United Nations Population Fund). 1980. *Sri Lanka: Report of a Mission on Needs Assessment for Population Assistance*. Report 36. New York: UNFPA.

UNICEF (United Nations Children's Fund). 1986. *Perinatal and Neonatal Mortality: Some Aspects of Maternal and Child Health in Sri Lanka*. Action Research Series, Monograph 1. Colombo: UNICEF and Department of Census and Statistics.

Vittachi, Tarzie. 1958. *Emergency 58, The Story of the Ceylon Race Riots*. London: Andre Deutsch.

Wahren, Carl. 1968. "The Role of Family Planning in Sweden's Development Assistance Program." Paper prepared for the U.S. Information Service.

Wijesooriya, N. G. 1971. "Report on Some Aspects of the Family Planning Program in 21 Health Areas." In *Family Planning in the Field*, ed. Gunnel Nycander, appendix 6, 1–9. Report prepared for the Swedish International Development Cooperation Agency, Colombo.

World Fellowship of Buddhists. 1969. "Family Planning" (editorial). *News Bulletin*, April 13, pp. 43–45.

World Health Organization. 1978. *Terminal Report on Family Health Project, 1973–77.* Geneva: World Health Organization.

Wright, Nicholas H. 1968. "Recent Fertility Change in Ceylon and Prospects for the National Family Program." *Demography* 5 (2): 745–56.

———. 1970a. "Ceylon: The Relationship of Demographic Factors and Marital Fertility to the Recent Fertility Decline." *Studies in Family Planning* 1 (59): 17–20.

———. 1970b. "Status of the Family Planning Program, End of 1969." Memorandum to C. Balasingham, Permanent Secretary, Ministry of Health.

———. 1984. *Report on the Sri Lankan Incentive Program for Voluntary Sterilization.* New York: Association for Voluntary Sterilization.

———. 1985. *Observations and Recommendations on Voluntarism and Medical Quality in Sri Lanka's Surgical Contraception Program.* Report 85-26-014. Colombia: U.S. Agency for International Development and Ministry of Plan Implementation, Office of Population.

Wright, Nicholas H., and Terrence Perera 1973. "Ceylon: Continuing Practice of Contraception by Acceptors of Oral Contraception and Intrauterine Devices in a Field Program." *Bulletin of the World Health Organization* 48 (6): 639–47.

21 Emergence and Development of Nepal's Family Planning Program

JAYANTI M. TULADHAR

Nepal, a relatively small country in comparison with its neighbors, is bounded by China to the north and India to the south. It has three distinct ecological zones: mountains, hills, and plains. The three zones are different not only in terms of climatic conditions, but also in terms of population density, living conditions, livelihoods, and economic conditions. The country is predominantly rural, and its people are mainly farmers who belong to more than 75 castes and ethnic groups.

Because of the harsh terrain, the mountain areas are less developed and have limited transportation and communication facilities, which restricts movement by people and also hinders their products from reaching marketplaces. Only 7 percent of the population resides in the mountain areas. The hills region is relatively more advanced on all development fronts and accounts for about 44 percent of the population. It has a number of fertile valleys and places of interest that attract foreign tourists, who bring revenue into the country. Almost half of the population (49 percent) lives in the plains region, which accounts for 23 percent of the total land area and is the most fertile part of the country. The region became livable after the eradication of malaria, and many people from the hills moved to settle there. This region is better off than the other two in terms of transportation and communication facilities and has attracted investors to establish industries.

The country's population doubled from 11.6 million in 1971 to 23.2 million in 2001, and is likely to have doubled again by 2031 given the current rate of population growth (2.3 percent per year in 2001). The urban population has increased at a much faster pace than the general population because of internal migration, and according to the 2001 census, it accounted for 14 percent of the total population (table 21.1).

Emergence of Family Planning, 1959–75

Family planning emerged both in the public (government) sector and in the private sector. The following subsections discuss each of these in turn.

363

TABLE 21.1 Selected Demographic Indicators, Selected Years

Category	1971	1981	1991	2001
Population (millions)	11.6	15.0	18.5	23.2
Percentage of the population by age group				
0–14 years	40.5	41.4	42.4	—
15–64 years	56.4	55.4	54.1	—
65+ years	3.1	3.2	3.5	—
Population density per square kilometer	79	102	126	158
Percentage of the population living in urban areas	4.0	6.4	9.2	14.2
Crude birth rate (live births per 1,000 population)	42	44	42	34
Total fertility rate (number of births per woman)	6.3	6.3	5.6	4.1
Infant mortality rate (deaths per 1,000 births)	172	117	97	64
Life expectancy (years)				
Male	42.0	50.9	55.0	—
Female	40.0	48.1	53.5	—
Mean age at marriage (years)				
Males	20.8	20.7	21.4	—
Females	16.8	17.2	18.2	—

Source: Central Bureau of Statistics 1995, 2001.

Note: — = not available.

Public Sector

Government-provided family planning services became available in 1965, soon after King Mahendra's address to parliament in support of the Third Five-Year Plan (1965–70). He stated, "In order to bring equilibrium between the population growth and economic output of the country, my Government has adopted a policy of family planning." The family planning program started offering its services in Kathmandu and then extended to cover the whole Kathmandu Valley as part of the maternal and child health program run by the Department of Health Services (DHS). Box 21.1 presents a timeline of major events in relation to family planning in Nepal.

The family planning program accelerated in 1968 with the formation of a semi-autonomous board, the Nepal Family Planning and Maternal and Child Health (FP/MCH) Board, chaired by the minister of health. The board's mandate was to make FP/MCH services and information available throughout the country. The board was soon reshuffled, with the director general of health services becoming chair; one representative each from the ministries of Health, Finance, and Education as members; and the chief of the Nepal FP/MCH Project as an ex-officio member secretary. The board was responsible for setting its own project policies, including in relation to human resources and activities. Implementation of the board's policies and activities was done through the Nepal FP/MCH Project, which was not autonomous like the board, but was administratively under the Ministry of Health.

Expansion of the family planning program was gradual outside the Kathmandu Valley with the establishment of 25 district-level family planning offices in 1969,

BOX 21.1 Timeline of Major Events

1959:	Family Planning Association of Nepal is founded.
1965:	The government begins to offer family planning services.
1968:	The national program accelerates with the formation of the Family Planning and Maternal and Child Health Board, chaired by the minister of health.
	The U.S. Agency for International Development begins to provide assistance.
1968–69:	Payments begin to providers for intrauterine devices and sterilizations and to clients choosing sterilization for work time lost.
1969:	Twenty-five district-level family planning offices are established.
1970:	The Integrated Community Health Services Development Project is established to provide health services, including family planning, by means of an integrated approach.
1972:	Thirty more district-level family planning offices are added.
1973:	Forty more district-level family planning offices are added.
Mid-1970s:	The Family Planning and Maternal and Child Health Project initiates sterilization and other services by means of mobile camps and also begins door-to-door visits.
	Alternative field approaches are tested experimentally.
1975:	The Fifth Five-Year Plan (1975–80) set targets to reduce the total fertility rate from 6.3 to 5.8 births per woman and the infant mortality rate from 200 deaths per 1,000 population to 150 during the plan period.
1976:	The United Nations Population Fund begins to provide assistance. Other donors help subsequently.
	The first nationally representative survey is conducted under the world fertility survey series. Subsequent surveys are carried out every five years.
1978:	The Nepal Contraceptive Retail Sales Company initiates social marketing of condoms and contraceptive pills through pharmacies and general stores.
1980:	The Sixth Five-Year Plan (1980–85) aims to reduce the population growth rate to 2.6 percent per year by 1985 and 1.2 percent per year by 2000 and to reduce the total fertility rate from 5.4 births per woman in 1985 to 4.0 by 1990 and 2.5 by 2000.
1982:	The Family Planning Association began small-scale integrated projects for health, agricultural development, and rural improvement.
1987:	The government decides that all health services, including family planning, must be integrated in all 75 districts. The Ministry of Health is restructured.
1993:	The 1987 changes are largely reversed.

30 more in 1972, and another 40 in 1973, through which a number of FP/MCH centers provided information and services. While district offices concentrated on program administration, the FP/MCH centers and clinics provided services. Depending on the availability of staff members, the typical FP/MCH clinic inserted intrauterine devices (IUDs), distributed contraceptive pills and condoms, and prepared patients for vasectomies, in addition to undertaking maternal and child health activities (prenatal and postnatal care). Outside the clinic setting, health aides were the program's key workers, making home visits to create demand and to follow up with family planning clients. Health aides were local women aged 20 years or older with at least eight years of schooling followed by six weeks of paramedical training (Taylor and Thapa 1972).

In the mid-1970s, the Nepal FP/MCH Project started providing services through mobile camps, especially sterilization (Nepal FP/MCH Project 1976), and through door-to-door services using *panchayat*-based health workers from the mid-1970s onward (Nepal FP/MCH Project 1988).[1]

During the 1970s, the project was also experimenting with various approaches for providing family planning services in rural areas. The following experimental programs were tested (Gubahju and others 1975):

- Use of village-based fieldworkers with multiple responsibilities

- Use of husband-and-wife teams and older women as family planning workers

- Use of an intensive worker approach using other government extension workers and female volunteers, supported by mass media and education campaigns

- Distribution of contraceptives using commercial outlets

- Tests of FP/MCH service delivery methods in areas where communication was difficult because of the terrain.

An especially significant experimental venture involved a type of integration. The family planning program was established from the beginning in a spirit of integrating its work with maternal and child health services. This approach was partly in response to Nepal's high child mortality rate, which in turn led to a greater focus on providing services for current children rather than reducing the number of future children (Taylor and Thapa 1972).

Thus, while the family planning program was receiving significant attention during the 1960s and 1970s, the government was also committed to providing basic health services, which included family planning, at the community level using an integrated approach.[2] As a trial, the government started providing family planning services as well as other services through the Community Health and Integration Division of the DHS with the idea of integrating all vertical projects in the two districts of Bara and Kaski. One appeal of this approach was a possible reduction in overhead and service delivery costs, resulting in a more cost-effective way to provide services in rural areas (Justice 1989). The pilot project was designed and funded by international donor agencies.

In the Kaski district, three health posts were chosen to examine whether malaria workers could perform additional tasks, including providing information on family planning during home visits. In the Bara district, 11 health posts were each divided into 3 to 7 localities with an average population of 5,000. Each locality was staffed with a village health worker, who received six weeks of basic health training and was responsible for providing ambulatory medical care, including family planning information and services and basic maternal health information and services (prenatal care, delivery, postnatal care). Each health post had an auxiliary nurse-midwife who provided FP/MCH services at the health post and during home visits.

Although the evaluation of this pilot project revealed problems in relation to both its concept and its implementation (Justice 1989), the integration process was extended to 4 more districts in 1975 and then to 23 of the country's 75 districts by fiscal 1986/87. (The FP/MCH Project was only operational in 52 districts.)

Private Sector

The Family Planning Association of Nepal, a nongovernmental organization (NGO) established in 1959, was responsible for pioneering work and is still one of the largest NGOs in Nepal, providing information and services in close cooperation and collaboration with the government. In 1982, the Family Planning Association of Nepal started operating a number of small-scale, integrated projects. These projects offered family planning information and services, as well as health, agricultural development, and rural improvement programs in selected districts.

Other nonprofit NGOs, both local and international, also operated in the country, such as mothers' clubs, the organization for ex-servicemen, the Nepal Red Cross, the Save the Children Fund USA, and Save the Children UK. All these organizations operated in selected areas, covering small target populations as pilot projects and concentrating on the educational and motivational aspects of family planning with limited service delivery components (contraceptive pills and condoms).

In addition, the Nepal Contraceptive Retail Sales Company, a nonprofit social marketing organization, was established in 1978 to distribute condoms and pills at nominal cost through existing retail outlets, such as pharmacies and general stores (Hamal 1986). After four years of operations, its products were available through 10,000 retail shops in 60 districts.

Goals of the National Family Planning Program

The family planning program was introduced with the objective of balancing population growth and economic growth (Tuladhar 1989). Each five-year plan contained specific goals. At the beginning of the program, the goal was to maintain the population at 16 to 22 million (Nepal FP/MCH n.d.). Demographic targets were set in the Fifth Five-Year Plan (1975–80), with the aim of reducing the crude birth rate from 40 live births per 1,000 population to 38 and the infant mortality rate from 200 deaths per 1,000 births to 150 over the five-year period. The total fertility rate was targeted to decline from 6.3 births per woman to 5.8 during the same period.

In the Sixth Five-Year Plan (1980–85), the aim was to stabilize the annual population growth rate at 2.6 percent per year. To supplement the plan, the government also came up with the long-term goal of reducing the population growth rate to 1.2 percent by 2000 and the total fertility rate from 5.4 births per woman in 1985 to 4.0 by 1990 and 2.5 by 2000 (Pant 1983).

Later, the government translated its long-term goal of reaching a total fertility rate of 2.5 by 2000 into numbers of new family planning acceptors, with a method mix among acceptors of contraceptive pills (15 percent of all contraceptive users), condoms (64 percent), sterilization (20 percent), IUD (0.4 percent), and injectables (0.9 percent) by 1982/83, with increasing shares over the years for all methods except condoms, which would lose share (Tuladhar 1989).

In time, additional changes took place. For the period from 1997 to 2017, the government's second long-term health plan (Ministry of Health 1999) states the following targets: reducing the total fertility rate to 3.05 births per woman, lowering the crude birth rate to 26.6 live births per 1,000 population, and increasing contraceptive use to 58.2 percent of couples.

Policies and Strategies for Reaching the Goals

In the early days of the family planning program, during the 1970–75 plan, the strategy was to develop basic infrastructure, such as building facilities, establishing district administrative centers, training paramedics, developing a supply system, and collecting data for program evaluation. The FP/MCH Board adopted the following five basic strategies to make services available (Nepal FP/MCH n.d.):

- Integrating maternal and child health services and family planning at all service delivery points

- Providing financial incentives to part-time medical and paramedical staff members involved in providing family planning services

- Selling contraceptives at a nominal rate where possible

- Distributing nonclinical contraceptives (condoms) through commercial channels

- Using mobile teams to provide family planning services in remote places on demand.

The program had incentives for both providers and clients. Providers were given cash payments for sterilizing clients and for inserting IUDs starting in 1968–69, while clients who had undergone sterilization were compensated for wages or work time lost.

As the family planning program began to mature and develop momentum, its policies became an integral part of Nepal's development plans, with a focus on encouraging a small family norm through education and employment programs (that is, on dealing with long-term concerns). The intent of the education and employment programs was to raise women's status and decrease infant mortality.

Program Assistance

The family planning program started with a budget of just US$3,000 in fiscal 1966, followed by US$369,000 in fiscal 1970, US$639,000 in fiscal 1974, and US$1.04 million in fiscal 1975 (Tuladhar and Stoeckel 1977). This government-initiated program received financial and technical support from the U.S. Agency for International Development as early as 1968, while the United Nations Population Fund provided financial support from 1976 onward. The World Health Organization provided technical support for family planning that was directed toward the integration of health services. Subsequently, a number of multilateral partners such as the World Bank also provided assistance, as did bilateral partners such as the German Agency for Technical Cooperation, the U.K. Department for International Development, and the Japan International Cooperation Agency. International NGOs were also actively involved, providing technical as well as financial support to the program.

Organizational Structure and Functions

As explained earlier, the Nepal FP/MCH Project fell under the auspices of the semi-autonomous Nepal FP/MCH Board, which was responsible for making family planning services and information available, undertaking research and training, and managing all required inputs. Even though the project was under the direction of the board, administratively it was under the Ministry of Health and operated through its field structures. Thus, it was decentralized through a four-tier system involving (a) the project's central office, (b) 5 regional offices, (c) 40 district offices serving 52 of the country's 75 administrative districts, and (d) 258 clinics and 2,596 *panchayat*-based centers.

In the 52 districts, the project provided information and family planning services through its clinics, which were attached to various preexisting health institutions that were already staffed by *panchayat*-based health workers. In addition to the resident staff members of the health institutions, the FP/MCH Project assigned a minimum of two workers full time to deliver information and services on FP/MCH activities (Tuladhar 1989).

Each FP/MCH clinic distributed condoms and contraceptive pills and provided information to those who came to the clinics. At the same time, the clinics provided maternal and child health services, including education on nutrition and sanitation. Some clinics were attached to hospitals and provided additional services, such as sterilization, IUD insertion, and injectables, depending on the availability of equipment and trained doctors. Most workers involved in service delivery activities provided follow-up services at users' homes, as well as motivation for potential clients within a radius of 3 miles from the clinic where they worked. Selected FP/MCH clinics, particularly those attached to a hospital, operated satellite clinics in nearby areas to provide information on FP/MCH and to distribute pills and condoms.

Panchayat-based health centers were run by *panchayat*-based health workers, who provided door-to-door services and information and were also responsible for the following (Tuladhar 1989):

- Maintaining ward registers to identify potential acceptors in village *panchayats* and dates of acceptance and methods used by acceptors

- Providing information, motivation, and education on family planning

- Distributing condoms and contraceptive pills

- Distributing oral rehydration solution for the treatment of dehydration resulting from diarrhea, as well as iron tablets for mothers

- Providing education on hygiene

- Referring sick mothers and children to health posts, health centers, or hospitals

- Disseminating information about voluntary sterilization camps.

The *panchayat*-based health workers program was a unique feature of the FP/MCH Project. First initiated as a pilot, its success was mainly due to the appointment of one worker per *panchayat*, regular supervision by more senior staff members, regular training and retraining, and a strong monitoring system. The program was expanded after the successful pilot to address the need to expand services in close proximity to potential users. *Panchayat*-based health workers were recruited locally on a one-year contractual basis with the recommendation of the village *panchayat* head and were supervised by so-called intermediate supervisors, who worked directly under district family planning officers.

In 20 of Nepal's 75 districts, the family planning program fell under the Community Health and Integration Project of the DHS, which was established in 1969. In 1970, this project was transferred to the Integration Board constituted in the Ministry of Health.

The task of integration was complex and involved a number of governmental and nongovernmental agencies. Various kinds of coordination mechanisms were needed as project activities and resources were moved from one organization to another. In 1987, the government decided that all health services, including family planning, would be provided by merging all vertical projects in all 75 districts. The Ministry of Health was restructured to accommodate most staff members in the vertical projects. With this restructuring, the Integrated Community Health Services Development Project was abolished and converted into the Public Health Division. All other vertical projects ceased having a separate identity by 1990. Integrated health services, including family planning, have been made available through district public health offices. The implementation of any family planning activity is to be done by district public health offices through regional health directorate offices and the Public Health Division.

Under the new structure of the Ministry of Health, the FP/MCH Project was given a new role to play in relation to family planning. The *panchayat*-based health workers were gradually phased out and were replaced by village health workers, who were responsible for all basic health services, including family planning and maternal and child health. The FP/MCH Project was limited to the following tasks (Nepal FP/MCH Project 1988):

- Developing policies and programs for family planning activities

- Carrying out central-level supervision and monitoring of family planning activities

- Helping implementing units to develop supervision and monitoring systems

- Negotiating with donors for program assistance

- Assisting local officials in establishing district-level family planning targets and programs

- Providing financial and logistical support to district public health offices and regional health directorate offices

- Helping to develop the trained manpower required for the program

- Providing information, education, and communication support

- Providing technical support to district public health offices and regional health directorate offices

- Evaluating the family planning program.

Family Planning under the Current Health Service Structure

In 1993, the 1987 changes were largely reversed. The responsibilities of the DHS now include implementing, monitoring, and supervising the various preventive, promotional, rehabilitative, and curative health programs. These functions are carried out through the department's divisions, centers, regional health directorates, and district health offices.

The family planning program has been fully subsumed under the DHS as one of eight essential components for reproductive health, all within the context of primary health care (DHS 1998). The Logistics Management Division of the DHS is responsible for procurement, warehousing, and distribution of reproductive health commodities, including family planning supplies.

Reproductive health services are provided throughout the country under the directives of the DHS, which delivers preventive and curative health services, including promotional activities. The subhealth post is the first contact point for basic health care and referral services, and in practice, it is also the referral center for traditional birth attendants, female community health volunteers, and community-based activities such as immunizations and primary health care. Each level above the subhealth post is a referral point in a hierarchical network designed to ensure the availability of basic health services and to make minor treatment accessible and affordable. Logistical, financial, supervisory, and technical support is provided to each lower level from the one above.

The institutions involved in the delivery of basic health services during 2001 to 2002 included 78 hospitals, 188 primary health centers or health centers, 608 health posts, and 3,129 subhealth posts. At the community level, Nepal had 48,307 female community health volunteers, 15,553 traditional birth attendants, and 14,769 primary health care outreach clinics. All these are to some extent involved in providing family planning information, services, or both to clients.

Family Planning Program Performance

Over the past four decades, the family planning program has experienced many challenges and has dealt with them by experimenting with different service delivery modalities, by increasing the program's coverage, and by improving the quality of services. It has also conducted various studies and has gathered extensive data through such means as national fertility and family planning surveys. The following subsection briefly reviews the program's performance based on the national surveys. The first was in 1976 and was conducted by the Nepal FP/MCH Project as part of the world fertility survey series. Subsequently, surveys of this type have taken place every five years, namely, the contraceptive prevalence survey (1981); the Nepal fertility and family planning survey (1986); and the demographic and health survey (1991, 1996, 2001, 2006).

Knowledge

Knowledge is a prerequisite for changed attitudes and behavior, and like other national programs, Nepal's program focused on information, education, and communication activities from the beginning. Table 21.2 presents information about knowledge of various family planning methods among currently married women during 1976 to 2001. In 1976, only 21.3 percent of currently married women knew of at least one family planning method. This figure increased remarkably to more than 50 percent by 1981 and to 99 percent by 2001. Knowledge about both temporary and permanent methods increased over the period. The percentage increases were greatest between 1986 and 1991 for all methods. This suggests that information, education, and communication activities were more intense and effective during that period. Among the modern methods, sterilization (male and female), followed by injectables, the pill, and condoms, are now the best known. The IUD, even though it was one of the first modern methods introduced into the program, is among the least well known.

TABLE 21.2 Knowledge of Family Planning Methods, Selected Years
percentage of currently married women who know about each modern method of contraception

Method	1976	1981	1986	1991	1996	2001
Any modern method	21.3	51.9	55.9	92.7	98.3	99.5
Female sterilization	13.0	44.4	51.2	88.8	96.3	99.1
Male sterilization	15.7	38.1	43.1	85.3	89.7	98.2
Pill	12.0	25.1	27.8	65.8	80.5	93.4
IUD	6.0	8.4	6.7	24.1	35.9	54.7
Injectable	n.a.	9.0	13.5	64.7	85.0	97.3
Condom	4.8	13.6	16.8	51.6	75.3	91.0
Implant	n.a.	n.a.	n.a.	34.6	57.3	79.8
Diaphragm, foam, jelly	n.a.	n.a.	n.a.	19.0	28.3	40.2

Source: 1976–96: 1996 Nepal Family Health Survey (table 4.2); 2001: 2001 Nepal Demographic and Health Survey (table 5.1).

Note: n.a. = not applicable.

TABLE 21.3 Use of Modern Contraceptive Methods, Selected Years
percentage of currently married women using modern contraceptive methods

Method	1976	1981	1986	1991	1996	2001
Any modern method	2.9	7.6	15.1	24.1	28.8	38.9
Female sterilization	0.1	2.6	6.8	12.1	13.3	16.5
Male sterilization	1.9	3.2	6.2	7.5	6.0	7.0
IUD	0.1	0.1	0.1	0.2	0.3	0.4
Pill	0.5	1.2	0.9	1.1	1.5	1.8
Injectable	0.0	0.1	0.5	2.3	5.0	9.3
Condom	0.3	0.4	0.6	0.6	2.1	3.2
Implant	n.a.	n.a.	n.a.	0.3	0.5	0.7

Source: Ministry of Health, New ERA, and ORC Macro 2002.

Current Use

During 1976 to 2001, the percentage of currently married women using modern contraceptives increased from 2.9 to 38.9 (table 21.3), an average annual increase of 1.44 percentage points per year, a relatively impressive pace compared with international experience. Female sterilization has continued to be the dominant method. At the beginning of the program, it offered couples only five modern methods of contraception: female sterilization, male sterilization, the pill, the IUD, and the condom. Since then, the injectable has become important. The implant is also available, while use of the IUD has remained low. As of 2001, the most widely used methods were female sterilization (16.5 percent), injectables (9.3 percent), and male sterilization (7.0 percent). Traditional methods are not popular in Nepal.

Sterilization Regret and Quality of Care

Sterilization has been, and continues to be, the major thrust of the family planning program. Mobile sterilization camps are organized around the country each year and those who are sterilized receive some financial compensation. Almost two-thirds of contraceptive users (60 percent) are using sterilization (male or female). The extent of regret about opting for sterilization may serve as an indicator of the quality of care (informed choice, choice of method, counseling, and provision of good quality services) offered by the program. Overall sterilization regret among currently married women who are sterilized or whose husbands are sterilized is about 8 percent according to the 2001 survey. The percentage was slightly higher in 1996 (9 percent). (Older international studies have indicated that sterilization regret ranges from about 7 to 17 percent.[3]) Both the 1996 and the 2001 surveys suggested that sterilization regret was due to side effects after the procedure. The declines in sterilization regret and in regret because of side effects between 1996 and 2001, while small, suggest that the quality of care might have improved slightly during the period.

Family planning users are largely dependent on the public sector for services and supplies (table 21.4). Between 1996 and 2001, there were only small changes in the

Table 21.4 Sources of Supply for Users of Modern Methods, 1996 and 2001
percentage of users of modern methods of contraception

Method	Public 1996	Public 2001	Private medical 1996	Private medical 2001	Other private 1996	Other private 2001
Female sterilization	87.7	85.8	9.1	6.8	3.1	7.3
Male sterilization	85.2	84.6	11.1	11.7	3.8	3.7
Pill	39.7	55.3	36.4	7.6	23.9	37.2
IUD	60.8	65.4	29.2	11.2	10.0	23.4
Injectables	85.9	86.0	13.5	5.1	0.6	9.0
Condom	34.1	46.0	38.3	4.2	27.7	49.8
Implants	87.6	51.5	12.4	42.3	—	6.2

Source: 1996 and 2001 Demographic and Health Surveys.
Note: — = not available.

proportions of users who received services and supplies from the public sector except in the case of the pill, the condom, and the implant.

Availability and Accessibility

Access to contraception has improved over time because of the expansion of health institutions and the increased number of female community health volunteers, who distribute contraceptives, especially condoms and pills. According to available information, in 1976, half of married women said that it took more than a day to reach a service delivery point. This improved to 2 hours or more in 1991 and then to 30 minutes in 2001 (Thapa and Pandey 1994).

Unmet Need

The demand for family planning is quite high based on the level of current use plus the level of unmet need. Unmet need is defined as those who say that they do not want any more children or that they want to wait two or more years before having another child, but are not using contraception. In the 2001 survey, unmet need for family planning was approximately 28 percent, 11 percent for spacing, and 16 percent for those not wanting more children. At the same time, the survey revealed a substantial gap between the total wanted fertility rate (2.5 births per woman) and the total actual fertility rate (4.1 births per woman). This implies that Nepalese women want fewer children than they are currently having. More unwanted pregnancies could be avoided by having a more aggressive family planning program.

Conclusion

Nepal's family planning program has been part of the country's national five-year economic plans, with their fertility reduction objectives. The focus has been on marital fertility and contraceptive use, as distinct from changes in the age of marriage or the use of induced abortion. While the program's impact is difficult to assess, the country has been making progress in reducing fertility and increasing contraceptive use, with increased public awareness and enhanced accessibility of family planning services, which are still largely provided by government health institutions. The 2006 national survey showed remarkable advances: the TFR fell from 4.1 in 2001 to 3.1 in 2006, and 44 percent of married women were using a modern method, up from 26 percent in 1996 and 35 percent in 2001. Nevertheless, demand and unmet need are still high, and services need to be expanded and made more effective to further reduce unwanted pregnancies.

Some lessons learned include the following:

- The early program decision to focus on developing basic infrastructure, such as physical facilities and human resources, helped accelerate the implementation of services during the ensuing years.

- The numerous experimental programs that were initiated early helped in the search for effective mechanisms to improve performance.

- The integration of family planning into broader health services during the 1970s, while in theory a good concept, occurred too soon, possibly hampering acceleration of the program because of a dilution of human resources.

- The involvement of the private sector and of NGOs was insufficient until 1990, perhaps because of a nonconducive political and economic environment before that time (a multiparty democracy was established in 1990).

Notes

1. During most of the period under discussion, Nepal was divided geographically into more than 4,000 *panchayats*, each consisting of nine wards, with each ward made up of one or more villages. The *panchayat* system was also partly political, and thus the term resists translation.
2. Basic health services, which were offered through district hospitals and rural health posts, were defined as immunizations; assistance to mothers during pregnancy and delivery; postnatal care and health services for children; contraceptive advice and services; adequate, safe, and accessible water supplies; sanitation and vector control; health and nutrition education; diagnosis and treatment of simple diseases; first aid and emergency treatment; and referral facilities (Justice 1989).
3. For those studies, see http://www.engenderhealth.org/res/offc/steril/factbook/pdf/chapter_5.pdf#search = %22Philliber%20and%20Philliber%2C%201985%22.

References

Central Bureau of Statistics. 1995. *Population Monograph of Nepal*. Kathmandu: Central Bureau of Statistics.

———. 2001. *Population Census 2001 of Nepal*. Provisional Population Report 2001. Kathmandu: Central Bureau of Statistics.

DHS (Department of Health Services). 1998. *National Reproductive Health Strategy*. Kathmandu: Family Health Division of Department of Health Services, Ministry of Health.

Gubahju, B., B. R. Pande, J. Tuladhar, and J. Stoeckel. 1975. "Experimental Family Planning Program in Nepal." Paper presented at the "Seminar on Population, Family Planning and Development in Nepal," University of California, Berkeley, September 24–29.

Hamal, Hem B. 1986. *Marketing Family Planning in Nepal: A Study of Consumers and Retailers*. Kathmandu: Nepal Contraceptive Retail Sales Company.

Justice, Judith. 1989. *Policies, Plans and People—Foreign Aid and Health Development: Comparative Studies of Health Systems and Medical Care*. Berkeley, CA: University of California Press.

Ministry of Health. 1999. "Executive Summary." In *Second Long-Term Health Plan: 1997–2017*. Kathmandu: Ministry of Health.

Ministry of Health, New ERA, and ORC Macro. 2002. *Nepal Demographic and Health Survey 2001*. Calverton, MD: Ministry of Health, Family Health Division; New ERA; and ORC Macro.

Nepal FP/MCH (Family Planning/Maternal and Child Health) Project. 1976. *Annual Report: 1975–76*. Kathmandu: His Majesty's Government, Ministry of Health.

———. 1988. *Workplan for Family Planning Activities*. Kathmandu: His Majesty's Government, Ministry of Health.

———. N.d. "Draft of Fourth Five-Year Plan." Monograph, His Majesty's Government, Kathmandu.

Pant, Yadav P. 1983. *Population Growth and Employment Opportunities in Nepal*. New Delhi: Oxford University Press and IBH Publishing.

Taylor, Daniel, and Rita Thapa. 1972. *Nepal*. Country Profiles Series. New York: Population Council.

Thapa, Shyam, and Kalyan R. Pandey. 1994. "Family Planning in Nepal: An Update." *Journal of the Nepal Medical Association* 32 (111): 131–43.

Tuladhar, Jayanti Man. 1989. *The Persistence of High Fertility in Nepal*. New Delhi: Inter-India Publications.

Tuladhar, Jayanti Man, and John Stoeckel. 1977. "Nepal." In *Family Planning in the Developing World: A Review of Programs*, ed. Walter B. Watson. New York: Population Council, 35.

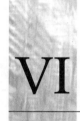

VI Sub-Saharan Africa

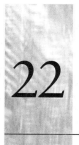

22 Family Planning in Ghana

JOHN C. CALDWELL AND FRED T. SAI

Among all the regions of the developing world, fertility decline and family planning programs came last to Sub-Saharan Africa. Good reasons account for this. Indeed, foundations and governments, and accordingly technical aid programs, doubted the value of introducing population programs to the region in the 1960s, as the countries were poor, attitudes were mostly pro-natalist, and independence was recent.

The early Population Council program in Ghana happened largely by accident, but Ghana turned out to be a fortunate setting. It was the earliest European colony in Sub-Saharan Africa to win its independence, doing so as early as 1957. It was also relatively rich, exporting large amounts of cocoa, gold, bauxite, industrial diamonds, and mahogany. In the early 1960s, its spending on education as a proportion of national income was the highest in the world. It was not riven by serious ethnic conflicts or demands to divide the country into separate nations. Above all, modernizing attitudes were widespread, both under President Kwame Nkrumah and under later regimes. Admittedly, Nkrumah's socialist beliefs led him to oppose family planning programs, but not the demographic research that implied the need for such programs.

Ghana had been a British colony, and in contrast to Belgian, French, Portuguese, and Spanish colonies, it had no history of official pro-natalism or attempts to prevent the sale of contraceptives (Caldwell 1966). Indeed, European officials and business people working or living in Ghana had been able to purchase condoms, diaphragms, jellies, and foaming tablets freely prior to Nkrumah's interference. In addition, at a time when family planning initiatives came predominantly from English-speaking countries, having English as the official language was advantageous. Not only were the first Population Council or U.S. Agency for International Development staff members likely to go to English-speaking countries, but so were early representatives of the Pathfinder Fund and the International Planned Parenthood Federation.

At the same time, a series of factors powerfully weighted the balance in the opposite direction (Caldwell 1968a, 1968b; Oppong 1977; Salway 1994). African families, at least in rural areas, tended to benefit from being large: the family was the production unit for farm work and children were considered a form of wealth and

BOX 22.1 Timeline of Main Events

1957: Ghana wins its independence from the United Kingdom, the first European colony in Sub-Saharan Africa to do so.

1959: St. Clair Drake visits President Nkrumah and encourages the creation of a demographic program, later provided by the Population Council with resident advisers from 1960 to 1966.

Late 1950s: Nkrumah decides that Ghana should be included in the 1960 round of censuses sponsored by the United Nations.

1962: Census data become available for analyses to inform policy development and demographic instruction.

1964: The Seven-Year Development Plan (1964–70) notes that national population growth may be excessive.

1965: Ghana participates in two key international conferences, one in Geneva sponsored by the Population Council and the Ford Foundation, and one in Belgrade sponsored by the United Nations and the International Union for the Scientific Study of Population.

1965–66: Representatives of the International Planned Parenthood Federation and other international agencies initiate regular contacts.

1966: Ghanaian representatives participate in the First African Population Conference in Ibadan, Nigeria.

The total fertility rate is estimated at the extremely high level of 7.0 births per woman, and the population growth rate is estimated at 3.0 percent per year.

1966: A military coup in February ends Nkrumah's government.

1967: The Planned Parenthood Association of Ghana is launched with one objective being lobbying for a national family planning policy and program.

1967: Ghana signs the World Leaders' Declaration on Population, the first Sub-Saharan African government to do so.

1968: The Two-Year Development Plan (1968–70) is published and promises a national population policy.

1969: A government policy paper, *Population Planning for National Progress*, is issued that outlines a broad set of demographic and social goals, including programs to provide advice and assistance to couples wishing to space or limit their reproduction.

1970: The new Family Planning Administration begins work. The only other country in Sub-Saharan Africa that had preceded such a move is Kenya.

Early 1970s: The National Family Planning Program takes shape under a formal secretariat that is designed to involve and coordinate various ministries, including the Ministry of Health. Coordination works only partially.

1972: The Danfa Comprehensive Health and Family Planning Project is enlarged with an experimental design to test four alternative field programs in collaboration with the University of California at Los Angeles.

1974: An international conference is held in Bucharest that encourages extensions of the National Family Planning Program beyond married women.

1985: The Abortion Law is liberalized, but is not well publicized, so unsafe abortions continue to account for substantial maternal mortality.

1986: HIV/AIDS arrives in Ghana.

1998: The total fertility rate is estimated to have fallen to 4.4 births per woman, though it probably remains stable during the next five years.

2003: A nationally representative survey shows that 25 percent of married women are using a contraceptive method; 19 percent are using a modern method.

Large rural-urban differentials exist in relation to fertility, as well as north–south differences in contraceptive use and fertility. Nationally, fertility has fallen substantially.

an insurance for old age. Female fertility was stressed, and children were considered as the guarantee of descendants and possible reincarnations of predecessors. Newly independent African countries were enthusiastic to develop and to promote national growth in terms of both the economy and the population. Indeed, until 1960, knowledge of demographic trends was sparse in Sub-Saharan Africa (Brass and others 1968; Gaisie 1969, 1975; Gaisie and Jones 1970). A census had been taken in Ghana in 1948, but a population undercount was suspected. As in most of Africa, Ghana had no comprehensive vital statistics.

In these circumstances, the clear priority was the need for demographic knowledge. Thus, the international population movement had little alternative to emphasizing demography rather than family planning. In retrospect, this emphasis was the right one, because it made many Ghanaians familiar with population concerns. When the regime changed, population knowledge was widespread, as was expertise.

Box 22.1 presents a timeline of the main events in relation to family planning in Ghana.

Beginnings, 1959–66

The first step was President Nkrumah's decision to accept the United Nations (UN) proposition that Ghana should be involved in the 1960 round of national censuses. This was in accord with his modernizing views. He was determined that Ghana should have the first modern African census. This was made easier by the possession of a good statistical office directed by a capable economics graduate, Emmanuel N. Omaboe, whose later positions included head of the ministry responsible for the family planning program. In addition, the UN provided a census expert, Dr. Benjamin Gil, who was on leave from Israel's statistical service. Gil was equal to the challenge and drove the census operation in a single-minded way. While he tended to see the staff members of the demography program at the University of Ghana as disloyal if they followed a course of academic independence, especially if their research aimed at testing the accuracy of the census, at the same time, the census data were invaluable to the teaching program as such data progressively became available from 1962. Unfortunately, the complex postenumeration survey was not easily reconciled with the census itself and was not available for analysis until 1971.

The University of Ghana's Population Council program at Legon, on the outskirts of Accra, was begun somewhat by accident. The eminent African-American sociologist Professor St. Clair Drake, one author of the famous study *Black Metropolis* (Drake and others 1993) and professor of sociology at Roosevelt University in Chicago, visited Nkrumah in 1959. He was studying the cinema in West Africa and called on Nkrumah, his former roommate at an American university. Nkrumah boasted of the first-rate census in preparation, and Drake advised that the university would need demographers to analyze it and to train Ghanaians in the discipline. He visited the Population Council in New York on his return to the United States to seek help with recruitment and funding. The council agreed to provide this partly because Frank Lorimer, who was at American University in Washington, D.C., but also had links with the Office of Population Research at Princeton University, had been urging the council to send him to Africa on a preliminary investigation of who and what would be available for the Princeton African project that eventually produced *The Demography of Tropical Africa* (Brass and others 1968).

From 1960 to 1966, the Population Council successively sent four demographers to teach at the University of Ghana. All sent graduate students on Population Council fellowships to overseas universities to undertake graduate degrees (at first to Princeton, the London School of Economics, and Australian National University). The four demographers were Jack Caldwell of Australian National University; Lorimer; Dov Friedlander of the London School of Economics; and Ian Pool, a Ph.D. graduate of Australian National University. Lorimer concentrated on the planned Princeton project, but the other three, while waiting for census data, carried out field research, planning the research as classroom projects and employing demography students as fieldworkers (Pool 1970).

Caldwell had two additional assignments. The first was a UN request to help set up a UN English-language demographic training center (which was held over to later years when it drew heavily on those trained by the University of Ghana program). The second was a request to contribute to *A Study of Contemporary Ghana* (Birmingham, Neustadt, and Omaboe 1967). This project was sponsored by the Ghana Academy of Sciences, funded by the Ford Foundation, and given high priority on the urging of President Nkrumah. Volume I concentrated on the economy, while volume II focused on Ghanaian society. More than three-quarters of volume II was devoted to demography and emerged largely from analyses undertaken as part of classroom work in the Population Council's survey program and from early census data. The study was important, because many of the students involved later became key personnel in Ghana's family planning program and because it was used heavily during the preparation of the planning paper that led to the National Family Planning Program (Government of Ghana 1969).

Many of those involved in the study also participated in the First African Population Conference in Ibadan, Nigeria, in 1966 and had their papers published in the ensuing volume (Caldwell and Okonjo 1968). Other important influences included visits from leaders of the International Planned Parenthood Federation and the Pathfinder Fund, as well as two international conferences held in 1965, one in Geneva on Family Planning and Population Programs sponsored by the Population Council and the Ford Foundation (Berelson and others 1966), and the other, the International Population Conference, held in Belgrade and sponsored by the UN and the International Union for the Scientific Study of Population (Smith 1968).

Caldwell (1966, 1968b) was asked to prepare reports for the conferences and wrote to all African national leaders seeking information on their population policies. Nkrumah set up a committee chaired by Omaboe to respond to Caldwell's request. This committee met briefly and replied that the government of Ghana did not intend to establish a family planning program, but it did put on record that population growth might well be too high, as was stated in the first draft of *A Study of Contemporary Ghana* (Birmingham, Neustadt, and Omaboe 1967) and the government's Seven-Year Development Plan (1964–70) (Government of Ghana 1964). By this time, Nkrumah had banned the importation of all contraceptives, and doctors providing them were doing so clandestinely.

This committee was to be renewed after Nkrumah's downfall and would come to quite different conclusions about family planning. *A Study of Contemporary Ghana,* the world fertility survey, another survey (Gaisie 1969), and the historical data published with the UN's population projections all came to a similar demographic conclusion, namely, that Ghana's total fertility rate had been around 7.0 births per woman until at least the 1960s, while its population growth rate had probably reached 3 percent per year. This was the situation when, in February 1966, a military coup overthrew Nkrumah and replaced him with the National Liberation Council.

Politics and Policy Making, 1967–70

Even though the coup was led by the military and the chair of the National Liberation Council was General Joseph Ankrah, the administration included civilians, with Omaboe responsible for the powerful economics portfolio. Before Nkrumah's overthrow, a small group of Ghanaians led by Dr. M. A. Barnor had been working quietly to establish a voluntary family planning association. The association, the Planned Parenthood Association of Ghana, was launched in 1967. One of its objectives was to lobby for a national family planning policy and program. Omaboe needed no convincing.

In 1967, the government signed the World Leaders' Declaration on Population and was the first Sub-Saharan African government to do so. In 1968, it published its Two-Year Development Plan, which promised a national population policy. The National Liberation Council was a modernizing body, but also a crisis administration that had to address the problem of economic decline and was determined to be strictly rational in terms of its policy. It set up a new committee, under Omaboe, to draw up plans for a national family planning program. The Ford Foundation provided a short-term adviser, Francis Sutton, and a longer-term one, A. S David, both of whom were attached to the University of Ghana (Harkavy 1995). The Ford Foundation also provided assistance both to the committee and for the establishment of the National Family Planning Program through Lyle Saunders and Gordon Perkin. They worked directly with the committee, with Gordon Perkin returning after the promulgation of the policy for a long-term assignment with the program. The Planned Parenthood Association of Ghana was represented on the committee by Fred T. Sai, professor of social and preventive Medicine in the University of Ghana Medical School.

In March 1969, the government produced a policy paper, *Population Planning for National Progress,* which was launched by its successor civilian government, and the Family Planning Administration began work in 1970. Its only predecessor in independent Sub-Saharan Africa was Kenya. The National Liberation Council handed power over to a democratically elected government in 1970, but that administration and all successive administrations retained the National Family Planning Program as a national institution and its existence was never challenged. Unfortunately, the strong and vocal political leadership needed for the success of such a program was not forthcoming from any of the administrations (Armar 1975; Armar and David 1977; Gaisie, Addo, and Jones 1975; Government of Ghana 1969; Hollander 1995; Jones 1972; Stanback and Twum-Baah 2001; UNFPA 1985).

Ghana's population policy received widespread international acclaim for its comprehensiveness and boldness, and the U.S. Agency for International Development used it as an example for many countries.

Policy Elements

The basic elements of the government's policy paper can be summarized as follows (Armar and David 1977: Gaisie and Jones 1970):

- The policy and program were to be integral parts of social and economic planning and development activity.

- The vigorous pursuit of ways to reduce the high rates of morbidity and mortality would be an important aspect of population policy and programs.

- The specific and quantitative population goals would be established on the basis of reliable demographic data and the determination of demographic trends.

- The government would encourage and itself undertake programs to provide information, advice, and assistance for couples wishing to space or limit their reproduction to do so safely and effectively.

- The government would seek to encourage and promote productive and gainful employment for women; to increase the proportion of girls entering and completing school; to develop a wider range of nondomestic roles for women; and to examine the structure of government perquisites and benefits and, if necessary, change them in such ways as to minimize their pro-natalist influences and maximize their anti-natalist effects.

- The government would adopt policies and establish programs to guide and regulate the flow of internal migration and influence the spatial distribution of the population in the interests of development progress, and would also reduce the scale and rate of immigration in the interests of national welfare.

- The government would make provisions to establish and maintain regular contact with other population programs throughout the world through intensified relationships with international public and private organizations concerned with population problems.

Program Structure

Because Sub-Saharan Africa introduced family planning programs later than Asia and North Africa, and because the National Liberation Council had been methodical in its planning, Ghana's program incorporated much that had been proven to work elsewhere. The program was to have an overall council, the National Family Planning Council, consisting of senior representatives from all lead agencies and civil society organizations working on family planning and related issues. One feature was that a high-level officer from each concerned agency would interact regularly with the secretariat to help ensure that the agency would carry out its assigned functions. The council was to provide policy guidance and supervise the National Family Planning Secretariat. Council members were also supposed to ensure that agreed policies and programs were appropriately acted upon and supported by the organizations they represented. Day-to-day activities were in the hands of the secretariat (Armar and David 1977). The secretariat's main activities were to be planning, coordination, evaluation, and funding. Such a structure required agencies' willingness to accept responsibilities and act accordingly. Unfortunately, agencies often had other priorities and, without adequate extra funding, did not always pursue family planning activities satisfactorily. The secretariat itself was often too ambitious and did not separate coordination from implementation in all circumstances, a situation that caused unnecessary conflicts. Thus, in practice, the structure worked only partially.

The Ministry of Finance and Economic Planning dominated the original structure of the National Family Planning Program. It attempted to bring the Ministry of Health completely on board, but was only partly successful. The aim was to bring all ministries and private organizations together through the establishment of a distinct national family planning program advised by the National Family Planning Council with representatives from a wide range of government and private organizations.

Initially, the program provided contraceptives for distribution to three groups: government hospitals and health centers; private family planning clinics; and outlets of the Ghana National Trading Corporation, formed earlier by the nationalization of Leventis Stores, a Greek-owned, pan-African retail network. Its aim was first to prevent the rate of natural population increase from rising and then to reduce it. This was a difficult struggle because of falling death rates, but natural population increase was probably less than 2.5 percent per year in 1970 (Agyei-Mensah, Aase, and Awusabo-Asare 2003; Agyei-Mensah and Casterline 2003; Central Bureau of Statistics 1983; Ghana Statistical Service, Noguchi Memorial Institute for Medical Research, and ORC Macro 2004; Tabutin and Schoumaker 2001; U.S. Bureau of the Census 1997). However, fertility did fall, with the total fertility rate declining from close to 7.0 births per woman in 1970 to 4.4 by 1998, but appears to have stagnated after that, as the 2003 figure was about the same. Furthermore, in contrast to the situation in much of the West African region, fertility was falling in rural as well as in urban Ghana. By 2003, the rural total fertility rate was down to 5.6 births per woman, and in Accra the rate was under 3.0. Nevertheless, major differentials in fertility were apparent between urban versus rural areas and across levels of education. The decline had been led by the educated urban elite, who in the capital were down to replacement-level fertility by 2003. This group had been worried about the costs of educating large families for decades, and various studies in the 1960s had shown them moving toward limiting the size of their families (Agyei-Mensah, Aase, and Awusabo-Asare 2003; Caldwell 1968a; Oppong 1977; Pool 1970).

Assessment of the program has been mixed. Many inside observers believe that it could have achieved more given the environment and the resources available. Others, mainly external observers, feel that enough was done to lay the foundation for future success. Perhaps the assessments depend on whether observers were looking at the decline in fertility alone or the changes in public perceptions and other variables that could precede fertility decline. That fertility did not fall appreciably in the early years was not solely the program's fault, but can be ascribed largely to limited, though slowly increasing, demand. Almost certainly, the later marked fertility decline would not have happened when it did but for the familiarization with contraception that occurred in the 1970s. Both the communication and the service delivery aspects of the program could have done better with stronger political support. The program has been evaluated frequently and has been the first to point out limitations arising from budget and other constraints. The basic model has remained intact while the program has tried to bring in more private doctors, nurses, midwives, and retailers.

The National Family Planning Program learned from the experience of other countries in the 1960s. For example, it established appropriate training courses for everyone involved with the program. Two other points are also relevant in this connection. First, the program was up-to-date in its view that family planning was more than a health service, and therefore it should not be run by the Ministry of Health. This decision allowed many other ministries to provide information and services. At the same time, however, this meant that the Ministry of Health did not regard the family planning activities of government health staff members, especially doctors, as being of foremost importance in personnel assessments, especially for promotions. Hence, many government health workers dragged their feet when it came to such activities.

Second, even though the program aimed at emphasizing the provision of information as well as of contraceptive services, the government was perceived as providing services rather than as placing moral pressure on the population to accept them. Indeed, during the program's early period it withdrew media advertising of contraception, especially on the radio and television, after protests that this was indecent and might encourage sexual immorality among the unmarried population, and even among wives. The public service and other sections of the establishment did not follow Asia in portraying contraception as a national duty. The private clinics, mostly Planned Parenthood Association of Ghana and various Christian groups, had many fewer outlets than the government, but their clinics were larger and existed mostly in urban areas, with the result that private clinics, with support from the program, provided almost half of all services.

Opposition to the Program

Ghana, though not ethnically homogeneous, does not have the ideological and cultural divisiveness found in many African countries. The only real ideological opposition to family planning came in Nkrumah's time from his socialist ideology. Almost 66 percent of Ghana's population are Protestant Christians (including evangelical African churches), with only 14 percent being Catholic and 16 percent being Muslim.

A country's religious composition is important in Africa, and the high percentage of Protestants made acceptance of the program more likely. Some opposition came from more conservative sections of the population, who had the unfounded fear that family planning would cause sexual immorality, but the opposition has not been powerful.

Technical Assistance

The role of foreign agencies has been important and welcomed. In Nkrumah's time, the Population Council's demography program was of fundamental importance. Later, the council also supported demographic training and research at the University of Cape Coast. UN advice and support for the 1960 census was also important. As the National Family Planning Program developed, the Ford Foundation provided both direct and indirect assistance and the Population Council provided a medical adviser. In due course, both the U.S. Agency for International Development and the UN Population Fund assumed significant roles, and in all cases, the provision of financial and contraceptive supplies was of key importance. The International Planned Parenthood Federation also provided assistance by way of training and supplies through the Planned Parenthood Association of Ghana. Ghana also had a good deal of expertise of its own.

Lessons Learned

The program was well planned. Perhaps not making the Ministry of Health an equal partner was an error, but on the whole, the ministry's approach largely appears to have aligned with the overall policies adopted. What was unfortunate was that the secretariat moved beyond its mandate and assumed roles that belonged to the Ministry of Health. While in general the program was well planned, the separation of roles, especially between coordination and execution of tasks, was too poorly clarified to make for smooth relationships between the secretariat and the lead ministries.

By the time the program started, it employed several contraceptive methods. Evidence from elsewhere, especially South Africa, indicates that greater emphasis on the injectable would have been useful. Ghana liberalized its abortion laws in 1985 and expanded the basis for exceptions. Unfortunately, because doctors, lawyers, and the general population did not know about these exceptions, many women died from unsafe abortions. The country might now be able to tolerate a more liberal approach to abortion, and efforts are currently under way to expand safe abortion services to the extent permitted by the law. In addition, perhaps more efforts are needed, and should have been made earlier, to discourage the view that family planning services are only for the married population, especially married women.

As the program developed, so did the new medical school at Korle Bu in Accra, where Sai conceived and implemented the Danfa Comprehensive Health and Family Planning Project in collaboration with the University of California (Los Angeles) School of Public Health. The main purpose of the project was to test the thesis that a comprehensive health approach to family planning delivery would be more successful in Ghana than a vertical approach. The findings were to be fed into the National Family Planning Program. An early evaluation (Ampofo and others 1976; Belcher and others 1978) in the Danfa project area showed that far more Ghanaians had heard of family planning than were practicing it. A 1976 report (USAID 1976) argued that family planning fieldworkers needed to visit households, because each clinic served at most only a population within a 5-mile radius; however, this finding may have underestimated people's mobility. A more serious problem, as government succeeded government, was shortages of contraceptive supplies at both the national and the clinic levels (Monteith 1981).

Ghana's early independence and relatively high education levels were important. Ghanaian elites, and to some degree the whole population, saw the country as being a trailblazer in African modernization. What the program mostly showed is that the effort to reduce fertility in Sub-Saharan Africa is not going to be easy. The National Family Planning Program was well organized in a country sobered by repeated economic shocks, yet it has taken decades to bring down fertility levels significantly. Patience is needed along with continued funding.

Conclusion

The control of fertility in Sub-Saharan African is by far the major challenge facing the international family planning movement. By the end of the century, the population could well quadruple in this region, with its limited natural resources, especially the lack of good soils. Apart from southern Africa, where the bulk of rural incomes is remitted from towns, and also the commercial farming areas of central Kenya, the advantages of fertility control are not apparent to rural, poorly educated, and largely subsistence populations. The driving forces for both mortality and fertility decline are urbanization, education, and the conversion of subsistence farming to commercial farming, all of which depend on continued economic growth.

Looking at the case of Ghana from a regional perspective, the reduction of the country's total fertility rate from around 7.0 births per woman per year to 4.4 in less than three decades should be regarded as a success story. The drop of about 2.5 in the total fertility rate is greater than what most Western European countries achieved in the late 19th and early 20th centuries and greater than what India accomplished in the late 20th century. Sub-Saharan Africa's greatest problem has been its initial extremely high fertility.

The program's successes have been notable, despite considerable constraints. Although the total fertility rate has not yet fallen below 4.4 births per woman, and seems to have ceased falling in recent years, the fertility differentials point in a hopeful direction. In contrast to a total fertility rate of 7.0 in the northern region of the country and 5.6 in rural areas, it has fallen to 3.1 in urban areas and to 2.9 in Greater Accra. In a country where a quarter of the women have had at least a middle school education, the total fertility rate is 3.5 for such women and 2.5 for those with a secondary or higher education.

The fertility reduction reflects the rise in use by married women of modern (18.7 percent) and all contraceptives (25.2 percent), as of 2003. This is only one quarter or less of the level that has been needed in the industrial countries to achieve replacement-level fertility. While no particular method of contraception has been predominant, three methods are used to roughly the same extent and together account for the majority of contraceptive users, namely, the contraceptive pill, injectable, and condoms. The relative rise in the use of the injectable suggests that it may be of increasing importance in achieving lower fertility.

The constraints include an average age of female marriage of only 20, an increase of less than two years since the program began. The infant mortality rate is 65 deaths per 1,000 births and the mortality rate among children under age five is 110 deaths per 1,000 births. While the infant mortality rate compares favorably with that in the West during the early years of the 20th century when fertility there was already low, mortality during the next four years of life is much higher in Ghana, and in Sub-Saharan Africa as a whole.

The startling contrast between significant levels of fertility control in southern Ghana and much lower levels further north emphasizes the importance of low child mortality, high education levels, and a diversified economy in encouraging contraceptive use. Ghana's program has been the most successful in West Africa, and indeed the most successful in Sub-Saharan Africa north of the Limpopo River. Nevertheless, an annual population growth rate of 2.7 percent is no lower than the West African average and remains a threat to continued economic growth.

The arrival of HIV/AIDS in 1986 introduced another reproductive health problem. Currently, it is managed by a structure similar to that of the National Family Planning Program, but it is reasonably funded, allowing it to play its coordination role well. Efforts to harmonize its activities with those of the National Population Council are under way. Some benefits for the National Family Planning Program include the increase in condom use and the emphasis on youth and adolescent education and the role of men. The major lessons of the HIV/AIDS program for the reproductive health field generally are the importance of visible, vocal, and consistent political leadership and the assurance of dependable funding. Unlike the National Family Planning Program, the HIV/AIDS program has had both.

The attention being paid to unsafe abortion and to reducing maternal mortality are also helping to reposition family planning as a national development priority. All things considered, Ghana is probably poised to make a much greater effort to lower its fertility now than at any time in the past.

References

Agyei-Mensah, Samuel, Asbjorn Aase, and Kofi Awusabo-Asare. 2003. "Social Setting, Birth Timing and Subsequent Fertility in the Ghanaian South." In *Reproduction and Social Context in Sub-Saharan Africa*, ed. Samuel Agyei-Mensah and John B. Casterline, 89–108. Westport, CT: Greenwood Press.

Agyei-Mensah, Samuel, and John B. Casterline, eds. 2003. *Reproduction and Social Context in Sub-Saharan Africa*. Westport, CT: Greenwood Press.

Ampofo, Daniel A., David D. Nicholas, S. Ofosu-Amaah, Stewart Blumenfield, and Alfred K. Neumann. 1976. "The Danfa Family Planning Program in Rural Ghana." *Studies in Family Planning* 7 (10): 266–74.

Armar, A. A. 1975. "Ghana." In *Family Planning Programs: World Review 1974*, ed. Hervé Gauthier and George F. Brown, 283–86. *Studies in Family Planning* 6 (8) (suppl.).

Armar, A. A. and A. S. David. 1977. *Ghana*. Country Profiles Series. New York: Population Council.

Belcher, D. W., A. K. Neumann, S. Ofosu-Amaah, D. D. Nicholas, and S. N. Blumenfield. 1978. "Attitudes towards Family Size and Family Planning in Rural Ghana-Danfa Project: 1972 Survey Findings." *Journal of Biosocial Science* 10 (1): 59–79.

Berelson, Bernard, Richmond K. Anderson, Oscar Harkavy, John Maier, W. Parker Mauldin, and Sheldon Segal. 1966. *Family Planning and Population Programs*. Chicago: University of Chicago Press.

Birmingham, Walter, Ilya Neustadt, and Emmanuel N. Omaboe. 1967. *A Study of Contemporary Ghana*, 2 vols. London: Allen and Unwin.

Brass, William, Ansley J. Coale, P. Demeny, D. F. Heisel, F. Lorimer, A. Romaniuk, and E. van de Walle, eds. 1968. *The Demography of Tropical Africa*. Princeton, NJ: Princeton University Press.

Caldwell, John C. 1966. "Africa." In *Family Planning and Population Programs: A Review of World Developments*, ed. Bernard Berelson, Richmond K. Anderson, Oscar Harkavy, John Maier, W. Parker Mauldin, and Sheldon Segal, 163–81. Chicago: University of Chicago Press.

———. 1968a. *Population Growth and Family Change in Africa: The New Urban Elite in Ghana*. Canberra: Australian National University Press.

———. 1968b. "Population Policy: A Survey of Commonwealth Africa." In *The Population of Tropical Africa*, ed. John C. Caldwell and Chukuka Okonjo, 368–75. London: Longmans.

Caldwell, John C., and Chukuka Okonjo, eds. 1968. *The Population of Tropical Africa*. London: Longmans.

Central Bureau of Statistics with the collaboration of the World Fertility Survey. 1983. *Ghana Fertility Survey, 1979–80*. Accra: Central Bureau of Statistics.

Drake, St. Clair, Horace R. Cayton, William J. Wilson, and Richard Wright. 1993. *Black Metropolis*. Chicago: University of Chicago Press.

Gaisie, S. K. 1969. "Estimation of Vital Rates for Ghana." *Population Studies* 23 (1): 21–42.

———. 1975. "Ghana: Fertility Trends and Differentials" and "Ghana: Population Growth and Its Components." In *Population Growth and Socioeconomics in West Africa*, ed. John C. Caldwell, 339–67. New York: Columbia University Press.

Gaisie, S. K., N. O. Addo, and S. B. Jones. 1975. "Ghana: Population Policy and Its Implementation." In *Population Growth and Socioeconomics in West Africa*, ed. John C. Caldwell, 408–24. New York: Columbia University Press.

Gaisie, S. K., and S. B. Jones. 1970. *Ghana*. Country Profiles Series. New York: Population Council.

Ghana Statistical Service, Noguchi Memorial Institute for Medical Research, and ORC Macro. 2004. *Ghana Demographic and Health Survey 2003*. Calverton, MD: ORC Macro.

Government of Ghana. 1964. *Seven Year Development Plan, 1963–1964 to 1969–1970*. Accra: Government Printing Department.

———. 1969. "Ghana: Official Policy Statement." *Studies in Family Planning* 1 (44): 1–7.

Harkavy, Oscar. 1995. *Curbing Population Growth: An Insider's Perspective on the Population Movement*. New York: Plenum.

Hollander, D. 1995. "Despite Desire for Smaller Families, Few Ghanaians Practice Contraception." *International Family Planning Perspectives* 21 (3): 121–23.

Jones, S. B. 1972. "Population Policies and Family Planning Programs." In *Population Growth and Economic Development in Africa*, ed. S. H. Ominde and C. N. Ejiogu, 369–73. London: Heinemann.

Monteith, Richard S. 1981. "Evaluation of the Ghana Family Planning Program." Unpublished report, Washington, DC.

Oppong, Christine. 1977. "A Note from Ghana on Chains of Change in Family System and Family Size." *Journal of Marriage and the Family* 39 (3): 615–21.

Pool, Ian D. 1970. "Social Change and Interest in Family Planning in Ghana: An Exploratory Analysis." *Canadian Journal of African Studies* 4 (2): 207–27.

Salway, Sarah. 1994. "How Attitudes toward Family Planning and Discussion between Wives and Husbands Affect Contraceptive Use in Ghana." *International Family Planning Perspectives* 20 (2): 44–47, 74.

Smith, T. E. 1968. "Africa and the World Population Conference." In *The Population of Tropical Africa*, ed. John C. Caldwell and Chukuka Okonjo, 345–50. London: Longmans.

Stanback, John, and K. A. Twum-Baah. 2001. "Why Do Family Planning Providers Restrict Access to Services? An Examination in Ghana." *International Family Planning Perspectives* 27 (1): 37–41.

Tabutin, Dominique, and Bruno Schoumaker. 2001. "Une analyse régionale des transitione de fécondité en Afrique sub-saharienne." Paper presented at the 24th International Union for the Scientific Study of Population General Population Conference, August 18–24, Salvador, Brazil.

UNFPA (United Nations Population Fund). 1985. "Ghana." In *Inventory of Population Projects in Developing Countries around the World, 1984/85*, 197–98. New York: United Nations.

USAID (U.S. Agency for International Development). 1976. Ghana Office unpublished report on population program support. USAID Ghana Office, Accra, Ghana.

U.S. Bureau of the Census. 1997. *Ghana*. Country Demographic Profiles 5. Washington, DC: U.S. Bureau of the Census.

23 Family Planning in Kenya in the 1960s and 1970s

DONALD F. HEISEL

In the 1960s, motivated by a desire to lower the rate of natural population increase, Kenya became the first nation in Sub-Saharan Africa to formally adopt a national family planning program. Yet more than 10 years after the adoption of its policy, Kenya was reporting the highest total fertility rate in the world, eight births per woman, resulting in a population growth rate of around 4 percent per year.

After a decade of experience with a family planning program that the international donor community supported relatively well, but that was universally described as weak and ineffectual (Lapham and Mauldin 1984; Mauldin and Berelson 1978), fertility began to decline (Kelley and Nobbe 1990; Robinson 1992). A few years later, the family planning program improved and enjoyed support at the highest political levels in the Kenyan government and among the international donor community. By the end of the century, the total fertility rate had fallen between 35 and 40 percent to about five births per women. The fertility transition was clearly under way.

Box 23.1 provides a timeline of major events.

Political, Economic, and Social Context

Kenya gained recognition as an independent nation in December 1963 following the transfer of majority power in parliament from the white settler minority to the black majority. In a purely formal sense, the transfer and independence took place through an orderly legal process, similar to the way it had occurred in the other former British and French colonies of Sub-Saharan Africa. However, in Kenya the transfer of power had been preceded by a deadly struggle during the 1950s, the Mau Mau revolt, referred to as the "Emergency," which was fought almost entirely in the areas occupied by the largest tribe, the Kikuyu, and two closely related tribes, the Embu and the Meru. The organized revolt began in 1952 and did not formally end until 1960. Estimates indicate that some 12,000 to 15,000 people were killed as a result of the fighting (Kyle 1999; Maloba 1993). The entire Kikuyu community, which had

---

BOX 23.1 Timeline for Population and Family Planning

1958: Local family planning associations receive international financial assistance from the Pathfinder Fund.

1960: Local family planning associations open clinics to serve multiracial populations in Nairobi and Mombasa.

1962: The Family Planning Association of Kenya is established and becomes affiliated with the International Planned Parenthood Federation.

The first postindependence census reveals an extremely high rate of population growth.

1965: A key economic planning document—*Sessional Paper Number 10*—is issued and includes a call for moderating the rate of population growth.

The government invites the Population Council to send an advisory mission on population policy.

The Population Council fields a mission and recommends a national family planning program, with the lead role to be taken by the Ministry of Health.

1966: The Ministry of Health issues a circular to provincial and district medical officers announcing the establishment of the national family planning program.

1967: The Ministry of Health issues a second circular on family planning stipulating that family planning service providers should be trained and that the services should be offered free of charge.

1969: A new census indicates that the rate of population growth is extremely high.

1971: The government asks the World Bank to help develop an enlarged national family planning program.

1975: The five-year (1975–79) enlarged national family planning program is started with an overall budget of US$39 million.

1979: A new census indicates that the annual population growth rate is approaching 4 percent.

---

traditionally lived dispersed in rural areas, was resettled in new, armed villages by government order—an extreme version of land reform.

Discussion of events connected with the Mau Mau experience was rare during the early years of independence. The struggle had been between a segment of the Kikuyu, Embu, and Meru and the white settler community along with the imperial and colonial armed forces, but also between the Mau Mau and other Kikuyu, Embu, and Meru who remained aloof from the struggle or supported the government. Indeed, most of the Home Guard and other military and paramilitary forces used to suppress the Mau Mau were recruited from among the Kikuyu. Thus, Kenyans felt that the events surrounding the revolt were too recent, too complex, and too wrenching to easily come out into the open and almost universally shared a powerful and fervent desire to forget that past and to move on with the tasks of development.

One important consequence of the Mau Mau experience was that it, in effect, canonized Jomo Kenyatta as the *mzee* (elder), the father of the nation. Kenyatta had been a leader of Kenya's nationalist movement from the mid-1940s, and for 14 years before that, its voice in the United Kingdom. In 1952–53, Kenyatta was tried and convicted by the British authorities on the grounds (now mostly considered highly dubious) that he was a senior Mau Mau leader. He was interned for the remainder of the Emergency. As the country moved toward African rule and independence, he was released in 1961 and elected president of the new nation. He served as president until his death in 1978. His heroic past meant that his authority was almost unchallengeable, and he defined the issues and set the government's priorities throughout most of the 1960s and 1970s. Rapid population growth and extremely high fertility were manifestly not high on his list of issues calling for urgent action (Holmberg and others 1984). The gossip in Nairobi at the time was that the president viewed family planning as a kind of foolishness, of interest to some of his younger colleagues, but nothing he needed to take seriously. However, various observers held different views of Kenyatta's opinions on the importance of population growth and of family planning, as described in Chimbweteàà, Zulu, and Watkins (2003).

At the same time, Kenyatta brought stability to a country that had recently been politically transformed and had suffered from armed conflict. He made a concerted effort to calm intertribal rivalries. He made an equally concerted effort to reassure the European and Asian minorities that their presence was welcome and secure. The latter was crucial, because at the time that he was elected president, Kenya was socially and economically sharply segmented along racial lines. A highly productive modern sector existed that was primarily focused on agricultural exports, along with a small but growing industrial base, both largely owned and managed by the white settler community. A flourishing trade network operated throughout the country that was largely in the hands of the Asian community. Yet together, the Europeans and Asians (and a smaller number of Arabs who lived along the coast) accounted for less than 5 percent of the total population. At the same time, 80 percent of the population were African rural subsistence smallholders. Other members of the African population included a tiny, highly educated elite; a small but growing number of landowners increasingly engaged in commercial farming; a larger number of skilled and unskilled industrial workers; rural laborers; and a growing number of unemployed.

At the macroeconomic level, Kenya's economy continued to grow at a satisfactory rate during the 1960s and 1970s, not unduly disturbed by the political transformation that was taking place. Per capita gross domestic product was estimated at about US$750 in 1960 (Maddison 2003), rising to more than US$900 by 1970 and more than US$1,000 by 1980. The rise was comparatively steady, with a few reversals along the way, such as the first oil shock in the mid-1970s. The steady economic growth may well have served to diminish any sense of urgency about the impact of population growth on the part of those other than population specialists.

The economic issue that did generate a sense of urgency was the increasing unemployment and inequality. The talk was of growth without development. During 1970 to 1977, employment in the high wage sector grew by 4.8 percent, but that sector absorbed only 17 percent of total labor force growth. The rest of the growth had to be absorbed in the low-productivity traditional and informal sectors. By the late 1970s, 30 percent of all households were living in absolute poverty and 70 percent of the poor were small, near-subsistence farmers (Faruqee 1980).

Development specialists in Nairobi at that time tended to compare Kenya rather unfavorably with Tanzania, which had placed greater emphasis on maintaining income equality and had adopted a generally communitarian approach to planning for development. For many, Tanzania's President Julius Nyerere—the *mwalimu* (teacher)—was the most admired leader in Sub-Saharan Africa.

A series of documents issued by the powerful Ministry for Economic Planning illustrates Kenya's broad approach to development. These include *Sessional Paper Number 10* (Republic of Kenya 1965) and the three successive five-year development plans that covered the years from 1966 to 1978. The sessional paper provided the basic development strategy that guided Kenya throughout the 1960s, 1970s, and thereafter. It almost certainly reflected the thinking of Tom Mboya, the minister for economic planning and development (Ajayo and Kekovole 1998), one of Kenya's most brilliant and effective political leaders during the early days of independence. The paper sets forth the leading goals of development policy: freedom from want, disease, ignorance, and exploitation. The means to achieve these goals were economic growth, a mixed economy, and self-reliance (Faruqee 1980). The paper also explicitly called for steps to moderate the rate of population growth.

While calling for a mixed economy, the sessional paper set forth a more conservative economic path than that of most of its African neighbors. Private ownership of land and other capital goods was assured (Leys 1974). At the same time, Kenya's approach to development assigned the central government a leading role in directing action. Both government and donor community development specialists generally agreed that the national government was the only institution capable of effective action to achieve the country's development goals. The great mass of the population were seen as poor, with widespread unmet health needs; uneducated; and until recently, exploited by a colonial landowning class. Members of the great rural majority were unlikely to be able to produce the resources or entrepreneurship needed to develop the country. The European and Asian minorities did have considerable resources and entrepreneurial skills, but they were not universally trusted to use their resources and skills in the country's best interests. Finally, the decade of Kenya's independence was also a time when both national and international development specialists tended to be self-confident about their ability to devise economic plans that a strong government could implement successfully, and thereby achieve rapid growth.

The key operational documents used to plan Kenya's development strategies were the successive five-year plans. The evolution of development planning priorities during the 1960s and 1970s is interesting (Ghai, Godfrey, and Lisk 1979). The First Five-Year Development Plan (1966–70) emphasized support for growth in the modern sector. Those preparing the Second Five-Year Development Plan (1970–74) increasingly recognized that the modern sector alone could not produce the number of new jobs needed, and the emphasis shifted to more broadly based growth, and especially to agriculture. The Third Five-Year Development Plan (1974–78) demonstrated a growing realization that income inequality was increasing at an unacceptable pace and that a still more broadly based development strategy was called for. Thus, the plan moved strongly in the direction of a basic needs approach.

The successive five-year plans implicitly recognized the importance of the high and increasing rate of population growth for Kenya's economic development (Henin 1986). The plans did not set forth programs of action to deal with population growth or with high fertility as such, possibly on the grounds that other documents more narrowly focused on population dealt with these matters. However, they did refer explicitly to the links between population and development, with increasing reference to job creation. They also provided a planning context within which the family planning program fit nicely. The emphasis was on centralized planning with responsibility for action largely vested in the hands of the national government.

Meanwhile, Kenya remained a predominantly rural country. In the early 1960s, about 7.5 percent of the population lived in urban areas. The capital, Nairobi, was home to about 33 percent of the urban population. The proportion of the population that lived in urban areas rose to around 16 percent by 1980, a moderately rapid rate of urban growth, but still a comparatively low level of urbanization. Because Kenya was a mainly agricultural country, the issue of access to land had been on the public agenda, among both Europeans and Africans, since at least the 1920s, and was widely seen as becoming increasingly serious.

Two crucially important policy initiatives took up the issue of land tenure in the 1960s and 1970s. The first was the consolidation and registration of small landholdings. This program had its origins in the colonial period (Leys 1974; Maloba 1993), with the goal of establishing a class of small proprietors. It gained considerable impetus in the regions members of the Kikuyu tribe inhabited following the end of compulsory villagization. Consolidation and registration then became the official policy goal for all rural landholdings with the aim of converting agricultural land from the traditional system of lineage-based landholding to individual household ownership. The second major initiative was the buying out of some of the estates owned by white settlers (using funds provided by the British government) and dividing their lands, plus some state-owned lands, for settlement by African smallholders, who were given title to their smallholdings if they settled them and took steps to develop them. This was something of a revolutionary process, as ownership and leasehold of land in these highly fertile areas had been restricted to whites during the colonial period. Along with registering their titles to the land, the new proprietors were encouraged to produce cash crops, including coffee, tea, pyrethrum, and a variety of other more valuable crops. This also was something of a revolutionary process: during the colonial era, African farmers had been prohibited from growing or marketing cash crops such as coffee.

Both initiatives provided economic opportunities that, in turn, absorbed some additional numbers of the growing population. They certainly made a net positive contribution to the economic well-being of those African farmers who were able to benefit from them. They also probably brought some real psychological benefits. Prior to the time when African farmers were permitted to produce and market cash crops, the large-scale commercial producers (settlers or multinational corporations) expressed concern that African smallholders would be incapable of meeting the high quality standards that brought premium prices for Kenyan coffee on the world market. However, once the African producers entered the market, their product was shown to be of excellent quality. The ability of the African smallholders to meet the standards set by international commercial producers provided reassurance for all concerned.

Nevertheless, the positive impact of these land reform initiatives was not without problems. In the first place, observers noted that implementation of the resettlement scheme had in some cases led to rising tribal competition for resettlement lands. The demand was far greater than available supply, which meant that a choice had be made among the tribal applicants. Second, as much of the land involved in the resettlement process was sold, those Africans who could not secure sufficient credit or did not have enough savings to buy it were at greater risk of being left landless. Third, the process was vulnerable to corruption. Finally, titles to land, whether acquired through resettlement or through consolidation and registration, were almost inevitably issued in the name of a male householder, a practice that seriously disadvantaged women, who lived on the land and were the chief source of farm labor.

Thus, if land reform is a leading precondition for fertility decline, as McNicoll (2006) recently observed, Kenya made an important start in that direction during the 1960s and 1970s. The process was, however, far from complete; although the traditional lineage ownership system retained a powerful hold on people's thinking about landholding, the issue was high on the public agenda, and change was under way.

Like nearly every other country in Sub-Saharan Africa, Kenya was and remains a multiethnic society. As mentioned earlier, around the time of independence, Kenya had a small but economically powerful minority of Europeans, Asians (almost all from India), and Arabs. More than 95 percent of the population were Africans of one tribe or another. The largest tribe was the Kikuyu, who accounted for just over 20 percent of the total population. They were followed in size by the Luhya and the Luo (around 13 percent each); the Kamba and the Kalenjin (about 11 percent each); and the Meru, Embu, and Gusii (around 7 percent each), plus a large number of smaller groups. In all, the country recognized more than 70 different tribes.

An important consequence of the ethnic heterogeneity was the resulting linguistic heterogeneity. Each tribe spoke its own language, and the languages were to a greater or lesser extent mutually incomprehensible. Indeed, the African languages of Kenya fall into three different linguistic families, which in some cases are as structurally and historically unrelated as, say, English and Arabic. Moreover, many of the tribal languages lacked a written form, and even in the case of the larger tribes, their existing written literature was limited.

To some extent, the country attempted to overcome the linguistic barriers by the use of a common language, either English or Swahili. For the vast majority of Kenyans, use of English was dependent on formal education. Kenya made a major investment in formal education: as of about 1965, just over half of all children were enrolled in primary school, but only some 4 percent were attending secondary school (Kelley and Nobbe 1990). In addition, literacy was still at moderate levels: in 1976, less than half of all Kenyans aged 15 or older were literate (Bunyi 2006).

Swahili had the advantage of being somewhat more widely known as a spoken language. Many Kenyans of all races, but especially those in urban areas, inevitably picked up some Swahili. Newspapers were published in Swahili, although in some cases they depended heavily on translated material from the much more highly developed English press. Swahili had one additional important virtue: its contemporary written form was purely phonetic in the Latin alphabet. As a result, basic literacy could be achieved in just a couple of days by anyone who already knew spoken Swahili. It is the mother tongue of a comparatively small number of people who live mainly along the Indian Ocean coast and has its roots in the Bantu family of languages (which also includes Kikuyu, Luhya, Embu, Meru, and others) and in Arabic.

However, wider use of Swahili faced two constraints. First, for many up-country tribes, Swahili had a somewhat negative political reputation. It was historically associated with the slave trade, which persisted to a small extent even into the first half of the 20th century, and then with colonialism and the white settlers. It was said that some white settlers felt strongly that all whites should learn at least basic Swahili and should use that language exclusively in dealing with Africans to keep them from learning enough English to challenge white authority. The second and more important constraint was that fluency in Swahili was far from universal. Indeed, in more remote villages, especially in western Kenya, the majority spoke neither English nor Swahili. Watkins (2000) reports that in a Luo community in the 1990s, a substantial majority said that they could not carry on a conversation in Swahili. Furthermore, she observed that the use of family planning posters in Swahili contributed to the image of contraception as something alien to the Luo tradition.

Kenya's linguistic and educational environment in the 1960s and 1970s had at least two important consequences for its development efforts. First, to achieve some sense of a unified national identity and to reach the majority of the population with any kind of informational messages, the government had to make a large investment in formal and informal education. Kenya has made such investments. In the early 1970s, the percentage of gross national product spent on education was about 2.7 times the amount spent on health (Kelley and Nobbe 1990). Indeed, Ajayo and Kekovole (1998) demonstrate how seriously disfavored health was. Second, virtually all written information and education had to be presented in what was for nearly everyone a second language, either Swahili or English. The precise extent to which the linguistic heterogeneity created difficulties for an issue such as family planning is difficult to say, but it certainly did not help.

Another distinctive feature of Kenyan society that may have to some unknown extent impeded fertility change was the traditional family structure. In a widely discussed article, Frank and McNicoll (1987) argue that those who designed the family planning program had unduly ignored some unique features of the way traditional families were organized and that this, in turn, had been an important factor in sustaining fertility at high levels.

As described by Frank and McNicoll, the core of the traditional, rural, Kenyan family was not the husband and wife dyad. Rather, the key familial institution was male lineage. Male members of a lineage gained access to a given plot of land, assigned to them by their lineage elders, when they married, and then provided their wife's labor to make the land productive. The husband gained control over his wife's labor, and that of her children, by paying a bride price. The wife did not become a member of her husband's lineage at the time of her marriage and remained forever a member of her own birth lineage. However, her children belonged to her husband's lineage. Thus, from a woman's perspective, bearing an additional child could bring her three significant advantages. First, the child would eventually add to the farm's labor force. Second, by adding an additional member to her husband's lineage, she solidified her claim on continuing access to her home on that farm. Third, she could hope that in the event that she became a widow, her own children, albeit members of their father's lineage, would support her.

In addition, under the traditional system, the mother was expected above all to cover the cost of feeding her children. Men had been expected to do the occasional hard physical labor required for the farm, such as clearing the land under the system of swidden agriculture. As the economy became increasingly monetized, more men sought paid employment off the land. Fathers were expected to provide school fees for their children, pay taxes, and help pay their sons' bride price when reaching marriageable age, but the division of family responsibilities did not have many junctures where husband and wife were expected to jointly make decisions about childbearing. Most husbands saw having babies as their wives' business, not theirs. Access to land for her children was the responsibility of the husband's lineage and completely outside the wife's control. Similarly, the cost of education was not her affair.

As a result, the traditional family structure appeared to have few points of leverage where the pressure of high fertility would be felt and would lead to a joint parental decision to reduce that fertility. This system may well have contributed to sustaining Kenya's high fertility. At the same time, Kenya's land tenure system had already undergone profound changes by the 1960s and was continuing to do so in the 1970s as a consequence of the national consolidation and registration policy and of the resettlement program. The lineage-based land tenure system may have continued to play a powerful role, especially in many people's thinking about the proper way to behave in family affairs, but it was not immune to equally powerful economic and legal trends. The Kenyan family, like all other social institutions, began to undergo profound changes around the middle of the past century. Cultural barriers to fertility limitation quietly began to weaken.

The speed and intensity of social, political, and economic upheaval, followed by success in gaining national independence after the trauma of the Emergency, generated an atmosphere of widespread optimism in the 1960s, along with a highly pragmatic willingness to change. This is the context in which the question of population was taken up.

Population Policy and Family Planning

Basic information on population is available from the series of national censuses taken in 1948, 1962, 1969, and 1979. Information from the censuses of 1962, 1969, and 1979 is summarized in the report of the 1989 census (Central Bureau of Statistics 1996). The 1948 census enumerated a total population of some 5.4 million. The total had increased to 8.6 million by 1962, 10.9 million by 1969, and 15.3 million by 1979. Earlier censuses are believed to be highly unlikely to have underenumerated the population, especially in 1948. The United Nations Population Division, which produces back estimates for all countries to 1950 that are consistent with estimates and enumerations to the present, implies an undercount of less than 10 percent in 1948 (United Nations 2004).

The census findings were highly influential in the formulation of the nation's population policy. In the early 1960s, as independence was approaching, the World Bank commissioned an overall review of Kenya's economy (Leavey and others 1962). At the time of the writing of the review, the results of the 1962 census were not yet available, and the report had to be based on the 1948 results. It estimated that Kenya's population was growing at 2.25 percent per year and, by implication, that the country would have no great difficulty in meeting the needs of its growing population. Subsequent World Bank assessments grew increasingly less optimistic.

Burrows' (1975) overall review of Kenya's economy noted that economic growth as such had done quite well and that the government had provided the necessary political stability for continuing growth, but that income was badly distributed; many were being left behind; unemployment and poverty were growing; and the landholding situation was such that "in many densely settled districts, able-bodied men are migrating in search of work in other rural areas or in urban centers, and whole families are moving into the lower potential areas" (p. 455). The report went on to suggest that the primary development goal would have to shift from macroeconomic growth toward agricultural development (thus echoing the government's five-year plan for the early 1970s) and job creation.

Burrows' report explicitly recognized that population growth was seriously exacerbating the difficulties. It documented demographic conditions using data based on the 1969 census: natural population increase of 3.5 percent annually and urban population growth of 7 percent per year. It also described in detail the organization and goals of Kenya's national family planning program. What the report did not do was to propose any active role for the World Bank in that program. The grounds for inaction were set forth in the concluding paragraph of the report's chapter on "Emerging Issues and Options":

> The final word must be reserved for population growth. In this report, which looks ahead a decade, the population growth rate is not an important variable, since all the labor force we are trying to provide for during this decade is already in the homes and shambas of Kenya. No conceivable thrust of population control would significantly affect our major conclusions. But as we look ahead to the eighties, we are moving into a period where effective curbs on population growth instituted now, could start to have a real impact. More than anything else, a slower population growth getting under way in the seventies could relieve the burden on rural land and would allow an acceleration in rural household incomes towards the end of the century (Burrows 1975, pp. 49–50).

The paragraph is noteworthy in showing a clear appreciation for just how crucial population growth was, but also as an example of the widespread tendency for development specialists to focus on their own issues. In the case of Kenya, those issues in almost every instance were indeed crucial, and fully justified the specialists' undivided attention.

In 1980, the World Bank published a report that closely examined population and its social and economic consequences in Kenya (Faruqee 1980). It was able to draw on data from the 1979 census and on the 1977–78 fertility survey. The report documented Kenya's status as having one of the highest total fertility rates and rates of natural population increase in the world—a total fertility rate of about eight births per woman and a population that was growing at around 4 percent per year.

The report thoroughly summarized what was known about Kenya's population and the experience of the national family planning program through the 1960s and most of the 1970s. It went on to present a set of population projections to the end of the 20th century showing the social and economic consequences of continuing high fertility or of declining fertility. With respect to the family planning program, the report recognized its weak performance and diagnosed problems on both the supply and demand sides.

Three supply-side constraints were identified. First, the number of trained medical personnel was grossly insufficient. Second, institutional and managerial capabilities to administer the program were seriously lacking. Third, medical facilities were inadequate, especially in rural areas, where the vast unmet demand for curative health services made providing any preventive and promotive services, notably including family planning, extremely difficult.

The demand for family planning services was recognized as weak, again especially in rural areas. At the same time, active demand for children was high, as demonstrated by previous research (Dow 1967; Heisel 1968; Molnos 1972), as confirmed by the fertility survey (Lightbourne 1985), and as verified by the persistence of the high total fertility rate. The demand for children was ascribed to the needs for old-age economic security and for child labor in subsistence agricultural, and also to the low cost of education. The demand for children was sustained, among other things, by the weakness of the information and education components of the family planning program.

The report makes some broad recommendations of policy initiatives to reduce fertility. First, the delivery of family planning services would have to be improved. Second, the program should consider the use of incentives and disincentives, a suggestion probably arising from Asian experience at about that time. Third, priority should be given to socioeconomic development initiatives that are valuable in their own right, but that would accelerate the adoption of smaller family size norms.

The World Bank's position in the area of population evolved from that of a satisfied onlooker to a proactive leadership role among international donors.

Launch of the Family Planning Program

Family planning became available in Kenya in the 1950s, and possibly even earlier, through private medical practitioners and through the use of condoms available in pharmacies (Chimbweteàà, Zulu, and Watkins 2003; Gachuhi 1972). However, its use was almost entirely limited to members of the European and Asian communities. Few Africans would have been able to make use of the private physicians or pharmacies.

In the 1950s, family planning associations that provided service to Africans were established in Nairobi and Mombasa. Their leadership consisted of Africans, Asians, and Europeans. They obtained external financial support from the Pathfinder Fund in 1958. The Family Planning Association of Kenya (FPAK) was formally established in 1962 and became affiliated with the International Planned Parenthood Federation shortly thereafter.

Family planning received a much sharper impetus following the release of the findings of the 1962 census. As noted earlier, the drafters of the sessional paper drew explicit attention to rapid population growth as a matter of urgency for economic development. The leading participants involved in the inclusion of population in the paper were Mboya, the minister for economic planning and development; Mwai Kibaki, another senior official who is currently president of Kenya; and two international experts, John Blacker, who had directed the analysis of the 1962 census, and Edgar O. Edwards, a Ford Foundation senior economic adviser. All indications are that both Mboya and Kibaki were strongly and personally committed to the goal of reducing what they saw as Kenya's excessive rate of population growth and of achieving that goal through a national family planning program. Thus, the original initiative for family planning came from specialists whose primary concern was with economic growth and demographic issues, and the approach was in line with what has come to be known as neo-Malthusian.

In addition to the discussion in the sessional paper, Mboya apparently was the leading force behind a request addressed to the Population Council for an expert mission to visit the country and advise the government on the following:

- What would be an ideal rate of population growth
- What kind of program the government should adopt to achieve the ideal growth rate
- How to administer the program
- How to obtain the technical assistance needed to implement the program.

The request was sent in April 1965, and the Population Council sent the requested mission in June of that year. The Population Council's mission report (Ministry of Economic Planning and Development 1967) served as the intellectual and programmatic foundation of much of Kenya's approach to population policy questions in the following decades.

The mission members were Richmond Anderson (chair), director of the Technical Assistance Division of the Population Council; Ansley Coale, director of the Office of Population Research at Princeton University; Lyle Saunders, population programs associate at the Ford Foundation; and Howard Taylor, chair of the Department of Obstetrics and Gynecology at Columbia University. During the mission's three weeks in Kenya, mission members met with senior officials in the Ministry of Economic Planning and Development; the Ministry of Health; and the ministries of Information and Broadcasting, Education, Labor, and Cooperatives and Social Services. In addition, they met with representatives of the FPAK, private and public medical associations, municipal health services, and key informants from six of Kenya's seven provinces. In particular, they held discussions with Mboya and Kibaki of the Ministry of Economic Planning and Development and with Dr. J. C. Likimani, director of medical services of the Ministry of Health.

The mission reviewed the demographic estimates and projections prepared by Blacker, who had used the results of the 1962 census. Their working estimates were that Kenya had a crude birthrate of about 50 live births per 1,000 population, a crude death rate of 20 deaths per 1,000 population, and, as a result, a population growth rate of about 3 percent per year. Blacker produced a set of projections for the mission indicating that if fertility did not change, Kenya's total population would reach 30 million by 2000. The current United Nations medium estimate for Kenya for 2000 is 30.7 million (United Nations 2004). Blacker also projected that, if fertility could be reduced by 50 percent during the next 15 years, the country's population in 2000 would be about 19 million. He then elaborated a series of projections for education, the labor force, and individual income to demonstrate the potential impact of various levels of fertility. Thus, for example, if fertility remained unchanged and if the increase in school placement were to grow at the rate projected by the Ministry of Education, Kenya would have 1.59 million children aged 6 to 12 who could not be enrolled in school in 1990. If fertility were to decline by 50 percent in 15 years, all children in that age group could be enrolled. He set forth similar projections for the numbers entering the labor force. Furthermore, he indicated that per capita incomes could be expected to rise by 40 to 50 percent more by around the end of the century if fertility were reduced than if it remained unchanged.

The mission estimated that the cost of preventing a birth would be miniscule compared with the government's cost for providing medical care at the time of birth; for providing 3.5 years of education per child, the prevailing average at that time; and for making the investments needed to provide jobs.

Finally, in summarizing the rationale for a family planning program, the mission observed that both mothers and their children would benefit in terms of health gains, as a result of both better spacing of children and avoidance of unwanted births among high-parity women. It concluded by noting that contrary to appearances, Kenya was not underpopulated, as its high-quality land was already densely settled.

Thus, the arguments in favor of a national family planning program were essentially within the then widely accepted demographic and economic—neo-Malthusian—framework. They were clearly influenced by experience gained in other regions of the world, especially East Asia. The mission proposed a set of goals for a population program based on the following broad principles:

- The population program should be integrated with national development planning.

- The family planning program should have a clear link to health programs in general.

- The participation by couples in the family planning program must be wholly voluntary and must respect their wishes and religious beliefs.

The mission went on to, in effect, reject its original terms of reference. It argued that setting an ideal rate of population growth was impossible and proposed that a better goal was to aim for the lowest possible mortality level and a level of fertility such that each and every child was a wanted child. It then took the extremely optimistic view that if all children were wanted, fertility might decline by 50 percent in 10 to 15 years.

The mission went on to make detailed recommendations for implementing a family planning program that included the following key points:

- The government should adopt a policy to reduce the rate of population growth that had more specific terms than that presented in the sessional paper.

- The government should provide some of the necessary funding and should involve all relevant ministries.

- The method of choice should be the intrauterine device (IUD).

- A knowledge, attitudes, and practice survey and a field test of IUD use and acceptability should be the first steps in relation to supporting research.

- The government should emphasize the training of medical staff in family planning service delivery.

- The government should assure the availability of supplies.

- The government should launch a public education program on family planning.

- The government should take the lead role in providing family planning, with the FPAK playing a supporting role.

- The government should strengthen the collection and compilation of national statistics, especially vital statistics.

- The various political parties should be asked to support the program.

- The government could use foreign advisers to help implement the program.

The ministries called upon to support the Ministry of Health in its lead role were the Ministry of Economic Planning and Development and the ministries of Finance, Education, Cooperation and Social Services, and Information and Broadcasting. The efforts of the various ministries were to be coordinated by the National Family Planning Council, jointly convened by the Ministry of Economic Planning and Development and the Ministry of Health. In addition to the ministries, each of the seven provincial governments would be represented.

The mission reviewed the available medical resources that would provide the base on which primary program activities would have to be built. At that time, Kenya had some 800 doctors, but just 20 percent of them were located in rural areas. Moreover, only about 10 percent of doctors were African. The country also had 159 public and private (including mission-based) hospitals, 160 health centers, and 400 dispensaries. Clearly, the health centers and dispensaries would have to be the primary means for providing family planning. Under the plan, each health center was to be led by a medical assistant who was expected to have 10 years of basic education, 3 years of training in nursing, and 1 year of training in medicine and public health. The center's support staff members should all have at least two years of formal health training. The mission suggested adding a dedicated family planning worker to the staff of each health center and training medical assistants or midwives to insert IUDs.

The mission recommended that the FPAK should play an active supporting role, but made explicit its view that the association was too weak to take the lead. It suggested that the FPAK be encouraged to provide family planning services in its own clinics.

The mission also recommended that the government should launch a family planning information and education program through existing medical and health facilities from the outset and that other government adult education programs should add family planning to their curricula. Eventually, the government might make use of the mass media, but this step should be taken cautiously, because family planning remained a sensitive issue in Kenya.

Despite the daunting nature of the tasks to be achieved by the family planning program and the limited human and material resources available, the mission expressed confidence that the program could be set up. It argued that the family planning experience of the municipalities of Nairobi and Mombasa and of the FPAK had demonstrated that contraception was acceptable.

Regarding costs, the mission estimated that by using existing Ministry of Health personnel at the outset, the program could be undertaken with an additional expenditure of some US$300,000 for the first year, rising to US$500,000 per year in the next five years. It assumed that external funding could cover most of the early additional costs, but that the government should take over the financing after the first five years. The mission suggested that sources of external funding could include the Population Council, the Ford and Rockefeller foundations, the International Planned Parenthood Federation, the Swedish International Development Cooperation Agency (SIDA), and the United Kingdom's Ministry of Overseas Development. It added that at some point, the U.S. Agency for International Development might also be willing to provide support.

The government accepted the mission's report and formally adopted a national family planning program, albeit without public fanfare, and the Ministry of Health issued an official circular to provincial and district medical officers announcing the establishment of the national family planning program (Henin 1986). Kenya thus had a formal policy and the outline of a program. The circular stated the ministry's intention that family planning would be an integral part of health services and that training in family planning for medical personnel would begin in the near future. In 1967, the ministry sent a second circular to all government medical officers, local authorities, and mission hospitals stating that family planning services should be made available to the public, that personnel should be trained, and that the services should be provided free of charge. The ministry reached a working agreement with the FPAK that the provision of family planning services would be largely left to the Ministry of Health, while the FPAK would focus the work of its 50-person field staff on motivating and recruiting contraceptive acceptors (Gachuhi 1972). Apart from these initiatives by the ministry, no other activities related to family planning or population growth appear to have taken place in any other ministry in the late 1960s.

Limited overt opposition to the population policy initiatives was apparent. Chimbweteàà, Zulu, and Watkins (2003) report that in 1967, the then vice president of Kenya, Oginga Odinga, publicly opposed family planning, reportedly asserting that family planning was simply a white racist plot to eliminate Africans. However, at that time, Odinga was on the verge of resigning from the national party, the Kenyan African National Union, and forming an opposition party, the Kenya People's Union. In the Cold War setting of the era, Odinga moved the Kenya People's Union closer to ties with the former Soviet Union (Kyle 1999), while the Kenyan African National Union was pro-Western. Odinga may thus have been anticipating the view forcefully put forth at the World Population Conference of 1974 that "development is the best contraceptive." Odinga's opposition may also have reflected the dynamics of local politics: if the Kenyan African National Union was in favor of a particular policy, then the Kenya People's Union would challenge it.

Gachuhi (1972), by contrast, describes opposition to the program as negligible and sporadic. In his view, the opposition was mostly based on the mistaken public perception of Kenya as an underpopulated country. He observes that the Catholic Church had offered little opposition, that Catholic mission hospitals were offering family planning services to non-Catholics who requested them, and that the FPAK had received support for family planning from Muslim leaders. He also reports that the military supported the national family planning program. Indeed, in informal conversations among intellectuals and others in Nairobi in the late 1960s, the most commonly voiced objection to family planning was that it would encourage immorality, because if women gained control over their own fertility, they would be more likely to engage in extramarital affairs.

According to Gachuhi (1972) and Henin (1986), the Ministry of Health's director of Medical Services had overall responsibility for the family planning program, which was closely linked to the delivery of maternal and child health services. Program statistics were to be assembled and reported by the Ministry of Health's Section on Epidemiology, while staff training was the responsibility of the ministry's Health Education Unit. Comparatively little activity was reported in the way of information and education activities.

In the late 1960s and early 1970s, the program received useful, but somewhat fragmented, international support. The Population Council provided a medical adviser to the Ministry of Health and a demographer to the University of Nairobi; SIDA funded an administrative adviser in the Ministry of Health and covered the cost of contraceptive pills and IUDs for the program; the Ford Foundation awarded grants for training and travel; the International Planned Parenthood Federation supported the FPAK, including the cost of fielding mobile teams that offered family planning services; the government of the Netherlands provided two obstetrician-gynecologists, two nurse-midwives, one cytologist, one demographer, and a statistician; the government of Norway supplied clinical equipment for 50 clinics; the U.S. Agency for International Development provided a health education expert and audiovisual equipment; the Food and Agriculture Organization of the United Nations funded a program in family life training that included family planning; and Family Health International launched a social marketing scheme for contraceptives (Ajayo and Kekovole 1998).

Table 23.1 presents figures on family planning clinic activities from the program's inception. As the table shows, the program grew rapidly in the first few years, and

TABLE 23.1 Attendance at Family Planning Clinics, 1967–82

Year	First visits		Repeat visits		Acceptors	
	Number (thousands)	Percentage change	Number (thousands)	Percentage change	Number (thousands)	Percentage change
1967	6.4	—	13.9	—	—	—
1968	13.1	106	28.8	108	—	—
1969	29.8	127	72.9	153	—	—
1970	35.1	18	113.7	56	—	—
1971	41.1	17	138.7	22	—	—
1972	45.2	10	172.3	24	—	—
1973	50.1	11	211.2	23	47.3	—
1974	51.4	3	236.4	12	48.5	2
1975	53.5	4	244.2	3	51.0	5
1976	61.2	15	271.5	11	52.5	3
1977	72.6	19	283.7	4	71.4	36
1978	74.7	3	302.8	8	74.7	5
1979	64.8	−13	308.3	2	63.8	−15
1980	65.4	1	350.4	14	53.2	−16
1981	58.7	−10	296.9	−15	57.7	8
1982	54.5	−7	296.9	0	54.1	−7

Source: Ministry of Finance and Planning 1984.
Note: — = not available.

then stabilized with an intake of initial acceptors of about 50,000 per year. The number of acceptors increased again in 1976–78, followed by a return to the previous plateau in the late 1970s and early 1980s. Given the highly optimistic expectations for program performance at the outset, and the fact that during this period Kenya had some 500,000 or more births each year, the results were no doubt frustrating and disappointing.

Efforts to Revitalize the Program

Clearly the women of Kenya were more than successful in having the comparatively large numbers of children they said they wanted (around six) in response to the question on ideal family size in the early knowledge, attitudes, and practice surveys (Dow 1967; Heisel 1968) and in the later fertility survey (Lightbourne 1985), which was part of the world fertility survey.

The lackluster performance of the national family planning program into the early 1970s and the high rates of population growth and fertility revealed by the 1969 census stimulated the government and donors to try to revitalize the program. In 1971, the government formally requested the World Bank to help it mount a renewed and enlarged program (Faruqee 1980; Henin 1986; Holmberg and others 1984; UNFPA 1979). The primary focus was to be on training support-level medical staff, strengthening information and education, and improving program management, or doing a better job of implementing the Population Council's earlier recommendations, not changing them.

The government prepared a five-year plan for 1975–79. The budget for family planning was US$39 million, with 32 percent of the cost to be covered by the government and the remainder to be provided by international multilateral, bilateral, and nongovernmental donors. The World Bank's International Development Association provided US$12 million. Other major donors included SIDA (US$5.4 million), the United Nations Population Fund (US$3.3 million), the U.S. Agency for International Development (US$3.5 million), the government of the Federal Republic of Germany (US$1.8 million), and the British Overseas Development Ministry (US$0.9 million). The International Development Association funds were to be used to cover capital costs: 8 community nurse training schools, 30 new rural health centers, a headquarters building for the National Family Welfare Center (NFWC), and a health education center (Faruqee 1980).

Along with capital costs, a key program initiative in 1975–79 was the establishment of the NFWC to provide overall management for the family planning program. The center's director was to be a deputy director of medical services in the Ministry of Health. Its mandate included administration and planning, clinical services, training, information and education, and evaluation and research.

Other program goals for 1975–79 included a large-scale increase in the number of family planning service delivery points, especially in rural areas; a similar large-scale increase in the number of nurses and midwives enrolled in the program; the recruitment and training of a new cadre of fieldworkers, the family health field educators; and the provision of vehicles and other means of transportation.

Program Issues and Problems

Program support from multiple sources made a welcome contribution to the program, but it was not without problems. In its needs assessment report, the United Nations Population Fund (UNFPA 1979) indicated that, in all, 24 international agencies were actively participating in the program in the mid-1970s, and a 1977 SIDA evaluation mission called attention to the lack of coordination among the international donors, although it recognized that such coordination would have to be done in a way that would not undermine the lead authority of the Ministry of Health (Holmberg and others 1984).

In addition to the weakness of donor coordination, other failures were also identified. Henin (1986) enumerates a depressing series of recruitment failures for senior management posts in the NFWC and notes that it was not until 1982 that the first full-time director of the NFWC was appointed, that is, eight years after the initiation of the 1975–79 Five-Year Plan. Performance was similarly troubled in each of the NFWC's divisions. For example, it never put an effective monitoring and evaluation system in place. Service statistics were based on limited information gathered from new acceptors. These data were then incompletely reported to the NFWC's centralized program management. The NFWC's Evaluation and Research Division, in turn, was never staffed with sufficient expertise to fully analyze and report on the data received during the five-year plan period. Similarly, the ineffectiveness of the Information and Education Division was such that SIDA terminated its support for that activity in the mid-1970s.

Finally, Henin (1986, p. 38) provides a melancholy description of transport facilities: in 1977, the center had a total of 23 vehicles, of which 12 were off the road. Authority to repair the remaining vehicles was given in July 1982. However, when the original Five-Year Plan was agreed on, reference had been made to the provision of 87 vehicles.

By contrast, Faruqee (1980) cites some noteworthy achievements at the operational level. Some 300 service delivery points had been added during the plan period; the target for nurses, midwives, and other field staff members enrolled in the program had been met; and 300 family health field educators had been recruited, trained, and put in place. Finally, as indicated in table 23.1, by the end of the 1970s, the program had served more than 600,000 new acceptors.

At the same time, the good personnel news reported by Faruqee has to be tempered. A much later Population Council (1992) report indicated that less than half of all Ministry of Health workers who received training in maternal and child health and family planning between 1972 and 1989 were actually providing such services. Whether the poor staff retention record was a problem unique to these workers, to all Ministry of Health staff members, or indeed was common to the civil service can only be surmised.

Quantitative targets had been suggested for the 1975–79 plan: the goal was to recruit some 700,000 new acceptors during the plan period and avert 150,000 births. If the plan succeeded, those involved suggested that the total fertility rate would fall to 4.7 births per woman by 1999 (Henin 1986). As noted earlier, the United Nations (2004) estimated total fertility rate for that year was 5.0. That is, Kenya was off by less than 7 percent in reaching the goal set in 1974—a noteworthy achievement.

Assessments made during the late 1970s showed little evidence of confidence that the program would come so close to reaching its long-term goals. Rather, an atmosphere of dismay and discouragement was prevalent. Various evaluations carried out during the 1970s determined that the national family planning program was significantly underperforming and was seriously adrift (Henin 1986; Holmberg and others 1984; UNFPA 1979). In general, the early assessments tended to focus on specific areas of operational weakness rather than to question the validity of the program's original formulation. The most notable weaknesses identified were meeting personnel needs; managing the program; and fostering the growth of demand for family planning, especially in rural areas.

Observers noted that shortages of trained staff members were seriously impeding the program. At some point during the first five years of the program, the Ministry of Health recognized that the shortage of doctors (to some extent probably exacerbated by the retirement of foreign staff members and moves toward "Kenyanization") led to the decision to authorize nurses, medical assistants, and midwives to dispense contraceptives, including IUD insertion (Gachuhi 1972). Doctors were to function in a supervisory capacity.

A commonly observed problem was that the enormous demand for immediate curative services left staff members little time for preventive services, including family planning. A widely, although not universally, shared consensus among medical professionals was that one simply could not allow patients to continue to suffer, and perhaps risk death, in order to achieve demographic goals. That was the case even among many who could easily see that in the long run, reducing the rate of population growth and fertility levels was essential.

Confrontation with the reality of unmet needs led to a melting away of the optimism of the first years of independence. Realization of the extent of unmet needs in health and in all other development fields as well led to growing dismay. After the Emergency had been brought under control, independence had been won, and the economy was surging, optimism was widespread, but by the early 1970s, the majority was making its voice heard and demanding services that had never previously been provided, or even recognized. In some respects, the rising demand for medical services in Kenya was not unlike the experience of most countries, developed as well as developing. However, in Kenya, the process was starting from an extremely low level. For example, the infant mortality rate was nearly 150 deaths per 1,000 population in the early 1950s and did not fall below 100 until the early 1970s.

An analogous situation existed in most other fields where action in support of family planning had been called for. In the field of agriculture, for example, a great many specialists, from foreign advisers and program supervisors to field demonstrators, fully recognized the need to deal with rapid population growth and welcomed the family planning program. However, they also were committed above all to their own area of expertise. Their concern was to increase farms' productivity, and they were satisfied to leave family planning to the Ministry of Health. Although reducing Kenya's rate of population growth was widely accepted as a crucial necessity, to the agricultural specialists, bringing in this year's and next year's harvest had to take priority—those already born had to be fed. A similar situation prevailed in other areas such as education and basic literacy training.

In addition to the lack of active support for the program from institutions and specialists in other development fields, the family planning program suffered from a variety of additional weaknesses. A leading problem was that Ministry of Health staff lacked training in the provision of family planning and in the reasons for offering such services. For medical professionals working in the late 1960s and early 1970s, such topics had rarely been part of the curriculum when they had trained. Again, making up for the deficiency in training called for additional resources at a time when the Ministry of Health was thinly stretched just to meet the most basic curative needs.

Another major area of weakness identified in evaluations was in overall program management. Senior management posts associated with the program remained vacant for long periods; decisions could not be made in a timely fashion; experts often found that they could make little use of their expertise because they were forced to act as substitute program managers; monitoring and supervision of field staff was seriously deficient; and administrative tasks such as assuring the continuing flow of clinical supplies, especially to rural centers and subcenters, were neglected. A sufficient number of skilled and dedicated program managers to keep the system running smoothly was simply not available. The outcome at the clinic level was, not surprisingly, that program performance clearly failed to live up to expectations.

At the same time that demand for services was rising in the 1960s, there were strong expectations in government circles that Kenyanization of the civil service would quickly occur. Many expatriate civil servants left as quickly as they could find opportunities out of the country; their longer-term career opportunities were clearly not going to be enhanced by the recent political changes. At the same time, the late 1960s and early 1970s were a period of moderately healthy economic growth in the United Kingdom, and even better growth in Australia, Canada, and the United States, so that posts elsewhere were available. Of course, not all wanted to leave. Some civil servants of European origin were deeply committed to continuing to work in the new Kenya, to make whatever contribution they could, and to become part of the new multiracial society. Many were truly outstanding in terms of the quality of their work, but their numbers were small.

Nevertheless, Kenyans recognized that rapid Kenyanization was essential. The new nation could not feel secure if its civil service remained overly dependent on expatriates. The process faced two challenges. First, the supply of candidates was insufficient to fill the vacancies that were arising with the departure of the expatriates and the need to staff the new posts being added to meet escalating public demand for services. Second, Kenyanization of the higher levels of the civil service required that Kenyans be rapidly promoted to senior posts. In many cases, this was done without difficulty. In other cases, however, it gave the individuals little opportunity to gain management experience and self-assurance. Some were simply not qualified for the posts they were asked to fill.

The availability of technical assistance allowed the civil service to meet some of its management needs. Foreign donors were generally willing to supply expatriate specialists to work in Kenya as part of their program and project support. The Population Council's mission had explicitly recommended that such international expertise be used in the national family planning program. Thus, expatriate technical advisers played a crucial role in implementing and managing the family planning program. Most were highly dedicated and made outstanding contributions; however, the widespread use of expatriates resulted in some distinctive problems. First, they tended to come for fixed, and often rather short, periods of time: a two- or three-year stay was common. The comparatively high turnover inevitably resulted in less than optimum effectiveness. Second, most were recruited by an international organization and then seconded to a Kenyan institution. This meant that to some extent the expatriates had to be conscious of the demands and expectations of two institutions, one local, the other international.

A theme that grew in importance over the years was the need to strengthen information and education programs to stimulate demand for family planning. While the numbers of new acceptors had surged during the first few years of the program (table 23.1), it quickly reached a plateau. Most observers realized that more had to be done than simply adding new service delivery points.

When the program was first established, attention was focused primarily on direct contraceptive service provision, an activity for which the Ministry of Health was largely responsible. The FPAK was to take primary responsibility for motivation and for field activities to recruit new family planning acceptors. It would also, along with the municipalities of Nairobi and Mombasa, continue to provide family planning services in its clinics.

Henin (1986) reports that the FPAK made important contributions to such successes as the family planning program had during the late 1960s and early 1970s. FPAK mobile units recruited about one-third of all initial and repeat acceptors to the family planning clinics, a fairly strong contribution to a generally weak program.

The division of labor between the Ministry of Health and the FPAK was not rigorously maintained during the 1970s. Both institutions provided some direct contraceptive services and both undertook some information and education activities. However, the essential point is that both were relatively weak in relation to motivational activities in general. Virtually every assessment indicated that program performance in the area of information and education was significantly below expectations. For example, the SIDA evaluation indicated that in 1974–75, only 40 percent of the amount budgeted for information and 60 percent of the amount intended for education was actually used (Holmberg and others 1984).

The FPAK experienced its own managerial and program delivery weaknesses. It encountered management and accountability problems in the early 1970s, and in 1981, the International Planned Parenthood Federation, a primary source of external funding for the FPAK, found itself obligated to take over direct supervision of the association for a number of years (Holmberg and others 1984).

Added to the lack of effectiveness in relation to information and education on the part of both the Ministry of Health and the FPAK, realization was growing that creating demand for family planning was not going to be an easy task. Unlike the experience of some other regions of the world, little evidence pointed to any great unmet demand for contraceptive services. That realization led a number of commentators to suggest that Kenya should explore additional ways to increase demand for family planning.

Three approaches were frequently mentioned. First, the work of family planning motivators and educators should be supplemented by adding family planning and population education to the work of field specialists in other areas, such as teachers, social workers, and agricultural extension agents. Second, development planning in general should give priority to those initiatives that would be most likely to decrease the demand for children. Thus, criteria for adopting a given agricultural or educational policy should not simply be its impact on crop production or educational attainment, but also its impact on human fertility. Third, some commentators urged that the family planning program should adopt various kinds of direct incentives and disincentives. However, none of these proposals ever seemed to have moved much beyond the discussion stage.

As time went on, another more far-reaching form of program assessment began to appear. The emphasis here was not on the inadequacies of program implementation, but on flaws in the original formulation of the program. Two key points were made. First, the original program as formulated by the 1965 Population Council mission was unduly optimistic about what could be accomplished (Ajayo and Kekovole 1998).

As a result, the program became vulnerable to criticism by anyone who questioned the need or appropriateness of family planning in Kenya, for whatever reason. There well may be some truth to this view. The mid-1960s were indeed a time of considerable optimism in Kenya, as in other former African colonies, and not only in the field of population, and population was by no means the only area in which the optimism of the early days of independence failed to live up to expectations in Sub-Saharan Africa.

The second criticism was that the original policy prescription was fundamentally flawed in that it did not take unique Kenyan institutions sufficiently into account (Chimbweteàà, Zulu, and Watkins 2003; Frank and McNicoll 1987). That led to program failure, which, in turn, made the policy vulnerable to criticism, and even to rejection. Some commentators have described this flawed approach as a case of international advisers bringing in a "one size fits all" set of policy recommendations that failed to address Kenyan realities. The recommendations the international advisers brought to Kenya were certainly informed by the experience available at the time and were derived mostly from population programs in Asia. Facilitating the process whereby one country learns from what appear to be best practices in other countries is a role often played by professional experts. Whether it necessarily leads to bad practices is subject to debate.

Some have argued that Kenya's adoption of the international recommendations as it national population policy, with scant prior internal debate in parliament or at academic or other forums, provided insufficient opportunity to adapt the program to Kenya's unique needs and realities. However, the rapid adoption of the program may have been no more than a result of a sense of urgency about the high rate of population growth, coupled with what in hindsight appears to have been unwarranted confidence in the government's ability to plan for social and economic development using technocratic solutions. The process may indeed have made the policy more subject to later criticism.

Some critics have argued that an important factor in the family planning program's weakness was a result of deliberate stalling on the part of the Ministry of Health (Chimbweteàà, Zulu, and Watkins 2003). These critics suggest that senior ministry personnel were opposed to many aspects of the family planning program, that they accepted international assistance that was being pressed on the country, but then effectively held back on implementing those elements of the program that they saw as potentially troublesome. Whether deliberate stalling was indeed a significant factor in the program's overall weakness is difficult to say. Certainly there was a more than sufficient number of other problems to produce the same program weakness in the field of population as in many other sectors.

Conclusion of the First Phase of the Policy and Program

As the 1970s came to a close, three important events took place. First, in 1978, President Kenyatta died, to be replaced by Daniel Arap Moi, with Kibaki as his vice president. The era marked by the lack of strong leadership on population issues (which reflected Kenyatta's lack of interest and the absence of Mboya, who had been assassinated in 1969) came to an end. President Moi and Vice President Kibaki clearly recognized the urgent need to deal with Kenya's extremely high rate of population growth, seeing it as a serious impediment to economic and social development. During the 1980s, they took the issue to the public and made it a matter of high priority for the civil service and the country's political leadership.

Second, Kenya's robust economic growth at the macroeconomic level reached a plateau and stagnated in the late 1970s and early 1980s. The growth of the economy was clearly not going to eventually reach everyone, and job creation was obviously going to be completely insufficient to match the growing labor force.

Third, the 1979 census showed that population growth was continuing at a high rate, with a powerful demographic momentum underlying it. From 1969 to 1979, the total population had increased by just over 40 percent and stood at more than 15 million. While fertility now appeared to be so high—a total fertility rate of around eight children per woman—that it could not go much higher, that was of scant comfort. Moreover, no clear evidence existed that indicated that fertility was beginning to decline. The findings reminded all concerned that population growth such as that being experienced in Kenya was a development issue that could not be ignored. To do so would jeopardize all other development goals.

As a result, just as during the late 1960s when the population practitioners had tended to be excessively optimistic about what they could accomplish, during the late 1970s they tended to become overly pessimistic. Nevertheless, despite its failings and weaknesses, the first 10 years of Kenya's national family planning program laid an institutional foundation that could facilitate the beginnings of the nation's fertility transition. During the next 25 years, the total fertility rate would fall by about 38 percent.

References

Ajayo, Ayorinde, and John Kekovole. 1998. "Kenya's Population Policy: From Apathy to Effectiveness." In *Do Population Policies Matter? Fertility and Politics in Egypt, India, Kenya, and Mexico*, ed. Anrudh Jain, 113–56. New York: Population Council.

Bunyi, Grace. 2006. "Real Options for Literacy Policy and Practice in Kenya." Paper commissioned for the Education Foundation for Africa, Nairobi, Kenya.

Burrows, John. 1975. *Kenya: Into the Second Decade*. Baltimore, MD: Johns Hopkins University Press.

Central Bureau of Statistics. 1996. *Kenya Population Census, 1989*. Nairobi: Central Bureau of Statistics, Office of the Vice President, and Ministry of Planning and National Development.

Chimbweteàà, Chiweni, Eliya Zulu, and Susan Cotts Watkins. 2003. "The Evolution of Population Policies in Kenya and Malawi." Working Paper 27, African Population and Health Research Center, Nairobi. http://www.aphrc.org.

Dow, Thomas, Jr. 1967. "Attitudes toward Family Size and Family Planning in Nairobi." *Demography* 4 (2): 780–97.

Faruqee, Rashid. 1980. *Kenya: Population and Development*. Washington, DC: World Bank.

Frank, Odile, and Geoffrey McNicoll. 1987. "An Interpretation of Fertility and Population Policy in Kenya." *Population and Development Review* 13 (2): 209–43.

Gachuhi, J. Mugo. 1972. "Family Planning in Kenya: Program and Problems." Paper presented at the United Nations Educational, Scientific, and Cultural Organization and World Health Organization Consultation on Communication and Education in Family Planning, December 12, New Delhi.

Ghai, Dharam, Martin Godfrey, and Franklyn Lisk. 1979. *Planning for Basic Needs in Kenya: Performance, Policies and Prospects.* Geneva: International Labour Office.

Heisel, Donald. 1968. "Attitudes and Practice of Contraception in Kenya." *Demography* 5 (2): 632–41.

Henin, Roushdi. 1986. *Kenya's Population Program 1965–1985: An Evaluation.* Nairobi: Population Council.

Holmberg, Ingvar and others. 1984. *Evaluation of Swedish Assistance for Family Planning in Kenya.* Stockholm: Swedish International Development Cooperation Agency.

Kelley, Allen, and Charles Nobbe. 1990. "Kenya at the Demographic Turning Point? Hypotheses and a Proposed Research Agenda." Discussion Paper 107, World Bank, Washington, DC.

Kyle, Keith. 1999. *The Politics of the Independence of Kenya.* New York: Palgrave.

Lapham, Robert, and W. Parker Mauldin. 1984. "Family Planning Program Effort and Birth Rate Decline." *International Family Planning Perspectives* 10 (4): 109–18.

Leavey, Edmond and others. 1962. *The Economic Development of Kenya.* Baltimore, MD: Johns Hopkins University Press.

Leys, Colin. 1974. *Underdevelopment in Kenya: The Political Economy of Neo-Colonialism, 1964–1971.* Berkeley and Los Angeles: University of California Press.

Lightbourne, Robert E. 1985. "Individual Preferences and Fertility Behaviour." In *Reproductive Change in Developing Countries: Insights from the World Fertility Survey,* ed. John Cleland and John Hobcraff, Oxford, U.K.: Oxford University Press, 838–61.

Maddison, Angus. 2003. *The World Economy: Historical Statistics.* Paris: Organisation for Economic Co-operation and Development.

Maloba, Wunyabari, 1993. *Mau Mau and Kenya: An Analysis of a Peasant Revolt.* Bloomington and Indianapolis: Indiana University Press.

Mauldin, W. Parker, and Bernard Berelson. 1978. "Conditions of Fertility Decline in Developing Countries, 1965–1975." *Studies in Family Planning* 9 (5): 89–147.

McNicoll, Geoffrey. 2006. "Policy Lessons of the East Asian Demographic Transition." *Population and Development Review* 32 (1): 57–74.

Ministry of Economic Planning and Development. 1967. *Family Planning in Kenya: A Report Submitted to the Government of Kenya by an Advisory Mission of the Population Council of the United States of America.* Nairobi: Ministry of Economic Planning and Development.

Ministry of Finance and Planning. 1984. *1984 Economic Survey.* Nairobi: Central Bureau of Statistics.

Molnos, Angela, ed. 1972. *Cultural Source Materials for Population Planning in East Africa.* Nairobi: East African Publishing House.

Population Council. 1992. *Kenya: Evaluation, MOH In-Service Training. Final Report (Condensed).* African Operations Research and Technical Assistance Project. Nairobi: Population Council.

Republic of Kenya. 1965. *Sessional Paper No. 10: African Socialism and Its Application to Planning in Kenya*. Nairobi: Government Printer.

Robinson, Warren. 1992. "Kenya Enters the Fertility Transition." *Population Studies* 46 (2): 235–54.

UNFPA (United Nations Population Fund). 1979. *Kenya: Report of Mission on Needs Assessment for Population Assistance*. Report 15. New York: UNFPA.

United Nations. 2004. *World Population Prospects: The 2004 Revision*. New York: United Nations, Department of Economic and Social Affairs, Population Division. http://esa.un.org/unpp.

Watkins, Susan Cotts. 2000. "Local and Foreign Models of Reproduction in Nyanza Province, Kenya." *Population and Development Review* 26 (4): 725–59.

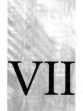

VII Conclusions and Lessons for the Future

24 Family Planning: The Quiet Revolution

WARREN C. ROBINSON AND JOHN A. ROSS

In 1960, few in the developing world used contraceptives. Fifteen years later it was common, and now the majority of couples use some method of contraception. During those early years, a quiet social innovation occurred: the official national program to implement contraceptive practice throughout the entire country. That innovation spread across much of the developing world, becoming a new determinant of fertility, and did much to reverse traditional pro-natalist attitudes. The story of that revolution deserves a new examination, as undertaken in this volume.

The 23 case studies presented here were the earliest national efforts to establish organized family planning programs for entire populations. Useful accounts of the history of the family planning movement are available (Donaldson and Tsui 1988; Mason 2001; Seltzer 1998; Watson 1977), but the wealth of early country studies and analyses has been largely forgotten (see, for example, Bogue 1968; Bulatao 1993; Freedman and Berelson 1976; Mauldin 1978; Mauldin and Berelson 1978; Nortman 1969; Watson 1977). Much of the history behind the creation of national programs has vanished, and young people entering the field have limited awareness of it. Planners of related reproductive health programs lack ready access to the lessons gained from the formative years of nationally oriented family planning efforts. It is useful therefore to fill these gaps by providing accounts of those experiences and their implications for today's concerns.

The selection of programs here touches on three continents and a diverse range of history, socioeconomic settings, and outcomes. The authors are senior professionals who had firsthand experience with the programs; regrettably, the gender bias of the period has resulted in predominantly male authorship. All the writers shaped their accounts independently, paying attention to policy origins, program structures, donor involvement, difficulties encountered, lessons learned, and implications for other countries and programs. The resulting chapters naturally vary in terms of their balance of history, analysis, and personal reflections given the wide diversity of national contexts and program types.

Our overall conclusion is that, for the most part, the family planning program "experiment" worked: policy and program interventions contributed substantially to the revolutionary rise of contraceptive use and to the decline in fertility that has occurred in the developing world in the past three decades. The results achieved did not come easily and were not uniform across all programs studied. In some cases, the optimists were initially too optimistic, but in almost all cases, the pessimists were too pessimistic. Culture and traditional pro-natalist values did not prove to be insuperable barriers to program achievements, although socioeconomic modernization was, as some had predicted, nearly as important as the programs themselves. Our task in this final chapter is to collate and simplify the complexity of the country-specific experience and to provide guidance for future program planners and managers.

The Policy-Program-Results Framework

No framework can capture the complexity of the process by which the national programs emerged, but the simple one shown in table 24.1 at least lays out certain of the elements. Policy may be taken to mean a formal position taken on an issue,

TABLE 24.1 Elements Affecting Policies and Outcomes

I. THE SETTING

Positive factors for policy adoption	General factors	Negative factors against policy adoption
• Economic imperative	• Socioeconomic setting	• Traditionalism
• Public support	• Communications	• Religious barriers
• Political leaders favorable	• Transport infrastructure	• Political barriers
• Nongovernmental organizations well established	• Mortality forces	
• Perceived abortion or maternal and child health problem	• Marriage patterns	

II. TYPE OF POLICY

Authoritarian

Consensus

Informal

III. IMPLEMENTATION

Delivery systems	Central capacity	Resources available
• Ministry of health or nongovernmental organization clinics or hospital-based facilities	• Program leadership	• Contraceptive technology
	• Management structure	• Ministry of health infrastructure
• Fieldworker- or health post–based system	• Program effort	• Ministry of health staff in place
• Mixed approach		• Foreign and local funds
• Information, education, and communication/behavior change communication system[a]		• Technical assistance
		• Statistical capacity

Source: Authors.

a. The literature uses the terms interchangeably.

usually by a government, that structures action and tries to change the future. It may generate a major program, leading to a set of results that can be monitored. Though in reality, the process is not always linear, sequential, or predictable. It is colored by background factors and is pushed in different directions by positive and negative forces in the environment, as well by structural features of the program itself. By simplifying some of this complexity, we can offer a framework to encompass some of the wealth of information in the 23 case studies.

Policy

Normally, the first step in the policy-program-results progression is the definition and adoption of a "policy," but this term has come to mean different things in different contexts, so we must be clear how we interpret the word.

Meaning of Policy

Policy usually means government policy, that is, a position taken to define the government's stance toward some large issue and one intended to influence future events. Governments generally implement policies by enacting laws, creating implementing agencies, and expending public resources (Demeny 2003; May 2005; Roberts 1990; UN 1973). This concept can be broadened, as positions taken by nongovernmental agencies may be well articulated and allied to the government's implementation efforts. Furthermore, the genesis of policies often rests on widespread, popular sentiments that constitute actual societal positions, with calls to action. (Several recent writers have suggested calling these implicit policies. See Johanssen 1991; Posner 2001.) Thus, the policies described in the case studies take various forms and do so in different degrees.

Positive Factors for Adopting a Policy

Following World War II, great political upheavals occurred in what had been colonial and semicolonial regions of Africa and Asia, creating dozens of new nation states. These soon faced population growth at troublesome rates as mortality fell, frustrating their hopes of raising living standards—the so-called revolution of rising expectations—that found sympathetic support among international agencies. Many of the political leaders and technical elites of the newly independent states were Western educated and had been exposed to the views of Malthus and the classical economists on population growth. The notion that population growth might require corrective action harked back to at least the anti-Malthusian leagues of the mid-19th century in England and elsewhere, which launched the modern family planning (or birth control) movement. International and nongovernmental organization (NGO) groups had been working in the colonial regions for many years and were already aware of the postwar population increase. An additional factor was the state-of-the-art macroeconomic models, most notably the Coale-Hoover model (Coale and Hoover 1958), which seemed to establish that rapid population growth was a serious obstacle to achieving increased capital investment and raising per capita incomes. As noted in chapter 1, most government economic planners were convinced of the model's truth.

Other, more humanistic arguments for family planning also existed, buttressed by the rise of unsafe, illegal abortions that had led to rising maternal mortality. Unwanted fertility also meant more births at both the lower and the higher ends of a woman's reproductive age span, which are high-risk for both infant and mother. It was generally accepted that rising infant and maternal mortality trends were a partial byproduct of high fertility and that abortion was linked to unwanted fertility. Abortion, both legal and illegal, continued to play a role in many countries even after programs were launched.

The weight attached to such considerations varied, and some countries placed great emphasis on central economic planning as the impetus for fertility reduction (Bangladesh, India, Indonesia, the Republic of Korea, Pakistan, Thailand). In other countries, the perception of a link between high fertility and health-related issues such as abortion and maternal mortality provided a key argument (Chile, Colombia, Guatemala, Jamaica, Malaysia). Nearly all countries in both groups had private voluntary birth control associations with influential members who were already making the case for a forward-looking policy. The humanistic elements combined with the macroeconomic models provided powerful arguments in favor of policies aimed at reducing fertility. A positive population policy seemed to be the overwhelmingly sensible course of action and was widely adopted starting in the mid-1960s.

Negative Factors against Adopting a Policy

In nearly all traditional cultures, the family unit is central to the social system, and high fertility both provides protection against high mortality and is useful for child labor and old-age economic security (Leibenstein 1954). Deep values are imbedded in such a system, which is generally stable because of the balance between fertility and mortality. A profound disturbance to that system occurred when mortality plummeted, leading to rapid natural population increase. Moreover, as economic transformations began to occur, people moved into cities, where children were both more expensive and less useful. Nevertheless, values did not change overnight, and the traditional allegiance to large family size was a drag on anti-natalist policy decisions.

Religious conservatism, especially by the Catholic Church, slowed policy development in Latin America and Francophone Africa and caused timidity in some ministries of health (Chile, Guatemala). Yet in other Latin American countries such as Colombia, programs thrived despite the church's position. Elsewhere, Muslim opposition to sterilization (Indonesia) and to family planning in general (early on in Iran and Morocco) was unhelpful, but other Muslim countries have been in the forefront of forward-looking policy (the Arab Republic of Egypt, Malaysia, Tunisia). Buddhism has been generally tolerant or indifferent to family planning (Thailand and the Subcontinent, except for Sri Lanka).

In the face of such opposition, real or potential, political hesitancy was understandable. Well into the post–World War II period, nearly all the programs in this study had either de facto or officially recognized pro-natalist policies enforced by religious and ethical sanctions, frequently with legal restrictions on contraceptive supplies and information. (So too did most European nations and many U.S. states.) In a few programs, family planning policy also ran into early opposition from the geopolitical and military notion that a large population meant national power and influence. Some faced serious opposition from left-wing political groups that perceived a U.S.-sponsored effort to reduce developing country autonomy and influence. This, combined with the traditional, negative, Marxist view of family planning, was particularly powerful in Latin America and the Caribbean (Guatemala and, to a lesser extent, Chile, Colombia, and Jamaica).

Political timidity was also a force in Francophone Sub-Saharan Africa, although not in Morocco and Tunisia in North Africa. Across Sub-Saharan Africa, the failure of Francophone governments to take action in large part explains their absence from our set of the 23 early programs.

The Decision to Adopt a Policy

The decision to establish a family planning policy represented a balancing of the negative and positive elements in each case. It was a political decision, and in many cases the open adoption of a national policy was controversial and required considerable political courage. Hostility in some quarters often persisted and some political risk was involved.

The actual decision to adopt a family planning policy came about in several ways. First, in some cases the decision reflected the judgment of a powerful, authoritarian, national government leader who could mandate policy without due concern about public opinion. In these authoritarian cases, the political leader became convinced of the dangers of rapid population growth and created a new policy and program. This appears to have been the case with nine of the programs discussed in this volume: Egypt (Gamal Abdel Nasser), Indonesia (Suharto), Pakistan (Mohammed Ayub Khan), the Philippines (Ferdinand Marcos), Singapore (Lee Kuan Yew), and Tunisia (Habib Bourguiba), as well in Iran, Morocco, and Nepal, where leaders were royal rulers or their key advisers. These programs were either "authoritarian" or "visionary," depending on one's point of view.

Second, some governments took action when they had broad support among the political and social elite, if not among the public at large, and we refer to these as consensus policies. This appears to have been the case in 10 of the programs: Bangladesh, Colombia, Hong Kong, India, Kenya, Korea, Malaysia, Sri Lanka, Thailand, and Turkey. In some of these cases, private groups and influential individuals took the lead, organized national seminars, wrote articles, and succeeded in generating enough social momentum and public support to lead to the adoption of a formal government policy and program. Key government leaders often worked quietly with the private groups. Some authoritarian policies became consensus ones with the passage of time.

Third, sometimes groups or institutions in the private sector were able to marshal enough resources and outreach to have an effect, and sometimes made the decision even when they lacked formal government support. Private family planning organizations played a role in nearly all the programs, but took the lead in four: Chile, Ghana, Guatemala, and Jamaica. What we therefore can call informal policies and programs were created outside the structure of formal government. In Chile, Ghana, and Jamaica, official policies followed within a decade, but in Guatemala, four decades passed before the government acted.

Programs

Large-scale programs contain fundamental features that profoundly affect their effectiveness. Several of these features are now discussed in turn, with attention to past experiences that offer guidelines to improved implementation.

Strong and Consistent Leadership

Political leadership was required to adopt a policy, but strong administrative leadership was the key to successful program implementation. The various chapters in this volume underscore the vital role strong, effective leaders played or the weaknesses created by their absence. Most of the early successful programs are intimately linked with the names of key program directors: Hong Kong (Ellen Li), Indonesia (Haryono Suyono), Korea (Taek Il Kim), Singapore (Wan Foo Kee), and Thailand (Somboon). Elsewhere, even when the program ultimately proved successful, frequent turnover of key personnel was harmful (Egypt, Pakistan, the Philippines). Poor leadership often dampened programs' achievements.

Program Management Structure

Large-scale program efforts have typically proceeded under the control of the ministry of health, but in the 1960s, some programs began largely as NGO activities (Colombia, Hong Kong, Malaysia, Singapore). With program growth, however, the burdens became untenable for some NGOs, and the health ministries assumed the primary role. Hybrid structures often persisted, with some functions remaining with the private associations (public information, research, demonstration projects, standards), while the health ministries were responsible for mainline services (Hong Kong, Korea). In any event, the transitions to health ministries proceeded unevenly, and remained limited to a degree in Colombia, and particularly in Guatemala.

Some ambivalence also existed within the ministries. Health was often the weakest ministry in the cabinet, with few resources and little political clout. In countries with severe endemic health problems, many medical professionals did not see family planning as a priority issue. Furthermore, "population control" was often more popular among economic planners than among health ministry staff members, who in some cases felt they were just being used as instruments for fertility reduction.

In those exploratory days, what should be done or how was not entirely clear. Public health behavioral interventions on the scale being contemplated were almost without precedent. Some saw an analogy with the World Health Organization's successful smallpox and bubonic plague eradication schemes, but as one-shot crash programs, they were poor guides to the unremitting tasks a long-term family planning program faced. The important "modern" contraceptive methods were still new, and the intrauterine device (IUD) and the pill were suffering much higher discontinuation rates in the field than had been predicted from their clinical trials. Berelson's (1974) formula that programs had to meet the three criteria of being acceptable, feasible, and effective was not a close guide in field programs, as they could only be gauged by trial and error, and error was costly.

Given the urgency of the problems and the weaknesses of health ministries, some family planning advocates felt that a crash program involving a new administrative structure was needed. Thus was born the family planning board or the population commission, a vertical structure created to supervise and coordinate all family planning activities by cutting across regular ministerial lines (Egypt, Ghana, India, Iran, Jamaica, Malaysia, Nepal, Pakistan, the Philippines). In some cases, the board was merely a coordinating body with little real authority, and with service delivery still remaining the province of the ministry of health (Iran, Jamaica, the Philippines), but in other cases, the family planning board directly supervised a network of field-workers and controlled logistics; information, education, and communication (IEC); and evaluation (Egypt, Indonesia, Nepal). Some structures of this sort built on pre-existing NGOs, and the government and the NGOs shared oversight (Colombia, Jamaica, Malaysia). Free-standing population and family planning boards had the advantage of being outside the government's normal personnel and accounting rules, which gave program leaders more flexibility. A downside was that this model could project the attitude that family planning was not particularly a health issue, but rather an economic or sociopolitical one, weakening commitment on the part of the health ministry.

Service Delivery Structures

Whatever the overall structure might be, services had to be delivered. Several approaches evolved, separately or in combination, namely:

- Clinic-based services were operated by the ministry of health or by NGOs. Typically, this system predominated where hospitals and urban-based clinics provided most health services (Chile, Hong Kong, India, Jamaica, Morocco, Singapore, Tunisia).

- Fieldworker-based networks by governments or NGOs were used to recruit and resupply clients (Iran, Kenya, Korea, Pakistan). These often included community-based commodity distribution programs and private sector distribution schemes.

- Combinations of the foregoing structures were used along with various other elements.

For most programs, reaching the countryside was difficult, and those that dispensed mostly clinical methods—the IUD and sterilization—attempted to take clinics to villages in the form of mobile health units (Egypt, Korea, Tunisia, Turkey), or else camps, which moved facilities through rural areas on a recurrent basis (India, Nepal). The former proved costly because of maintenance problems, and the latter fell out of favor because of the intermittent undue pressures on local staff to produce clients. A more effective way to reach rural areas was to train fieldworkers to insert IUDs (Thailand), to deal with side effects (Bangladesh), and to create health subposts from which to work. Providing access to services often required "de-medicalization," with a reduction in the power of established medical bureaucracies.

Contraceptive supplies were sometimes also provided under the government's integrated rural development program along with education, sanitation, and women's employment opportunities (Ghana, Iran, Turkey) and through the private commercial sector, including physicians, pharmacies, and shops (a vital part of the overall program in Chile and Iran). Government subsidies to contraceptive distribution schemes, known as social marketing, were also employed (India, Iran, Pakistan, the Philippines). All these approaches were typically add-ons to basic delivery schemes. Indeed, two or more approaches were often pursued simultaneously, and over time, programs tended to broaden service delivery by adding new delivery channels. To succeed, no program could use just a single structure for long.

Each program also had to choose a public information strategy, initially referred to as IEC and later as behavior change communication. Prominent types have included the following:

- Interpersonal communication with fieldworkers, often at group meetings, and usually linked to the distribution of supplies

- Community-based education involving village and neighborhood peer group activity, often linked to multipurpose development schemes

- Print media employing posters, leaflets, and other materials given to clients at clinics, hospitals, and elsewhere

- Electronic mass media using radio, films, and television.

Some economies employed no communication strategy in the belief that a low profile was the safest way for the program to proceed at first in the face of real or imagined opposition, which appears to have been the case in the beginning in Egypt, Guatemala, Iran, Morocco, Nepal, Pakistan, and the Philippines.

In most cases, several of these IEC strategies were implemented at the same time.

Resources Available to Programs

The list of structures and strategies suggests that countries could freely choose among numerous options. In reality, most faced severe constraints and the resources available dictated choices. Most ministry of health and NGO health services were in urban clinics and hospitals, which is where facilities and personnel were concentrated. A lack—in some cases, a nearly total absence—of service delivery facilities and personnel imposed hardships in the more disadvantaged countries where illiteracy was common. Barren infrastructure cramped all programs, whether for health, education, or agriculture, and this was particularly true in rural areas.

For a time at least, these initial shortages imposed sharp limitations on what was feasible, especially when the geography was already difficult and extraordinary efforts were required to reach out to rural populations. Nepal was an extreme case, but dispersed, small villages were common (Ghana, Guatemala, Kenya, Turkey), creating formidable logistics problems. Some rural populations lacked access to nearly all supplies, including contraceptives. Domestic infrastructure improved over time, especially roads and communication systems, but in many countries, the problem persisted. Civil unrest and lack of security also prevented some programs from working in certain rural areas (Guatemala, Ghana, Nepal, parts of the Philippines).

Technical Assistance

During the exploratory early years, as programs searched for workable approaches, donor agencies and technical advisers were often influential. They provided funds, but they also brought the experience of other countries and the results of applied research to bear. Initially, much of this came from private research and humanitarian groups, and through them programs obtained access to better contraceptive technology, IEC materials, and administrative techniques. Soon, as the general field grew, major foundations, national aid agencies, and multilateral agencies took the stage.

Donors, however, tended to favor their own models of how countries should organize efforts to use their funds, and this was not always helpful. The Ford Foundation favored the vertical, free-standing board or commission, which Ford's staff in the field encouraged. The Population Council began as a research-oriented group and favored research combined with action demonstration projects that moved on to larger-scale efforts. The World Bank was still in its bricks-and-mortar phase, which led it to emphasize clinic and hospital construction and the parallel service delivery mode. The U.S. Agency for International Development (USAID) model also generally favored free-standing commissions and large-scale contraceptive distribution schemes. The USAID's internal political dynamic demanded relatively quick results, and the agency often ignored the issue of absorptive capacity (Pakistan was an object lesson). During the programs' first two decades, family planning activities by the USAID were not yet the subject of the bitter domestic political quarrels that erupted in the 1980s and 1990s. When serious, organized resistance to U.S. government involvement in family planning from the conservative right and the feminist left became a reality, the U.S. government imposed many new rules on how funds could be used. This reduced the usefulness of U.S. support (Critchlow 1996), but such diminished usefulness had not yet come into play during the period with which this volume is most concerned. On balance, donors' close involvement in some programs affected the choices open to program planners, while the funds and some of the technical assistance they provided greatly expanded the possibilities for action.

As noted, technical assistance and financial aid were available for most countries largely from the international and NGO community during much of the pre-1975 period. The contraceptives themselves were less than ideal and placed heavy demands on services despite the historic breakthroughs they represented. The IUD was a clinical method and mobile teams could cover only limited parts of the countryside, the high-dose pill available then was under medical restrictions at the beginning, and the injectable was under suspicion of causing cancer and infertility. That situation left sterilization and the condom, each with its own drawbacks. In some cases, the IUD and the pill were brought online to clients without adequate local testing and without sufficient training of service providers. Even if such problems were resolved over time, they could cause a client backlash in the short run.

Finally, the capacities for data gathering and statistical analysis for program research and evaluation were primitive by today's standards. Personnel with quantitative skills were lacking, as were equipment and facilities. One of the major contributions the USAID made to development throughout the developing world was its work with the U.S. Census Bureau to create central statistical agencies to take censuses, collect survey data, and undertake analytical studies. Two decades later, the USAID's sponsorship of the world fertility survey and the still ongoing demographic and health survey program made an even more direct contribution to the programs. Without such efforts, recognizing mistakes or making needed corrections was difficult. These activities took time to get in place, and the many limitations were not easy to overcome in the short run.

Program Effort

A final feature of the programs concerns their actual levels of effort. The resources available to program managers could be used well, badly, or not at all, so the intensity of the program's effort and its choice of means have deserved careful attention. Here we explain the nature of available effort measures, and in later sections relate them to outcomes.

Researchers devised measures of program effort in 1972, and since that time have applied them periodically to most developing countries (Ross and Stover 2001; Ross, Stover, and Adelaja forthcoming). In these studies, independent, informed observers have rated the degree of program effort on 30 features, separately from the outcomes of fertility change or contraceptive use. The original measures were on a scale from 0 to 4 and were converted to percentages. As the studies began only in 1972, they are somewhat late for our purposes; nevertheless, they shed considerable light on the cumulative development of program capacity up to 1972 and later.

The 23 programs are divided into three groups (table 24.2, figure 24.1) according to their overall scores in 1972. They are tracked as cohorts to keep the same 1972 group membership over the years. As figure 24.1 shows, at only 18 percent of the maximum score, the lowest group of programs was low indeed in 1972, but improved markedly until 1989. The middle group began much higher, at 43 percent of the maximum, and also improved markedly until 1989. At 69 percent of the maximum, the high group was already high in 1972, and it remained there, rising only to 71 percent and then declining to 66 percent in 1999, partly by design as a few of the top scorers reversed their anti-natalist policies. The convergence of scores over the years was remarkable, with the low programs coming to resemble the middle and high ones. Note that the groups of programs according to overall effort remain much

TABLE 24.2 Groups and Mean Program Score Effort, 1972

Low	Medium	High
Bangladesh	Chile	Colombia
Egypt	Guatemala	Hong Kong
Ghana	Indonesia	India
Kenya	Iran	Jamaica
Morocco	Philippines	Korea, Rep. of
Nepal	Sri Lanka	Malaysia
Pakistan	Thailand	Singapore
Turkey	Tunisia	
Mean scores		
18	43	69

Source: Ross and Stover 2001.

FIGURE 24.1 Trends in Program Effort Score for the 1972 Cohorts, 1972–99

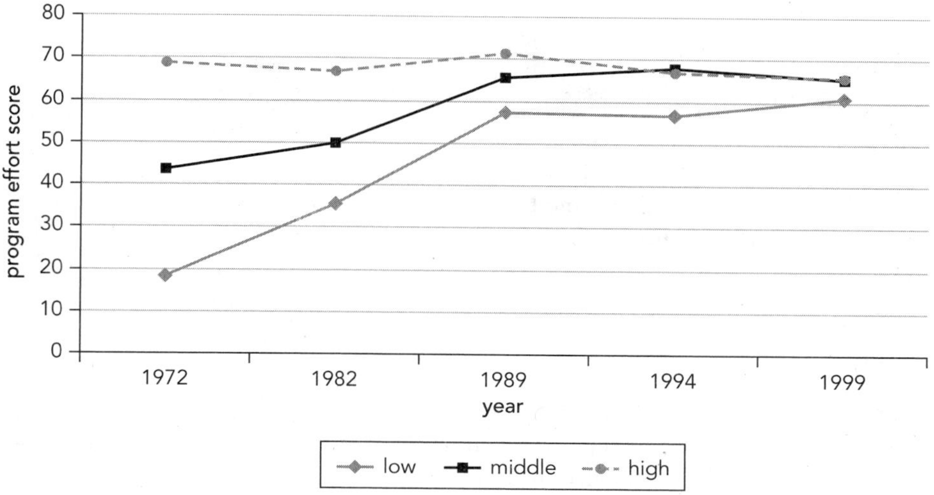

Source: Authors.

Note: Each line follows programs as grouped in 1972. X-axis not to scale.

the same as later, where the cohorts are defined by starting levels for contraception and fertility.

Regarding individual programs, the best performers stabilized at about 80 percent of maximum effort, while as of 1999, the others ranged between 60 and 75 percent. With the ceiling of 80 percent as par, they ranged from 75 percent (60/80) to 93 percent (75/80) of "best effort."[1] The percentages represent only partial effort compared with what might have been done, but it is encouraging that the programs that scored the lowest at the start moved up rapidly to close much of the gap with the best scorers. At the start, the difference between the lowest and highest mean scores was 77 points, which fell over the years to 68 points and then to 36 points.

Substantial diversity was apparent in how high scores were obtained. The total score was made up of the following four components:

• Policy and stage setting

• Services and service arrangements

• Evaluation and management use of information

• Availability of contraceptive methods, plus safe abortion.

In 1982, for example, the high scorers for official policy positions were the East Asian cases plus India, Indonesia, and Sri Lanka, while the low scorers included the African cases of Ghana, Kenya, and Morocco, as well as Iran, which scored lowest of all (but by 1999 scored extremely high). The services scores were only partly similar: Bangladesh and Colombia were strong on services, while Nepal, Pakistan, and Turkey scored low. High evaluation scorers included Colombia again, as well as the East Asian programs, while the lowest scores went to Egypt, as well as to Ghana, Iran, Kenya, and Turkey. For making methods actually available to whole populations, the picture was fairly uniform, showing parallel high or low scores for most of the programs that scored high or low on the other components. The programs that fell in the middle ranges shifted positions over time depending on the component.

After 1989, many changes in degree occurred, and some programs actually fell in overall strength because of deliberate policy reversals toward pro-natalism, as in Korea and Singapore. These later developments are interesting in what they reveal about the issue of campaigns "overshooting the mark" in relation to fertility reduction. Fertility declines cannot be fine-tuned, and in the most advanced cases, general modernization also took hold and produced its own momentum for small families beyond program effects.

Program Results

Program achievement follows from its own implementing measures, but to a large extent these are structured by the socioeconomic context in which the program finds itself. This must be taken into account in judging program results.

Contextual Features That Affect Program Results

All programs work against the background of major socioeconomic forces that shape the program's context, and those forces have their own effects on contraceptive use and fertility. Major contextual changes have been at work in essentially all the cases, most of which have helped the programs. The slow decline in mortality that occurred over many decades in Europe has been foreshortened drastically in the lead cases of the developing world; in particular, infant mortality declined rapidly, so that families no longer needed to have large numbers of births to guarantee their survival. Perhaps more important still have been changes in marriage patterns. A rising age at marriage is important in the long run, but it also involves a transition period during which first births, and some later births, are postponed. In the interim years, fewer births than normal take place, and those reductions represent lower fertility rates while the transition lasts. Even after that, the longer generation length means a lower annual crude birth rate.

Other contextual causes were also at work, although it is impossible to separate out the specific linkages between declining fertility and urban living, higher levels of female education and labor force involvement, and the secularization effects of Western media. These help make up what is meant by the socioeconomic setting (SES). All these factors were already at work before governments undertook deliberate policy and program efforts, and they help explain the initial differences in the levels of contraceptive practice and fertility among the three groups of programs shown later. Overall modernization and improved physical infrastructure made a large difference, easing movement about the country, accelerating communications, and furthering program operations.

Contraceptive Use

The most popular early evaluation paradigm in family planning research was the knowledge, attitudes, and practice framework. That is, programs aimed to

FIGURE 24.2 Contraceptive Prevalence Trends According to 1970 Prevalence Levels, 1970–85

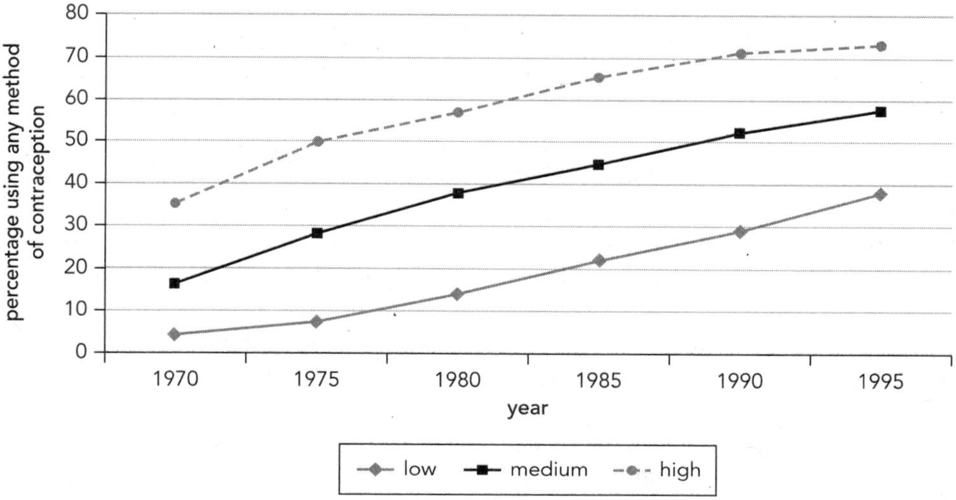

Source: Authors.

Note: Each line follows a group as defined in 1970.

supply knowledge of contraception, to change public attitudes toward their use, and to increase the practice of contraception. Early IEC efforts concentrated on the knowledge and attitudes elements, but program achievement was judged primarily with reference to practice, that is, increased contraceptive practice.

Research over the years has shown that a new national program is usually followed by an initiation or acceleration of contraceptive practice in the population. Use rose in most of the programs included here from the mid-1960s onward; however, the patterns varied by starting level, and figure 24.2 shows the result according to three levels of use in 1970 (we lack sufficient survey data for 1965 to estimate the levels then). The figure follows the three groups at five-year intervals to trace the upward movement. On average, the programs that started with the lowest prevalence levels remained the lowest, but use among all three groups rose steadily over the years.

The patterns for individual cases are also of interest, but are too detailed to be shown separately. Contraceptive use nearly everywhere rose in the early years, but the rise was uneven. Among the best performers, use finally leveled off at about 75 to 80 percent of couples using any method. (In no population do 100 percent of women practice contraception, as some believe themselves to be infertile, some are not sexually active, others are pregnant, and still others wish to become pregnant.) Once use started to rise, it continued to rise in every case, with almost no exception (however Kenya plateaued in the latest survey). In the early years, which are our focus, use rose in regular steps. The East Asian cases began their rise earliest and have risen to the highest levels. Generally speaking, the Sub-Saharan African cases have proven the most resistant to change.

Programs varied widely in the contraceptive methods they chose to emphasize, and those choices, in combination with public responses, generated differences in which methods were used the most. In the mid-1960s, when the IUD first appeared on the scene, programs emphasized it because it appeared to be a one-step, reversible, inexpensive method using inert materials—a technological breakthrough that seemed to promise historic change. However, continuation rates suffered by comparison with the experience of clinical trials, and for that and other reasons it faded in competition with other methods in some programs, and it was never a factor in Sub-Saharan Africa. Nevertheless, its use continued to grow in Egypt, Turkey, and numerous other countries. Sterilization played a large role in Asia and Latin America, but much less so in the Middle East and North Africa, where the IUD and the pill fared especially well. The percentage using sterilization rose slowly even in Asia and Latin America, as annual adoption rates were almost always low. However, the pool of users grew inexorably because the average age at adoption was only about 30, leaving women in the pool for a long time. Also, when a program introduced sterilization early in its history, that gave more time for the number of users to accumulate.

Some programs offered several methods, others only one. India and Nepal offered little but sterilization, while Colombia and Thailand gave people a choice among several modern methods. Total use tended to follow the number of available methods, as each one fitted the needs of a separate subgroup. Indonesia was interesting as the only case that implemented the contraceptive implant widely. It was also nearly unique in the vigor of its subsidization of the private sector. In most countries, the share of contraceptive use accounted for by the private sector has not been increased by deliberate public sector action, only by separate developments in the private sector itself.

Medical termination of pregnancy, or abortion, has been an important, if largely unacknowledged and unmeasured, element in many environments. The open and widespread resort to abortion was characteristic of East Asia, including, but not exclusively, in Hong Kong, Korea, Singapore, and Thailand. Even though it was not countenanced legally, it was generally safe and inexpensive. In Bangladesh, manual vacuum aspiration, or menstrual regulation as it was called, became quite prevalent, and as pregnancy was not confirmed, menstrual regulation was permitted because it could be legally distinguished from abortion. In most other countries, abortion was basically illegal and less prevalent. Its use was semisecretive, and the severe health problems caused by unsafe abortion in Latin America became a principal rationale for establishing national programs, as in Chile and Colombia. Interestingly, even Tunisia and Turkey made official provision for limited abortion services, with budget items to cover them.

Fertility Trends

In most programs, family planning policies and programs aimed at increasing contraceptive use to reduce fertility, and hence population growth, although in some cases fertility decline was an implicit rather than an explicit objective. A key question is what happened to fertility over the years, and then to relate those outcomes to program activities and efforts. However, the first thing to address is the close association between rising levels of contraceptive use and declining fertility. That link is

FIGURE 24.3 Total Fertility Rate and Contraceptive Use, Average Values for the 23 Cases, 1970–95

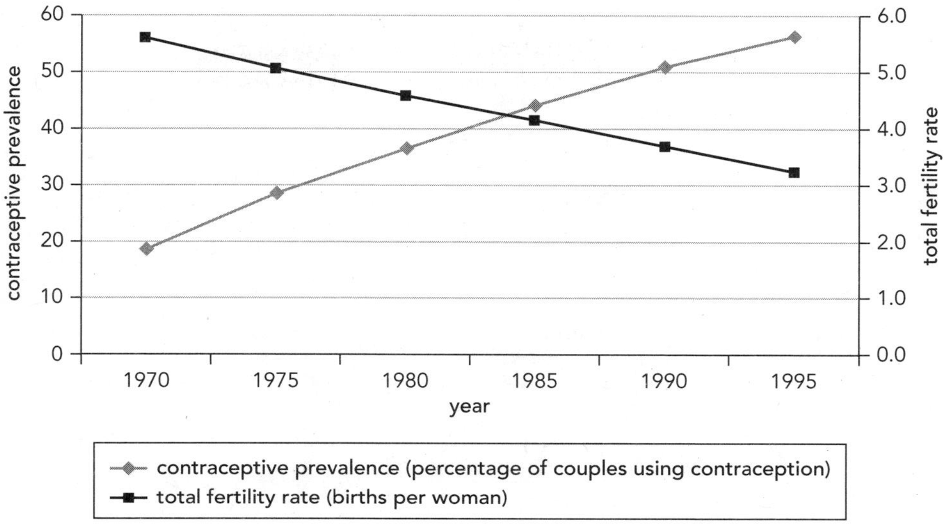

Source: Authors.

clear for the 23 cases included here (figure 24.3). Considering them together, over 25 years, contraceptive prevalence nearly tripled, and fertility was nearly halved (see Bongaarts and Potter [1983] for a general treatment of the relationship between contraception and fertility).

We can trace long-term fertility changes in the United Nations series of five-year total fertility rates (TFRs) (UN 2005) to cover the postwar period through 1995–2000. We employ these data for consistency and completeness of coverage; the individual surveys cited in the chapters are broadly consistent with the United Nations estimates. The 23 cases, taken together, began their fertility transition from an average TFR of 6.3 births per woman in 1960–65, falling to an average of 3.1, less than half, by 1995–2000.

The 23 cases are separated into three groups in figure 24.4, defined according to their starting levels. None showed much change until after 1960–65, when the figure begins. Declines then began for all three groups, which continued unbroken through the decades. The group of programs with the lowest starting TFRs showed the steepest decline, descending to an average of about 2.0 births per woman by 1995–2000. The other two groups fell to TFRs of about 3.5, but were continuing to decline at a sharper rate than the first group, for which the decline was leveling off. (As noted, the United Nations TFR values are given for five-years periods only.)

Fertility actually rose in some places at the start because of postwar baby booms, improved nutrition, and other factors, but by 1965–70, nearly every case showed a decline, attributable in part to program effects, but certainly to other influences as well. The subsequent declines were steep and unbroken nearly everywhere. The latest onsets of decline were not until 1985–90 for Ghana, Guatemala, Iran, and Pakistan, but once started, all declined, with Iran showing the steepest decline of all. The East

FIGURE 24.4 Trends for TFR Groups According to 1955–60 Levels, 1960–65 through 1995–2000

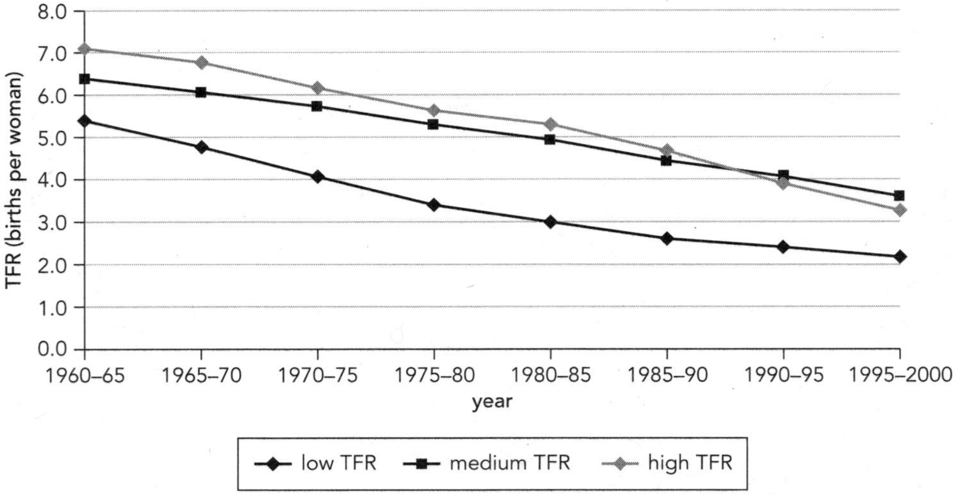

Source: Authors.

Note: Each line follows groups as defined in 1955–60.

Asian cases began with the lowest TFRs and fell first and fastest, reaching replacement level or going below it by 1975–1980 or 1980–85. These included Hong Kong, Korea, Singapore, and Thailand. At the high extreme was a mixed group: Ghana, Guatemala, Kenya, and Pakistan. The TFRs of the other 15 countries fell more moderately, with considerable scatter, but all ended up far below their starting points.

The literature has debated extensively the question of whether the organized programs themselves reduced fertility rates above and beyond what improving social settings would have done. Table 24.3 shows the relationship between program effort, social setting, and fertility for the 23 programs under consideration. Social setting in this instance is a composite index of six dimensions of social and economic development (see Freedman and Berelson [1976], who also review the debates on the programs' share of credit for fertility decline). Each cell shows the TFRs, and mean TFRs are shown in the final column. Strong programs showed a mean TFR of only 3.7, compared with 5.2 for moderately strong programs and a high 6.4 for the weakest programs. A similar gradient appeared for the strength of the social setting, for which the means are shown in the bottom row, with a change from a mean TFR of 3.7 for high social settings to 5.4 for moderate settings and 6.3 for weak settings. A sharp gradient also appears across the diagonal. An especially relevant feature is that the fertility level changes according to program effort within a given social setting. In the middle column, where the social setting is the same, the mean TFR is 5.2 for moderate program effort but higher, at 5.8, for weak program effort. In the third column, the average TFR is 5.7 for moderate effort and 6.5 for weak effort. These patterns are striking, and they create a presumption that program effort exerted some impact, independently from social setting.

TABLE 24.3 Estimated TFRs by Social Setting and Program Effort, 1970–75

	High social setting		Middle social setting		Low social setting		Mean
Strong program effort	Jamaica	5.0					
	Korea, Rep. of	4.3					
	Hong Kong	2.9					3.7
	Singapore	2.6					
	Mean	3.7					
Moderate program effort	Chile	3.6	Tunisia	6.2	Iran	6.4	
			Philippines	6.0	India	5.4	
			Malaysia	5.2	Indonesia	5.2	
			Colombia	5.0			5.2
			Thailand	5.0			
			Sri Lanka	4.1			
	Mean	3.6	Mean	5.2	Mean	5.7	
Weak program effort			Guatemala	6.2	Kenya	8.0	
			Turkey	5.3	Morocco	6.9	
					Ghana	6.7	
					Pakistan	6.6	
					Bangladesh	6.2	6.4
					Nepal	5.8	
					Egypt	5.7	
			Mean	5.8	Mean	6.5	
	Mean	3.7		5.4		6.3	5.4

Source: Adapted from an analysis by Freedman and Berelson 1976.

Table 24.4 adapts this approach to relate program effort to fertility change within different socioeconomic contexts. The patterns are quite marked: the mean decline for strong programs is 32 percent, compared with only 17 percent for moderate programs and 6 percent for weak programs. The decline across social settings changes identically, from 32 percent for high social settings to 17 percent for moderate settings and 6 percent for low settings. Across the diagonal, the change is from 32 percent to 5 percent.

Cross-tabulations like these, and multiple regression analyses, showed clearly that fertility and fertility declines moved with both social setting and program effort, and that each had an independent effect. The strongest effects occurred where both were favorable and the weakest ones where both were unfavorable. Within a given social setting, greater program effort meant lower fertility. (See Freedman and Freedman [1992] for a review of the various methods discussed here and later.)

Macro studies that used countries as the units of analysis have, on balance, supported the conclusion that programs and settings worked synergistically on fertility decline, with each having its own independent effect in addition to the joint effects.

TABLE 24.4 Percentage Declines in TFRs by Social Setting and Program Effort, 1960–65 through 1970–75

	High social setting		Middle social setting		Low social setting		Mean
Strong program effort	Hong Kong	47					
	Singapore	46					
	Korea, Rep. of	24					32
	Jamaica	11					
	Mean	32					
Moderate program effort	Chile	33	Colombia	26	Iran	9	
			Malaysia	23	India	7	
			Thailand	22	Indonesia	4	17
			Sri Lanka	20			
			Tunisia	14			
			Philippines	12			
	Mean	33	Mean	20	Mean	7	
Weak program effort			Turkey	14	Egypt, Arab Rep. of	19	
			Guatemala	5	Bangladesh	10	
					Morocco	4	
					Nepal	4	
					Kenya	1	6
					Ghana	0	
					Pakistan	0	
			Mean	10	Mean	5	
	Mean	32		17		6	15

Source: Adapted from an analysis by Freedman and Berelson 1976.

Multilevel analyses have demonstrated program effects on contraceptive use both within and between countries even after controlling for socioeconomic conditions. Moreover, program effort appeared to weaken socioeconomic differentials in use. Case studies have shown how program introduction of new contraceptive methods was followed by jumps in use. Intensive efforts in special cases, such as in the Matlab area in Bangladesh and Chogoria in Kenya, showed program effects even in extremely unfavorable environments. Within individual countries, greater effects were found in subareas where programs were stronger, controlling for socioeconomic differences. Bongaarts, Mauldin, and Phillips (1990) estimated that without the effects of family planning programs, fertility in developing countries would have been 5.4 births per women during 1980 to 1985 rather than the actual 4.2. These program effects reflect the buildup of program strength over the preceding years.

The weight of all this evidence is that the programs, taken as a whole, reduced fertility rates beyond what would have happened anyway as a result of general socioeconomic change. Of course, some programs were stronger than others, and the indices of program strength showed great variation, though progressively less over the years as the weakest programs tended to become stronger and resemble the effort levels of the more advanced cases.

Timing of Results

The case studies permit a separation between those that experienced early progress, those that achieved progress midway, and those that saw real progress only after some years. It is important to examine the conditions that distinguish the three groups to identify lessons for what worked more effectively during the early stages. On the basis of the timing of contraceptive prevalence increases with TFR declines, together with evidence from the case studies, we separate the 23 cases into three groups. Seven fall into the early group: Colombia, Hong Kong, Korea, Malaysia, Singapore, Sri Lanka, and Thailand. Eleven fall into the middle group, which emerged roughly a decade later: Bangladesh, Chile, Egypt, India, Indonesia, Iran, Jamaica, Kenya, Morocco, Tunisia, and Turkey. Five fall into the late group: Ghana, Guatemala, Nepal, Pakistan, and the Philippines.

To compare the three groups in relation to their program characteristics while holding the socioeconomic context constant, table A24.1 in the annex classifies the cases by SES level and by seven program characteristics following the outline of table 24.1. It also shows the timing of the achievement of results. Drawing on this information, table 24.5 shows the three achievement groups by their program characteristic profile and initial SES status.

No single profile of program and contextual elements fits all the early achievers, but a general pattern is apparent. Most began with a high (category 1) SES background, had strong support for the policy, had good program leadership, could draw on existing health facilities and personnel, and were operated as part of the health system. Such background elements were good predictors of both high program effort scores and speeded the pace of ultimate achievement. Strong, consistent program leadership was present in two-thirds of the better programs and in virtually none of the others.

None of the late achievers shared these features. Programs that initially faced serious opposition took a full decade or more to overcome it and achieve results. An authoritarian versus a more liberal policy adoption process did not have any clear effect on subsequent progress one way or the other. However, the adoption of an authoritarian approach in some cases, for example, Indonesia, led easily into strong program leadership. In the case of India, an overly centralized (if not authoritarian) administrative style probably delayed program achievements. Most of the early achieving programs were able to draw upon relatively strong existing health systems with facilities, personnel, and logistical systems in place. Family planning in the absence of such structures was more difficult and took longer to show results. Persistence in the face of discouraging early results was a vital part of achievements in the mid-range and late groups.

Finally, the cases with better levels of education, higher status of women, and modern transport and communications started from better positions and all achieved

TABLE 24.5 Programs by Characteristics and Timing of Results

Program features	Number of			
	Early achievers	Middle achievers	Delayed achievers	Total
Number of cases	7	11	5	23
Background to policy adoption				
Mostly positive	5	2	0	7
Mostly negative	0	2	3	5
Neither dominate	2	7	2	11
Policy adoption process				
Authoritarian	1	5	3	9
Consensus	6	4	0	10
Informal	0	2	2	4
Agency administering the overall program				
Health ministry	5	6	0	11
Vertical family planning board	1	5	4	10
No government agency	1	0	1	2
Strong program leadership				
Yes	7	6	1	14
No	0	5	4	9
Service delivery program structure				
Clinic- or hospital-based	4	2	0	6
Fieldworker- or health post–based	0	5	3	8
More than one structure	3	4	2	9
IEC strategy				
Adopted	7	7	2	16
Not adopted	0	4	3	7
Initial program effort score				
High	5	1	1	7
Medium	2	5	1	8
Low	0	5	3	8
Resources available to program at the outset				
Financial resources adequate	7	11	5	23
Health personnel, infrastructure, and other inputs available	6	2	1	9
Not available	1	9	4	14
Technical assistance available	7	11	5	23
Statistical and research capacity				
Available	7	2	0	9
Not available	0	9	5	14
Supporting context in relation to education, modernization, and social infrastructure				
SES category 1 (high)	3	2	0	5
SES category 2 (medium)	4	2	2	8
SES category 3 (low)	0	7	3	10

Source: Authors.

progress more rapidly than did those that lacked these elements of modernity. These ongoing transformations of the underlying economic and social structures helped lead to increasing client demand for fertility limitation. They also helped make the service delivery programs more efficient.

Similarly, a convergence of negatives was apparent around the programs listed as the late achievers, where only modest increases in contraceptive prevalence and declines in the TFR occurred, and then only decades after a policy was adopted and the program was launched. None of the five late programs had strong, widespread support for adopting the policy; none adopted the policy with a broad popular consensus; four of five had weak leadership (and the one with strong leadership was short-lived); and four of the five worked outside the ministry of health network and enjoyed little access to established facilities, personnel, or research and evaluation capacity. Finally, none of these programs was in SES category 1 or was able to benefit from favorable trends in women's education and employment. In short, both initial contextual factors and program features were negative.

Control of the programs by the ministry of health produced better outcomes than other structures, especially better than the vertical board or commission structure. Actual implementation seems to have worked well through either clinic- or hospital-based delivery, decentralized fieldworker approaches, or combinations of both plus other innovations. This had more to do with access to resources and facilities than with any inherent advantages of either structure. NGOs also proved to be a successful delivery structure. None of the programs seems to have been unduly limited by lack of funding, partly because of foreign donor assistance, although donors did not cover such mainline budget items as staff salaries and administration.

Another influence that affected the pace of achievements was the early role of such nongovernmental assistance groups as the Ford Foundation, the Rockefeller Foundation, the Population Council, the Pathfinder Fund, and the International Planned Parenthood Federation. In 1958, the Swedish International Development Cooperation Agency became the first official bilateral donor for family planning in Pakistan and Sri Lanka. All these were soon followed by the more massive inputs of the USAID, the United Nations Population Fund, and the World Bank, as well as some European agencies. Like the program directors themselves, the various international advisers were making up the rules as they went along, and not all donor suggestions were helpful. Although most donor influences were, on balance, positive, and their additional funding assisted substantially, in some cases donors' doctrines or rigidities were counterproductive. Also, not all recipients were prepared to absorb intensive donor inputs because of their weak infrastructure or a weak local commitment to a large-scale family planning venture. Over the ensuing decades, donor assistance remained a significant part of most of the national programs and one of the components important to program administration. In a few of the more advanced countries that attained low fertility and high contraceptive use, donors have now largely withdrawn.

Regional differences in the pace of achievement were prominent. Nearly all the early achievers (six of seven) were in East and Southeast Asia. The late achievers, however, were scattered globally (Ghana in Sub-Saharan Africa, Guatemala in Latin

America, Nepal and Pakistan in South Asia, and the Philippines in East Asia). The remaining 11 "midway" programs were also distributed across the regions. The East and Southeast Asian programs had, on average, better SES situations to start with than any of the other regions. However, among the five late achievers, three were in SES category 3 (Ghana, Nepal, and Pakistan).

Interesting anomalies were apparent within the regions. Indonesia was an early achiever despite being in SES category 3 and having poor health services to start with. The Philippines was the only East Asian program to be a late achiever despite being in SES category 2 and having a relatively favorable health services infrastructure to start with. In Latin America, Colombia and Guatemala began at roughly the same SES level and both employed an informal policy adoption and program implementation strategy to disarm opposition, but Colombia was much more successful than Guatemala. Strong, consistent program leadership in Colombia and Indonesia account partly for the difference. Ghana is the oldest program in Sub-Saharan Africa, yet seems to have been unable to overcome a low starting SES level, strong initial opposition, and lack of vigorous leadership. It was surpassed by Kenya and several North African countries. In South Asia, Pakistan fell behind Bangladesh (and all its neighbors) despite having comparable SES levels and infrastructure endowments. A special element in this comparison was the important role NGOs played in Bangladesh and the decision to work through the central ministries rather than a vertical, free-standing board. India, the oldest program of all, was not an early achiever and made several false starts in relation to tactics and organization because it continued with a strong medical establishment bias in delivering services and attempted to impose a single centrally directed model on an enormously diverse population. In later decades, it modified its policies and dealt with the vast disparities among states by sharing control between them and the central government.

The pace of change was affected on both sides of the equation. Programs with good initial infrastructure endowments, good leadership, and strong program effort could do well even when the setting was mostly negative. Similarly, weaker, less efficient programs could show some results in a positive, modernizing socioeconomic context. Where both constellations of factors were favorable, programs achieved early, strongly positive results. In turn, the programs themselves served to advance the process of socioeconomic change and modernization.

Impact of Delayed Fertility Decline

Given that all the programs could claim some success at least by the late 1990s, does the timing of their impact really matter? The answer is yes: early progress as compared with delayed progress is of considerable significance. Delays were followed by two to three decades of higher fertility and faster growth, producing a higher ultimate population size. For example, in 1970, Bangladesh had 5 million more people than Pakistan, but because the TFR in Pakistan remained some 50 percent higher for many years, by 2005, Bangladesh had 16 million fewer people than Pakistan (figure 24.5). That difference will continue to widen well into the future. Similar

FIGURE 24.5 TFR and Total Population, Bangladesh and Pakistan, 1970–2050

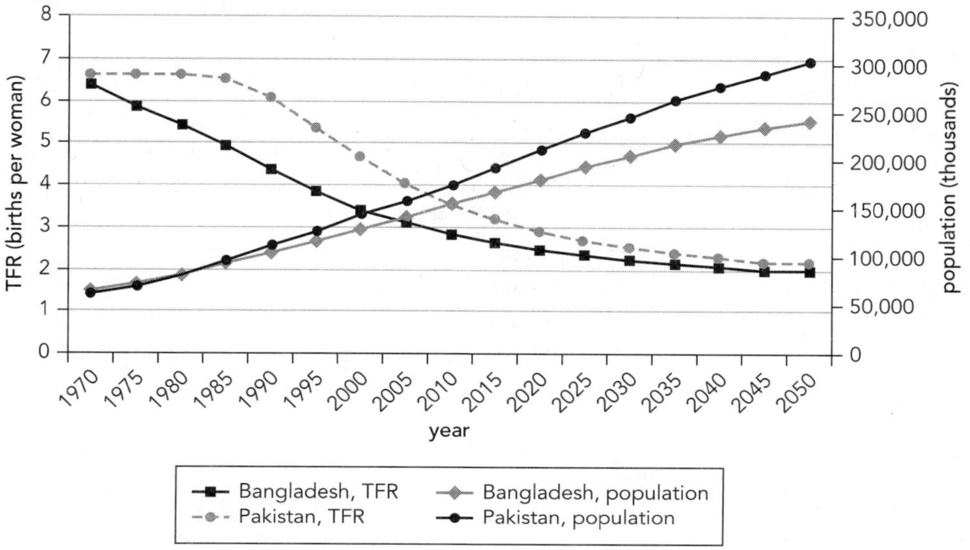

Source: Cleland and others 2006.

disadvantageous population growth has occurred regularly because of delayed fertility declines. Thus, the early program efforts were extremely important.

Lessons for Future Program Interventions

In most developing countries, the policies and programs aimed at reducing fertility were truly pioneering efforts aimed at modifying public services and health-seeking behavior on a large scale. While the short-run results were mixed, over the long run most programs have been relatively successful. What does this history tell us that can be of value as national and international agencies shape new policy and program interventions to deal with new emerging public health needs and challenges?

- *Policy adoption is a continuing process.* Various channels led national leaders and responsible professionals in the newly independent states of Asia and Africa to the conclusion that population growth posed a threat. Economic, political, and health considerations were typically intertwined. They continue to be so, as the 1994 Cairo conference amply demonstrated. Even while formal policies remain unchanged, their implementation can rise or fall, as the current competition with HIV/AIDS programs testifies. Patience and persistence must be the watchwords.

- *No one best pathway to policy adoption exists.* The mechanism by which adoption of family planning policies occurred was not critical: authoritarian, consensual, and informal (NGO-based) efforts all succeeded or, on occasion, failed. Public support by national leaders helped legitimize family planning, but could not guarantee its success, and withholding such support in some cases was a useful interim strategy.

- *Each new problem should not create a new administrative structure.* Donors and ardent local leaders frequently created new structures for family planning outside existing health agencies to bypass burdensome rules and to draw in multiple ministries. These commissions or boards were sometimes drawbacks, because they created overlapping authority and divisive rivalries, diluted scarce technical personnel, and blurred lines of responsibility. In most cases, the health system was the instrument through which family planning was administered, and threatening the health ministry with a separate budget and personnel and arguing for a vertical versus an integrated structure sometimes created resentment and sapped any sense of commitment by health staff. A few exceptions occurred however; also, the early vertical emphasis led to fuller integration as the years passed and programs matured.

- *Crash programs can entail dangers.* Most serious health problems are grounded in a behavioral context and are intertwined with other health issues. An entirely new vertical structure seemed merited for the classic malaria and smallpox eradication efforts, but those programs could truly hope for a short-run elimination of a given set of disease vectors over a finite time period. In the case of family planning, vertical structures were usually modified by using preexisting ministry of health systems to some extent. Nevertheless, some programs focused too narrowly on a single result and used excessive vigor in pursuit of it. The best ways to balance focus and vigor within health structures are not easily resolved, as is now apparent in the case of HIV/AIDS and other emerging diseases. Some of the mistakes that were made in service delivery programs—the neglect of quality of care, the rush of new methods into use without adequate testing, and the resort to quotas and even occasionally to outright coercion—flowed from the crash program paradigm: the honest, if misguided, conviction that extreme measures were justified in light of the urgency of the problem.

- *Initial SES levels are a good guide to program planning.* The NGOs typically found their first clients where urbanization, education, and nonagricultural economic activity had already taken hold. Early public sector programs found that clinics and hospitals were the natural outlets for early services. However, it soon became evident that well-run programs directed toward rural and less educated subgroups could find intensive interest among older, high-parity women, and that once established, effective programs could gradually reach down into younger, lower-parity subgroups. Such expansions could proceed apace with improvements in education and other social services.

- *The scale of the initial program must be realistic.* Some programs went national too soon, taking a bold gamble that a new and relatively sophisticated intervention into human behavior could be accomplished quickly among dispersed, illiterate, rural populations. Such large-scale efforts usually outstripped the capacity of existing health care delivery systems and scarce, overburdened personnel. In other cases, the shortcomings were poor planning and weak leadership, which led to a lack of vigor and outreach.

- *Financial resources are not a guarantee of success.* Funds are important when they are absent, but none of the cases reviewed here failed for want of financial resources to obtain commodities, facilities, or personnel. The obstacles were chiefly more general: backward infrastructure, inadequate equipment, poor training, and weak management. It takes time to acquire and put in place stronger human, physical, and institutional structures, and money can only do so much. Absorptive capacity is limited in the short run.

- *Consistency in program leadership and direction is important.* Many of the accounts in the chapters are also stories of great people who provided leadership and continuity to their programs. Saying that they were responsible for the successes goes too far, but it is tempting to ask whether programs would have succeeded even half as well without them, and whether better leadership or more consistent direction in some of the less successful cases would not have improved outcomes.

- *No single family planning approach worked everywhere.* Circumstances differed, and while best practices emerged to some extent, no two programs were identical. Donor pressures varied, and program planners rightly viewed many donor prescriptions with skepticism. The vast changes now taking place as a result of the decentralization of services, the HIV/AIDS pandemic, the disturbances of refugee movements and armed conflicts, together with uncertain funding prospects, mean that national programs require close tailoring to each set of local conditions and to the inevitable shifts they will undergo.

The best formula for program success is to make a full variety of methods available to the entire population through a wide variety of channels, with complete public information about all methods, and with the highest possible level of provider quality.

Final Note

On balance, the early efforts to bring contraceptive choices to much of the developing world constituted a pioneering social achievement. The pace and timing of success depended on the socioeconomic context as well as on the strength of the program and its leadership, but this was understood from the beginning of the effort. Some authors continue to be skeptical of the impact of family planning programs (Demeny 2001; McNicoll 2006; Watkins 2000), but the essays contained here suggest that this skepticism has not been well founded. No one realistically expected that policies and programs could bring down fertility overnight or that programs could work miracles. It was clear from the outset that some programs would take more time than others to yield results (Berelson 1978; Cassen 1970; Glass 1966; Robinson 1969) and that some risked failure. In the end, however, they did work, speeding the transition to lower fertility and reducing projected population sizes by many millions.

Four decades ago, in his concluding remarks to an early global conference on family planning programs, the then president of the Population Council, Frank W. Notestein, foresaw the future of the programs just beginning with remarkable prescience, and eloquently expressed his hope for what they might help bring about as follows.

I should like to hazard the guess that in two decades the major problems of overriding population growth may well be on the way to solution. . . . We have the policies, the interest, and the technology and are in the process of getting the organization. We are entitled to hope that population growth will not remain the almost insuperable obstacle to economic development that it appeared to be only a few short years ago. I am not suggesting that the task is done—it is scarcely started. But, we know now what to do, and in the first approximation how to go about the job. If we have learned in the past, it is reasonable to assume that we can learn even more in the future. If so, a generation that is chiefly conspicuous for conducting the most brutal wars in human history may yet redeem itself by creating for the first time in man's history a world in which health, education, and opportunity for individual fulfillment can be secured for all the world's people (Notestein 1966, pp. 829–30).

Annex: Major Program Features by Socioeconomic Level

TABLE A24.1 Initial Social Setting and Program Features

Program characteristics	SES category 1 (high)	SES category 2 (medium)	SES category 3 (low)
Number of cases	5	8	10
Policy background			
Strong opposition	Chile	**Guatemala, Philippines,**	**Ghana,** Iran
Strong support	Hong Kong; Korea, Rep. of; Singapore	Colombia, Malaysia, Sri Lanka, Thailand, Tunisia, Turkey	India, Indonesia
Neither	Jamaica	n.a.	Bangladesh; Egypt; Kenya; Morocco; **Nepal; Pakistan**
Policy adoption			
Authoritarian	Singapore	**Philippines,** Tunisia	Egypt; Indonesia; Iran; Morocco; **Nepal; Pakistan**
Consensus	Hong Kong; Korea, Rep. of	Colombia, Malaysia, Sri Lanka, Thailand, Turkey	Bangladesh, **Ghana,** India, Kenya
Informal	Chile, Jamaica	**Guatemala**	
Strong program leadership			
Yes	Chile; Hong Kong; Jamaica; Korea, Rep. of; Singapore	Colombia, Malaysia Thailand, Tunisia. Turkey	Bangladesh, India, Indonesia **Pakistan**
No	n.a.	**Guatemala, Philippines,** Sri Lanka	Egypt; **Ghana;** Iran; Kenya; Morocco; **Nepal**

TABLE A24.1 (*Continued*)

Program characteristics	SES category 1 (high)	SES category 2 (medium)	SES category 3 (low)
Management structure			
Health ministry	Chile; Korea, Rep. of; Singapore	Sri Lanka, Thailand, Tunisia, Turkey,	Bangladesh; Egypt, Ghana; Iran; Kenya; Morocco
Vertical board	Jamaica	Malaysia, **Philippines**	India, Indonesia, **Nepal, Pakistan**
No government agency	Hong Kong	Colombia, **Guatemala**	n.a.
Service delivery mode			
Clinic-based	Chile, Singapore	Malaysia, Sri Lanka, Tunisia	n.a.
Fieldworker-based	n.a.	**Guatemala**	Bangladesh, **Ghana,** Indonesia, Iran, Kenya, Morocco, **Pakistan,**
More than one mode	Hong Kong; Jamaica; Korea, Rep. of	Colombia, **Philippines,** Thailand, Turkey	Egypt; India; **Nepal**
Resources available at program outset			
Financial support and technical assistance available	Chile; Hong Kong; Jamaica; Korea, Rep. of; Singapore	Colombia, **Guatemala,** Malaysia, **Philippines,** Sri Lanka, Thailand, Tunisia, Turkey	Bangladesh; Egypt; **Ghana;** India; Indonesia; Iran; Kenya; Morocco; **Nepal; Pakistan**
Health personnel, facilities, and infrastructure in place			
Yes	Chile; Hong Kong; Korea, Rep. of; Singapore	Malaysia, **Philippines,** Sri Lanka, Thailand, Tunisia	n.a.
No	Jamaica	Colombia, **Guatemala,** Turkey	Bangladesh; Egypt; **Ghana;** India; Indonesia; Iran; Kenya; Morocco; **Nepal; Pakistan**
Statistical and research capacity in place			
Yes	Chile; Hong Kong; Korea, Rep. of; Singapore	Colombia, Malaysia, **Philippines,** Sri Lanka, Thailand, Tunisia	Bangladesh, Indonesia
No	Jamaica	**Guatemala,** Turkey	Egypt; **Ghana;** India; Iran; Kenya; Morocco; **Nepal; Pakistan**
IEC strategy adopted			
Yes	Hong Kong; Jamaica; Korea, Rep. of; Singapore	Colombia, Malaysia, Sri Lanka, Thailand, Tunisia, Turkey	Bangladesh, India, Indonesia, Iran, **Nepal, Pakistan**
No	Chile	**Guatemala, Philippines,**	Egypt; **Ghana;** Kenya; Morocco

Source: Authors' analysis based on the country-specific chapters.

Note: n.a. = not applicable. Early achiever economies are shown in regular type, midrange achievers are underlined, and late achievers are in bold italics.

Note

1. The entire series of data, which was for some 85 countries over time, shows that the mean total score rose in each round of the study and continued to do so through 2004. Within the set of 85 countries, the top scorers had leveled off, but the mean continued to rise as low scorers improved.

References

Berelson, Bernard. 1974. "An Evaluation of the Effects of Population Control Programs." *Studies in Family Planning* 5 (1): 1–12.

———. 1978. "Programs and Prospects for Fertility Reduction." *Population and Development Review* 4 (4): 579–616.

Bogue, Donald J., ed. 1968. "Progress and Problems of Fertility Control around the World" (special issue). *Demography*: 5 (3).

Bongaarts, John, W. Parker Mauldin, and James F. Phillips. 1990. "The Demographic Impact of Family Planning Programs." *Studies in Family Planning* 21 (6): 299–310.

Bongaarts, John, and Robert G. Potter. 1983. *Fertility, Biology, and Behavior.* New York: Academic Press.

Bulatao, Rodolfo A. 1993. *Effective Family Planning Programs.* Washington, DC: World Bank.

Cassen, Robert. 1978. "Current Trends in Population Change and Their Causes." *Population and Development Review* 4 (2): 331–53.

Cleland, John, Stan Bernstein, Alex Ezeh, Annibal Faundes, Anna Glaser, and Jolene Innis. 2006. "Family Planning: The Unfinished Agenda." *Lancet* (October): 44–64.

Coale, Ansley J., and Edgar M. Hoover. 1958. *Population Growth and Economic Development in Low-Income Countries: A Case Study of India's Prospects.* Princeton, NJ: Princeton University Press.

Critchlow, Donald T., ed. 1996. *The Politics of Abortion and Birth Control in Historical Perspective.* University Park, PA: Pennsylvania State University Press.

Demeny, Paul. 2001. "Intellectual Origins of Past-World War II Population Policies in South Asia." *Fertility Transition in South Asia,* ed. Zeba A. Sathar and James Phillips, 34–46, Oxford: Oxford University Press.

Demeny, Paul. 2003. "Population Policy." In *Encyclopedia of Population,* vol. II, ed. Paul Demeny and Geoffrey McNicoll, 752–57. New York: Macmillan.

Donaldson, Peter, and Amy Tsui. 1988. *The International Family Planning Movement.* Washington, DC: Population Reference Bureau.

Freedman, Ronald, and Bernard Berelson. 1976. "The Record of Family Planning Programs." Studies in Family Planning 7 (1): 1–40.

Freedman, Ronald, and Deborah Freedman. 1992. "The Role of Family Planning Programmes as a Fertility Determinant." In *Family Planning Programmes and Fertility,* ed. James F. Phillips and John A. Ross, 10–27. Oxford, U.K.: Oxford University Press.

Glass, David V. 1966. "Population Growth and Population Policy." In *Public Health and Population Change,* ed. M. Sheps and J. C. Ridley, 2–25. Pittsburgh, PA: University of Pittsburgh Press.

Johanssen, S. R. 1991. "Implicit Policy and Fertility Change during Development" *Population and Development Review* 17 (3): 388–414.

Liebenstein, Harvey M. 1954. *A Theory of Economic-Demographic Development*. Princeton: Princeton University Press.

Mason, A., ed. 2001. *Population Policies and Programs in East Asia*. Occasional Paper 123. Honolulu, HI: East-West Center.

Mauldin, W. Parker. 1978. "Patterns of Fertility Decline in Developing Countries, 1965–75." *Studies in Family Planning* 9 (4): 75–84.

Mauldin, W. Parker, Bernard Berelson, and Zenas Sykes. 1978. "Conditions of Fertility Decline in Developing Countries, 1965–75." *Studies in Family Planning* 9 (5): 89–147.

May, John F. 2005. "Population Policy." In *The Handbook of Population*, ed. D. Poston and M. Micklin, 827–52. New York: Kluwer.

McNicoll, Geoffrey. 2006. "Policy Lessons of the East Asian Fertility Transition." Working Paper 21, Population Council, New York.

Nortman, Dorothy. 1969. *Family Planning and Population Fact Book*. New York: Population Council.

Notestein, Frank W. 1966. "Closing Remarks." In *Family Planning and Population Programs: A Review of World Developments*, eds. B. Berelson, R. K. Anderson, O. Harkavy, J. Maier, W. P. Mauldin, and S. J. Segal, 827–30. Chicago: University of Chicago Press.

Posner, E. A. 2001. *Laws and Social Norms*. Cambridge, MA: Harvard University Press.

Roberts, Geoffrey, ed. 1990. *Population Policy*. New York: Greenwood Press.

Robinson, Warren C. 1969. "Population Control and Development Strategy." *Journal of Development Studies* 5 (2): 104–117.

Ross, John A., and John Stover. 2001. "The Family Planning Program Effort Index: 1999 Cycle." *International Family Planning Perspectives* 27 (3): 119–29.

Ross, John A., John Stover, and Demi Adelaja. Forthcoming. "Family Planning Programs in 2004: Efforts, Justifications, Influences, and Special Populations of Interest." *International Family Planning Perspectives*.

Sathar, Zeba, and James F. Phillips, eds. 2001. *Fertility Transition in South Asia*. Oxford: Oxford University Press.

Seltzer, Judith. 1998. *The Origins and Evolution of Family Planning Programs in Developing Countries*. Santa Monica, CA: RAND Corporation.

UN (United Nations). 1973. *The Determinants and Consequences of Population Trends*. Population Studies 50. New York: United Nations.

———. 2005. *World Population Prospects: The 2004 Revision*, vol. 1, *Comprehensive Tables*. New York: United Nations, Population Division.

Watkins, Susan C. 2000. "Local and Foreign Models of Reproduction in Nyanza Province, Kenya." *Population and Development Review* 26 (4): 725–59.

Watson, Walter B. 1977. "Historical Overview." In *Family Planning in the Developing World: A Review of Programs*, ed. Walter B. Watson, 1–9. New York: Population Council.

Index

Boxes, figures, notes, and tables are indicated by "b," "f," "n," and "t."

Eco-Audit

Environmental Benefits Statement

The World Bank is committed to preserving endangered forests and natural resources. The Office of the Publisher has chosen to print The *Global Family Planning Revolution* on recycled paper with 30 percent post-consumer waste, in accordance with the recommended standards for paper usage set by the Green Press Initiative, a nonprofit program supporting publishers in using fiber that is not sourced from endangered forests. Using this paper, the following were saved: 17 trees; 12 million BTUs of energy; 1,502 pounds CO_2 equivalent greenhouse gases; 6,235 gallons of waste water; 801 pounds of solid waste. For more information, visit www.greenpressinitiative.org.

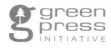